Administration, and other federal agencies. We still are on the waiting list for the FBI to answer our freedom-of-information request. We also have read dozens of books and reports, as well as hundreds of articles relating to the AMA and the issues we cover in the book.

In the end, the AMA agreed to grant an interview with Todd only if the AMA could review and comment on the section of the book in which this was used. The authors reluctantly agreed to that condition. After months of waiting, we interviewed Todd. The results of the interview are in the epilogue.

In *The Serpent on the Staff*, we have explored how the AMA has shaped our nation's health-care system and the role it has played in the major medical issues of our time. We have taken a historic look to trace the development of policy and to look for the organization's patterns of behavior over time. The AMA has played an important role in defining what health care is and how it is delivered in the United States. Before we can begin to talk about how to change our faltering health-care system, we should know how it got to be that way.

This book presents a critical view of the AMA. Our thesis is that the AMA is not a paternalistic Dr. Welby looking out after his patients. We see the AMA as more often than not a political entity that claims to be tending to the public's health, while in reality looking after doctors' interests. However, what's good for the AMA and its members is not necessarily good for the U.S.A. That's why our subtitle refers to the unhealthy politics of the AMA.

PREVIEW OF CHAPTERS

The first half of the book is devoted primarily to financial and political issues; the second half deals with how AMA politicos respond to health issues.

Chapter 1 provides an overview of the AMA, its organization, its membership, and how it works.

Chapter 2 describes the AMA's role in blocking, delaying, and weakening health-care reform. The AMA in the present as well as the past engaged in well-financed lobbying and scare tactics to fight and control reform.

Chapter 3 examines the one major battle the AMA lost when it tried to derail an idea whose time had come, Medicare, and how the AMA helped turned this defeat into a victory by ensuring that Medicare was a financial windfall for doctors. The AMA will try to repeat this success with whatever health reform comes.

Rorty wrote *American Medicine Mobilizes* in 1939. Historian James G. Burrow published a scholarly historical account, *AMA: Voice of American Medicine,* in 1963. Journalist Richard Harris wrote *A Sacred Trust* in 1966, providing an account of the AMA's efforts to block passage of the Medicare law. Although not specifically about the AMA, Paul Starr's 1982 opus, *The Social Transformation of American Medicine,* contains much of the history of the AMA in its excellent analysis of U.S. health care. We are indebted to these authors, and many, many others.

The most recent book about the AMA was an inside job, published in 1984. AMA public-relations executive and former *Life* magazine writer Frank D. Campion wrote an AMA-approved book tracing AMA activities from 1940 to the early 1980s. Campion had easy access to his colleagues and tells some revealing stories about the AMA.

This book is not authorized by the AMA and never was intended to receive the AMA's seal of approval. However, we approached the AMA in spring 1992 in hopes of getting some cooperation for this project. Chief Executive James S. Todd welcomed us, urging us to write about the AMA, its "warts and roses." But as is common in books like this, communications broke down. AMA officials did not like the nature of our questions and were unhappy that we did not provide them with a written outline of the book. Still, the AMA allowed us to use its library and gave us copies of its public statements.

However, AMA officials told us that our formal requests for interviews with AMA Board members and staffers would be at the bottom of the large stack of media inquiries. The AMA does not grant official interviews without approval from its public-relations office. In our case, the AMA said it would honor requests only when, as an AMA public-relations officer frankly said, "We can put a positive spin on it." Many of our requests essentially were ignored.

How the Book Was Done

We pushed on. We asked questions for the book during interviews on other subjects with AMA officials and at press conferences. All together, we interviewed more than one hundred people, including current and former AMA staffers and Board members, AMA critics, and academics from a host of disciplines including medicine, the law, ethics, history, and sociology. We have gone over thousands of pages of court documents and congressional testimony. We have pored over thousands of pages obtained under the Freedom of Information Act from the Centers for Disease Control, the Federal Election Commission, the General Services

Then, there was the story about how the AMA planned to print articles rejected by its journals in "educational" publications designed to bring in millions of dollars from drug companies. The AMA already is hooked on pharmaceutical-company advertising, which makes up about 20 percent of its operating revenue, second only to members' dues as a source of AMA funding. Consumerist Dr. Sidney Wolfe characterized this project as "massive prostitution." The AMA dropped this project. And there was the story that showed how the AMA's top brass tried to prevent friction with conservative members of Congress by ordering *JAMA*'s editor to back off on articles concerning three "particularly sensitive political" issues: abortion, tobacco, and nuclear war.

We broke a series of stories in 1989–90 on financial scandals involving the AMA's top managers. The articles resulted in the resignation in disgrace of the AMA's chief executive, Dr. James H. Sammons, then one of America's best-known medical politicians. The president of the AMA's for-profit subsidiary and a top investment executive also were forced out. Then we covered the organization's efforts to redefine itself as "The New AMA," a "friendlier, wiser" version of an organization notorious for confrontation, ultimatums, and hardball politics. The changes came at a fortunate time for the AMA, which was cultivating a new image when the country finally appeared to be trying to address the problems of access and high cost that have turned the health-care system into a nightmare for many Americans. But it looks like the New AMA is just the Old AMA in freshly laundered surgical scrubs.

No organization appreciates outside scrutiny by a news organization. The AMA, which largely has been left to its own devices by the general media, is no different. The AMA's press office and leadership prefer to choose how and when to enter the public spotlight. Our brand of adversarial journalism prompted the AMA communications director to refer to Wolinsky as "a snake" to the AMA Board of Trustees because of a story—based on AMA statistics—they did not like. As a result, "Snake" became the reporter's nickname among his medical-writer colleagues.

Having done this type of reporting over the years, we now have taken on the job of writing a book covering the AMA from a broader perspective. This book is a reporters' book, but we are going beyond reporting of news to analyzing how the AMA has affected the lives of Americans. The public should know more about a major organization that is attempting to play an important part in the health-reform effort that will affect all of us as well as coming generations.

There have been plenty of books about medicine over the years. But there has not been an independent book aimed at the general reader that examined the AMA on a wide range of topics since journalist James

Preface to the First Edition

THE HEADQUARTERS OF the American Medical Association is just down the block from the *Chicago Sun-Times*, where we have worked as reporters for the past decade. Howard Wolinsky is a medical reporter who probably knows the AMA as well, if not better, than most reporters. Before joining the *Sun-Times*, Wolinsky worked for one year on the AMA's weekly, American Medical News, where he learned how the AMA operates. Tom Brune is an investigative reporter who has teamed up with Wolinsky to ferret out hidden information for a variety of projects. Being in the AMA's backyard, we have covered the AMA the way some reporters cover City Hall.

We have reported on AMA policies as they have been formulated. We were there when the AMA announced its proposal to reform the health-care system and its first policies on AIDS. We wrote about controversies involving an *AMA Journal* article by an anonymous physician who wrote an account of a mercy killing. We have plumbed the AMA's own research for nuggets, such as the first time physicians' average pay exceeded $100,000 and $150,000. (That happened in 1983 and 1989, respectively.)

We have also reported on the internal foibles and hypocrisies of this large national institution. There was the 1981 piece on how AMA resident-physician members were upset over the incongruity of the AMA's Members Retirement Fund owning more than $1 million in tobacco stocks. After this was publicized, the AMA quietly sold the securities off. There was the story in 1985 about how the *AMA Journal*'s editor in chief knuckled under to pressure from a drug manufacturer, who had withdrawn advertising for several months, and ran an article extolling the virtues of one of the firm's products. The AMA fired the *Journal*'s news editor of fifteen years for speaking about the incident to the newspaper—even though she first obtained AMA permission to do so.

to sell its products, such as consumer books and bike helmets, and build its image.

Meanwhile, the AMA's political action committee continued to outspend all other individual health-care PACs, and its lobbying operation in Washington continued to be on the cutting edge of special-interest influence. If the Republicans succeed in pushing an agenda that further erodes federal oversight on health care, the AMA may have found it lost its best ally for protecting doctor income and independence.

As the AMA heads into its 150th year in 1997, it will be struggling to survive, at least in its present form. It will not vanish from lack of funds; despite some financial setbacks, it is laden with cash, real estate, a money-making journal, and products to license. But at some point, the question will arise: Who does the AMA really represent? And does anybody—doctors, the public—need the AMA anymore? These questions pose a challenge to the AMA for the coming years and century.

Chicago   Howard Wolinsky   Tom Brune
January 1995

But it could be an uneasy relationship. Only months earlier, during the final throes of the reform debate, the AMA had offended Gingrich and his conservative colleagues by joining with Big Labor and the senior citizens' lobby in a call for universal health coverage. On August 1 the irate Republicans sent a letter to members of the AMA House of Delegates to warn them to back off on "a misguided political agenda on the part of the AMA leadership" or else lose GOP support on legislation close to AMA hearts. Soon after the election, at its meeting in December in Hawaii, the AMA did back off on universal coverage.

Still, the AMA is concerned about Medicare, the federal program for the elderly, which it initially opposed but which most doctors now view as an economic mainstay and even birthright. AMA chief executive Dr. James S. Todd, who once noted that doctors fared better under the Democrats, acknowledged that organized medicine soon could be engaged in "the mother of all Medicare battles" in the next Congress under Republican rule.

Other AMA stands could cause it problems if it took some conservative litmus tests: The AMA talks tough—despite little action—about controlling tobacco, while some top Southern Republicans think too much has been said about tobacco already. The AMA also may have to do some fancy dancing on its essentially pro-choice positions, including its opposition to the gag rule, and its new gay-friendly policies.

In 1994, the AMA, challenged by external woes as well as civil war among doctors, again began to reshape its identity and image. As in the past, it resorted to smoke and mirrors. Annoyed at criticism of doctor pay—the average headed toward $200,000 a year—the AMA came up with a new formula for determining doctor compensation, making it lower by including the lower pay of physicians in training and those employed by the federal government.

As it has so often in the past, the AMA hired a high-powered consultant to chart the organization's future as it dealt with declines in full-dues-paying membership. Although the AMA declared in its 1994 strategic plan that members are its lifeblood, dues represent only one third of its revenue, while two thirds of its income comes from its businesses. As a result, the AMA introduced itself anew as, in effect, AMA Inc.

The AMA plan said the group intended to push its wares, especially information for and about physicians. Never shy about latching on to the latest business fads and buzzwords, the AMA said it was aiming to be an on-ramp to the so-called "information superhighway." And the AMA soon may be coming to a shopping mall near you—in fall 1994, as an experiment, the AMA opened a boutique in a Milwaukee department store

Preface

Iɴ ᴛʜᴇ ᴛɪᴍᴇ sɪɴᴄᴇ *The Serpent on the Staff* was first published in May 1994, the United States came closer than it had in nearly two decades to reforming its health-care system. But efforts faltered and finally collapsed, leaving the American Medical Association in an awkward position.

During the previous five years, the AMA had geared up for the coming health-care debate, pinning its star on being a major player.

But reform was a flop. The Clinton administration could not marshal its forces. An impotent Congress balked at tackling such a big job, as partisan politics overshadowed the public interest and public health. And this time, the AMA failed to have the clout and high profile that it demonstrated during reform campaigns throughout this century.

Ironically, health-care reform as envisioned by many Democrats could have created a role for the AMA as a negotiator for organized medicine. Instead, the AMA was left with an empty bowl, with many of its affiliated physician groups angry because the AMA had failed to deliver on health-system reform.

Now, the AMA is confronting antagonistic private-sector forces. During the debate on reform, the AMA criticized the insurance companies, the ultimate player in today's medical world, for bullying doctors by interfering with their traditional independence and their relationships with their patients.

And the AMA is facing an unclear fate in a Congress controlled by a new cadre of right-tilting and somewhat hostile Republicans. During a fly-in lobbying effort following the November election, AMA doctors stamped their feet and chanted, "Newt!" in homage to the new GOP majority leader, Representative Newt Gingrich (R-Ga.). Things would seem to be working in the AMA's favor because of shared political thinking.

We also owe thanks to the National Library on Money & Politics, especially Jacqueline Duobinis, for helping tame Federal Election Commission data, and to American Health Line and the Robert Wood Johnson Foundation for providing service for a year.

We wanted to show our appreciation to some staffers at the American Medical Association who shared documents and insights. However, they asked that their names not be mentioned. They feared retribution. Likewise, we are grateful to the AMA moles, people within the organization who over the years anonymously have passed along tips and leaked documents.

Acknowledgments

We ARE ESPECIALLY indebted to Beth Vesel, our agent, who came up with the idea for this book and then persuaded us to do it. We appreciate our publisher, Jeremy Tarcher, and his vision of the book's direction. Our editor, Rick Benzel, encouraged Tarcher/Putnam to take on the project and has steered us through the maze of publishing. Daniel Malvin, Tarcher/Putnam's Managing Editor, helped us on the homestretch with his consummate professionalism and good humor. Aileen Boyle, senior publicist, is a media maven who did a superb job of getting the word out. And Alice Evans, marketing coordinator, opened the doors to the right bookstores to promote this book.

The authors are responsible for the contents of the book, but owe a debt of gratitude to many people who have helped us over the years. We want to thank several generations of editors of the *Chicago Sun-Times*, particularly Mark Nadler, Dennis Britton, Mary Dedinsky, and Alan Mutter.

We are grateful to Ann Allen, Mark Bloom, Alan Blum, Arthur Caplan, David Carlson, Daniel Childs, Eugene Diamond, John Easton, Marc Edell, Norman Gevitz, Robert Graham, Robert King, Jane Larson, George McAndrews, Sharon McGowan, Jim McGowan, Kara McNamara, Joe Neel, Deborah Nelson, Chuck Neubauer, Peggy Peck, David Rogers, Benjamin Schatz, Eric Solberg, Ann Springer, Joseph Stanton, Patricia Spain Ward, Linda Johnson White, Judith Wolinsky, Quentin Young, and Tom Young.

We owe a debt to libraries, which we found are hothouses for more books. We want to thank the following libraries and their staffs: the American Medical Association library, the Homewood Public Library, the Suburban Library System, the Harold Washington Library (especially the Government Documents department), the *Chicago Sun-Times* Library, the John Crerar Library and Regenstein Library at the University of Chicago, and the University of Oregon Library.

Contents

HOWARD   WOLINSKY

This book is dedicated to my wife, Judith, and sons, Adam and David, whose support helped make this book possible. Also, to my late mother, Edith, who introduced me to the world of books, and my father, Sidney, who introduced me to the news and always can be found devouring a newspaper from cover to cover.

TOM   BRUNE

Dedicated to my wife, Deborah Nelson, and daughters, Molly and Anna, who were always there for me through long days and long nights.

A Jeremy P. Tarcher/Putnam Book
Published by G. P. Putnam's Sons
Publishers Since 1838
200 Madison Avenue
New York, NY 10016

First Trade Paperback Edition 1995

Library of Congress Cataloging-in-Publication Data

Wolinsky, Howard.
    The serpent on the staff : the unhealthy politics of the American
Medical Association / Howard Wolinsky and Tom Brune.
        p.   cm.
    "A Jeremy P. Tarcher/Putnam Book."
    Includes bibliographical references and index.
    ISBN 0-87477-800-X
    1. American Medical Association.   I. Brune, Tom.   II. Title.
R15.A55W58   1994
610 .6 073—dc20   93-47596   CIP

Design by Lee Fukui

Printed in the United States of America
1   2   3   4   5   6   7   8   9   10

This book is printed on acid-free paper.
∞

THE
SERPENT
ON THE
STAFF

The Unhealthy Politics of the
American Medical Association

HOWARD WOLINSKY
and
TOM BRUNE

A Jeremy P. Tarcher/Putnam Book
published by
G. P. Putnam's Sons
New York

Chapter 4 is devoted to AMPAC, the AMA's powerful political action committee, which has spent almost incomprehensible amounts of money to help the AMA get its way.

In *Chapter 5* we look at how the AMA has tried to keep alive the business ethic—and the opportunities to profit off patients—which ought to be antithetical to healers.

Next, in *Chapter 6,* AMA opposition to alternative medicine is explored. The evidence is presented here of how the AMA, in pursuing its own political and economic goals, has attempted to eradicate competing schools of medicine.

Chapter 7 is about one of the more egregious and callous cases of the AMA's unhealthy politics in action—its involvement with tobacco, the cause of the largest epidemic of our time. To this day, though the AMA has a solid antitobacco record on paper, many health advocates view the AMA as being "soft" on tobacco.

Next, in *Chapter 8,* abortion, perhaps the most contentious of medical-political issues, is studied by following the AMA's evolution from being an advocate for criminalizing abortion in the last century to its current efforts to duck this divisive issue with major moral and public-health implications.

Chapter 9 describes the AMA's role in another complicated and explosive issue, AIDS. After long ignoring the growing epidemic, the AMA often tried to promote political rather than scientific remedies with its AIDS policies.

THE SNAKE: SYMBOL OF HEALING

The title of this book, *The Serpent on the Staff,* is a reference to the AMA's symbol. In 1910 the AMA began using as its logo a snake entwined upon a knotty pine staff.

Since ancient times, the serpent has symbolized medicine. It is not the serpent of the Judeo-Christian culture, which viewed snakes as a symbol of evil, but of the ancient Greeks and Romans. To them, the snake's ability to shed its skin was a powerful image for renewal and healing. In Greek mythology, Asklepios, the son of the god Apollo and the mortal Coronis, had the ability to metamorphose into a snake. He was a potent healer who could bring the dead back to life, which angered Hades, god of the underworld. In one tale Asklepios changed into a serpent so he could be carried to Rome to end a plague. After this, the Romans made him a god too, Aesculapius, and built temples in his honor. The ruins of hundreds of these temples still can be found in Italy and Greece, some still populated by snakes. Asklepios also is credited with leading medicine toward science and away from primitive shamanistic practices. The modern medical doctor can be considered a descendant of Asklepios.

The AMA's logo featured an Asklepian viper, a wiry serpent, looking fierce with fangs and a forked tongue. But in 1990 the AMA decided it was time to go through its own transformation, to shed the skin of its past, to renew its image in the eyes of doctors and the public. It was a form of rebirth after the AMA was devastated by a financial scandal involving its top leaders. As part of an $800,000 image-building campaign, the AMA unveiled its new icon. The new serpent-on-the-staff appeared friendlier. The tongue and fangs were gone. The snake also appeared to be plumper and better-fed. And the AMA's new logo had added a slogan: "Physicians dedicated to the health of America."

The timing of the AMA's "rebirth" was important. The AMA was positioning itself for the great health-care debate. At the beginning of the 1990s, the United States entered into its sixth attempt in this century to reform the health-care system, to make it more accessible to those without the means to pay for their care, to make it more affordable for the country as a whole. Like all the other powerful special interests whose members provide care and profit from a huge industry, the AMA needed to put itself into a better bargaining position. To do this, it had to escape any scrap of a reputation it has as a trade association that put the political and economic interests of physicians ahead of all else.

As the citizens of the United States observe and participate in the drive for health-care reform, they owe it to themselves to know the players and what they stand for. Among the key players is the American Medical Association. Its power, though not nearly as great as it was a few decades ago, cannot be underestimated. In discussing the plight of those without health insurance, Princeton medical economist Uwe E. Reinhardt once said, "What the head of the AMA thinks in the shower in the morning is so much more important than the aspirations of 10 million Americans."

THE OTHER SNAKE: SYMBOL OF BUSINESS

There is another symbol of medicine that frequently is confused with the Asklepian serpent-on-the-staff. It is the caduceus, which has two snakes twisted around a short olive-tree wand with wings. The single-serpent and double-serpent symbols often are treated as if they are the same. Indeed, many physicians use these symbols interchangeably on their letterheads, prescription pads, or on signs in front of their office buildings. Newspapers and television stations often incorporate the two-snake symbol into their logos for medical stories, unaware of the history of the two symbols.

The two emblems have very different meanings. The caduceus is the shield of Mercury, the Roman god of communications, known as Hermes to the Greeks. Mercury has tenuous links to medicine. His symbol, with the two fighting snakes held at bay, is that of the messenger or herald, a peacemaker who was not to be attacked by warring parties. In the nineteenth century, some medical branches of the U.S. military dabbled with the caduceus as a symbol of their noncombatant status. The U.S. Army Medical Department made the double snake its emblem in 1902. From there, physicians and others involved in medicine, apparently thinking it represented healing, adopted the shield of Mercury. In fact, the AMA briefly flirted with the symbol itself, having it sculpted into a façade near the front entrance of its headquarters building constructed in 1902.

However, Mercury has some connotations that are rather unflattering for the healing professions. Mercury was a trickster, who often lied his way out of jams. He also was the protector of thieves and businessmen, dating from an era when profits were considered a form of stealing.

Despite their differences, the confusion about the two symbols is understandable. In reality, they represent two sides of medicine and the American Medical Association. There is no doubt that physicians, in the Asklepian tradition, are members of a healing profession, offering comfort, alleviating suffering, and saving lives. But doctors also are in the business of running offices and making money. Like all who are engaged in commerce, doctors face the temptations of Mercury's darker side to boost the bottom line and add to their personal gain.

The Serpent on the Staff is written for those readers who want to see through the imagery and mythology to discover the reality of the AMA.

Chicago   Howard Wolinsky   Tom Brune
February 1994

CHAPTER 1

The American Doctors' Association
Looking After Medicine's Special Interests

Mere mention of the American Medical Association's name elicits strong negative and positive reactions. Some doctors boast that they never have been AMA members and would never join that bunch of fossils. Others seem shocked anyone could think that the AMA is anything less than a noble organization defending what it is best for patient and doctor alike.

Some people hold AMA responsible for everything wrong with the health-care system. Conspiracy theorists consider the AMA to be at the center of all manner of plots to stifle alternative medicine, to keep cures for cancer from the public, and to restrict the availability of health foods and vitamins. Others think of the AMA as a group of medical elders looking out after us, a kindly Big Doctor who removes the bad apples and makes sure we get the latest medical miracles we have come to expect. Some think the AMA stands for high principles, but has let the country down by not campaigning for this cause or that. The author of one popular book, for instance, berates the AMA for not taking on the diet industry.

Despite the spirited reactions, most Americans have only the vaguest idea what the American Medical Association actually does. The AMA is much more and much less than what the public or even physicians think.

How the AMA Affects Our Lives

In point of fact, the American Medical Association, the nation's largest physician group, affects everyday life in America, often subtly. Your family doctor's training as a medical student and resident was influenced by standards the AMA helped shape. The AMA also has a hand in the doctor's continuing education to maintain *his* (though the number of female doctors is rising, most are still men) skills and knowledge after he is in practice. And the AMA's Principles of Medical Ethics and opinions from the AMA's Council on Ethical and Judicial Affairs guide the doctor's behavior as he cares for you.

The AMA is not the scientific authority it once was, when as recently as a few decades ago it ran the largest clinical meetings in medicine and operated its own laboratory. But it still has a huge impact on what physicians and the public know about medicine.

The AMA regularly issues positions on scientific matters and it conducts public-health campaigns on such subjects as adolescent health, domestic violence, and cholesterol reduction, typically with generous support from drug companies, food companies, and other corporate sponsors.

Perhaps the AMA's biggest influence is as a medical communicator. To try to keep up with the latest medical developments, many harried physicians rely on the *Journal of the American Medical Association (JAMA)*, a weekly that has been published since 1883. With a 700,000 circulation, a little over half of it in the United States, *JAMA* is the largest general medical journal in the world. Independent researchers who conduct the studies that appear in medical periodicals consider the AMA's flagship second only to the *New England Journal of Medicine* in prestige. The AMA also publishes ten medical specialty publications and a weekly newspaper, *American Medical News,* which focuses on political and economic developments in medicine. Each week, hungry for medical news, the mass media publish or broadcast reports based on studies appearing in *JAMA* or its sister publications.

To make sure the AMA message and news from its publications are not missed, the AMA has created a huge public-relations apparatus. Each week the PR staff sends news releases to 4,000 medical and science journalists. It also dispatches video news releases based on studies in *JAMA* via satellite to 340 TV outlets; this information is often incorporated into the broadcasts by the networks and local stations. And five days a week, the AMA sends one-minute medical reports to 5,000 radio stations via satellite or a toll-free phone number. In a joint project between the AMA and NBC, American Medical Television produces medical information aimed at physicians, but also can be viewed by lay people, on cable television. The AMA publishes a number of consumer books on health, such as the popular *American Medical Association Family Medical Guide.*

It is fair to say that no one on the planet disseminates more words on medicine to the profession and the public than the AMA. All of this influences what our doctors do to diagnose and treat us and helps establish what we expect from our physicians.

But the AMA's influence goes beyond mass communications into hands-on medicine. If you are admitted into the hospital to have a baby or undergo a bypass operation, or into a nursing home to recover from a stroke, or into a hospice to live out your days, the AMA is there. From birth through death, the AMA has a role, sanctioned by the U.S. government, in setting standards in these institutions through the Joint Commission on Accreditation of Health Care Organizations, of which the AMA is a major owner. The AMA determines the very language of medical practice: when the doctor submits your bill to the insurance company or government program for reimbursement, he or she writes down a code number for whatever the problem may be from a book written by the AMA.

THE AMERICAN DOCTORS' ASSOCIATION

But the AMA is far more than a benign arbiter of medical standards and a publisher of medical journals. Protection of the power, privilege, and pocketbooks of physicians is the AMA's compass. The AMA's name is pretentious and misleading, suggesting it is the guardian of all aspects of medicine. It would be the equivalent of the American Bar Association calling itself the American Justice Association. The American Medical Association more appropriately should be called the American Doctors' Association.

The AMA may accomplish things that help patients, but make no mistake, it is a doctor-first organization. If you believe the AMA's claims that your well-being as a patient is its first priority, then you probably believe that Marcus Welby was a real doctor. The AMA did not evolve into one of the wealthiest and most powerful political lobbies to protect our rights as patients, or as consumers, the more assertive term doctors hate. Rather, it has worked hard to look after physician income and interests.

It is because of the AMA, for instance, that consumers do not have access to the National Practitioner Data Bank run by the U.S. government that lists doctors who have committed malpractice, ethical breaches, or crimes. The AMA argued that the public would misunderstand this information, so it used its clout to keep the data away from us.

Doctors who perpetrated such wrongdoing historically had nothing to fear from the AMA. Until recently, the AMA never disciplined its errant members convicted of wrongdoing. In more of a symbolic move than anything else, the AMA began purging its membership rolls of doctors who had already lost their licenses, often years before. The AMA had its reasons for this token gesture. It was trying to obtain government approval for the profession to police itself, a responsibility doctors had botched in the past.

PRACTICING MEDICAL POLITICS

Some of the AMA's influence has been diminished in recent years as other groups representing medical specialists have risen in importance. But the AMA remains the premier practitioner of the art and science of medical politics. The AMA is the proverbial 800-pound gorilla on Capitol Hill.

No other group involved in health care—certainly none representing consumers—can touch the AMA in terms of influence or access to power brokers. The AMA pays dearly for this perk. It consistently outspends not only all other medical groups but virtually all other special interests.

American presidents seeking to make changes in the health system without consulting the AMA do so at their own risk. If nothing else, the AMA has great power as a spoiler, and can delay, derail, and destroy the best-laid plans of presidents, legislators, and consumer activists. In his address launching the Health Security Act, a reform on which he has seemingly staked his presidency, Bill Clinton gave a nod to the AMA. It was one of only two organizations he mentioned by name. He said nice things about doctors, and made out the insurance companies and drug manufacturers to be the villains in the health-care crisis. The Clinton administration seemed to fathom that the best way to get the legislation passed was to try to stay in the good graces of the AMA.

While Clinton said the system was badly in need of repair, the AMA considers it only partially broken. For the AMA the glass is 85 percent full. In the AMA mind, the 15 percent of the population without insurance is the primary problem. The AMA says it wants a "pluralistic system," one offering several choices to consumers. But what it really means is that it wants to preserve the fee-for-service component of the system in which doctors are paid for each service rendered instead of fixed average amounts per patient or some other financial arrangement.

One reason our system is in trouble is because the AMA historically has seen health care as a privilege rather than a fundamental right for Americans, a privilege all but the poor must pay for by themselves. At least until now, Congress has gone along. In part because health care is not a basic right, 38 million uninsured Americans do not have easy access to doctors. They often delay seeking medical attention until they are extremely sick, when their conditions are far more difficult and expensive to treat.

Another reason we are in trouble is because doctors in the AMA-endorsed fee-for-service system have had few incentives to hold down costs. As "captains" of the health-care team, physicians recommend whether we undergo expensive hospitalizations and the latest in costly high-tech testing and therapies. Because many physicians were not prudent, they now have insurers and the government more closely monitoring which medical services are provided to us. Doctors are not totally to blame because we as consumers, with expectations fed by the media, pressure physicians to give us the newest and best and to do everything they can. For these and a cascade of other complex reasons, we are paying the price as our nation's health-care bill soon will surpass $1 trillion, consuming nearly a fifth of our Gross National Product. Americans spend more per capita on health care than any other people in the world.

THE SHRINKING VOICE OF MEDICINE

Hillary Rodham Clinton, "navigator" of the president's health plan, came to make peace and common cause with the AMA at the physician group's annual meeting in 1993. The AMA official who introduced her attempted to demonstrate the group's authority and standing in American life when he said the AMA represents 90 percent of the doctors in the country and 100 percent of the patients.

Just as it is questionable that the AMA represents patients, its claim to represent such a high proportion of the nation's estimated 650,000 doctors is dubious. AMA membership numbers are an important aid in looking beyond the AMA's vast resources to evaluate its right to speak for the profession and determine how much weight to give its positions.

Historically, the AMA has proclaimed itself to be the Voice of Medicine. It is a catchy phrase, and one that fit in the 1960s when nearly three-quarters of American physicians were members. But with the defeat on

Medicare, rising dues, protests against its position on abortion, and other factors, the AMA has experienced a significant drop in membership.

The only way the AMA can claim to represent 90 percent of physicians is through its federation of medical specialty organizations. Most of the doctors whom the AMA calls members have not chosen to belong directly to the AMA. Instead, they are "members" because their specialty society, such as the American College of Physicians, the American College of Surgeons, and the American Academy of Family Physicians, sends a single delegate to AMA meetings. The AMA counts these physicians to boost its apparent membership and its prestige before Congress and the public. But this is a desperate move by an association that cannot compel doctors to become members and has considerable difficulty persuading them to join voluntarily. The different specialty groups often are warring factions whose own agendas and policies may not coincide with those of the AMA's.

The AMA's real membership figures undermine its title as being the Voice of Medicine. By its own reckoning the AMA has 41 percent "market share"—its term for the proportion of eligible physicians who are members. The AMA shouts that 90 percent of doctors are in its ranks, but more meekly has set a goal by the turn of the century to have 50 percent of physicians as members. And it will probably have trouble reaching it.

Membership Bloat

A closer examination shows that the AMA exaggerates its membership figures to inflate its significance. Even the AMA does not have the audacity to claim 576,000 members, which would be 90 percent of American doctors. Rather, in media reports, in its ad campaigns aimed at decision-makers, and other forums, the AMA often trumpets that its membership is "300,000 physicians strong." If there is strength in numbers, the AMA is far weaker than its press releases would have us believe.

When asked its membership figures in summer 1993, the AMA said it had 275,510 members. But closer examination reveals that the AMA doctors its figures. Subtract 32,045 medical students, who pay a nominal $20 a year in dues and who after all are not physicians, the membership falls to 243,465 physician members, and market share dips to 38 percent of physicians. Eliminate all physicians with reduced dues, such as residents, young physicians and military doctors, and also dues-exempt retirees, you are left with 153,268 members, just 24 percent of American doctors who pay full annual dues of $420.

The proportion of full-dues-paying members is less than half of what it was twenty years ago and a third of what it was thirty years ago. The "powerful" AMA of the 1990s is a shadow of the AMA of the golden age in the 1960s.

How the AMA Is Organized

The AMA is organized somewhat along the lines of federal and state governments. At its center is the House of Delegates, its legislative branch, often referred to as the House of Medicine. The House, the shorthand name for this body, represents a variety of viewpoints within medicine. Its delegates come from the fifty state medical societies and from the District of Columbia, Puerto Rico, the Virgin Islands, and Guam. Each of these groups gets one vote per 1,000 members, and delegates are elected by state or territorial societies' Houses of Delegates rather than by popular vote.

The next-largest contingent of delegates comes from about eighty medical specialty societies, such as the American College of Obstetricians and Gynecologists, the American Academy of Pediatrics, and the American Academy of Orthopaedic Surgeons. These delegates also are not elected by popular vote, but are appointed by the medical specialty groups' presidents or by their governing bodies. The smallest source of delegates is the ten special sections representing such areas as hospital medical staffs, medical schools, students, the Public Health Service, and military physicians. The military and Public Health Service groups are represented by their own surgeons general, while the other sections elect their delegates.[1] Within the House of Delegates, each specialty group and each section gets a single vote.

The House of Delegates meets twice a year to vote on hundreds of resolutions and reports prepared by the AMA's Board of Trustees and various councils and committees, dealing with such topics as medical education, science, ethics, public health, and delivery of medical services. The annual meeting is held in Chicago, AMA headquarters city, in June, and the interim or midyear meeting is held in December, typically in some vacation spot, such as Honolulu, Las Vegas, or San Francisco.

The AMA House of Delegates meetings open on a Sunday with pomp (an honor guard from a military group presents the colors), prayer (from rotating religious groups), and pomposity (with speeches by AMA leaders and sometimes a visiting dignitary). The politicking begins before the opening session, with early-morning breakfasts by state delegations or other groups. As the meeting wears on, various caucuses huddle to promote their special interests, such as those of medical schools, surgeons, or geographic areas. They hold hot dog lunches, cocktail parties, luaus, Texas barbecues, wine-and-cheese tastings, and other events to attract fellow delegates, whom they hope to persuade to vote this way or that on particular issues. The New Jersey delegation hands out boxes of saltwater taffy, the Washington delegation, apples, and the Hawaii delegation has distributed orchids. These groups and others do what they can to make friends and win votes for their favorite resolutions and to lobby for their slate of candidates for the AMA Board of Trustees or other posts. When expenditures on electioneering seemed to be getting out of hand in the 1980s, the House formally urged restraint.

The House on Sunday and Monday breaks into "reference committees," comparable to congressional committees, which conduct hearings at which any physician, AMA member or not, can speak. Outside groups, such as the National Rifle Association and the AIDS activist group ACT-UP, sometimes are permitted to express their opinions. The nine reference committees, each dealing with specific areas such as legislation, public health, and medical practice, typically are where issues are debated in the greatest detail in hopes of influencing the delegate-members serving on the reference committees. The individual reference committees, aided by AMA staff, then summarize the proceedings and prepare recommendations on how the House of Delegates should vote. Committees often work well into the night to reach a consensus and to prepare their reports.[2]

The full House of Delegates, consisting of about 440 members, convenes Tuesday morning to begin voting on these issues and meets until Thursday at annual meetings and Wednesday at interim meetings. The House may adopt, reject, or refer back various pieces of business. The meetings, directed by a parliamentarian known as the Speaker of the House, go on for hours and hours, sometimes disposing of the most serious issues without debate and other times endlessly discussing where to place a comma or semicolon. The AMA likes to refer to this as "democracy in action."

Positions taken at the meeting serve as AMA policy and help guide the AMA's more than 1,200-member staff on what direction to take in its day-to-day activities. AMA policy is not legally binding for society at large, but has influenced state and federal lawmakers and the courts.

Most policies pushed through by delegates will languish as a matter of record in the AMA *Policy Compendium,* a book listing several thousand AMA policies, including its concern about destructive themes in rock-

and-roll music, its questioning of the validity of studies that exclude women, its misgivings about the high cost of medications, and its opposition to the use of amphetamines as a weight-loss method. Every delegate with a pet project or pet peeve has a chance to make it part of the compendium. However, as large as it is, the AMA does not have the time or money to give all these policies its full attention. Furthermore, Dr. James S. Todd, who since 1990 has been AMA executive vice president, the AMA term for chief executive, has stressed that the AMA now has to do fewer things and to do them better.

One of the more important duties of the House is to elect the AMA's powerful Board of Trustees, a sort of executive branch that includes the AMA president. The AMA Board has the ultimate legal and financial responsibility for the association, a not-for-profit organization that runs on a $180-million-a-year budget and owns several for-profit subsidiaries involved in investments, real estate, and other businesses. The Trustees also travel regularly to Washington to present AMA views to Congress. The board members speak to state and local medical societies, to the auxiliaries, and to other related groups to keep them informed of new developments, to make them feel connected to the national organization, and to listen to their problems. Board members also explain AMA policies on all sorts of issues, such as euthanasia or health reform, to the public through the media. The board, which meets approximately every other month, determines AMA policy when the House of Delegates is not in session. The House later may affirm or reject board positions.

The board's real power rests with the chairman, who decides which members carry out what duties. If a member is on the outs for some reason, he or she may get few choice assignments. Chairmanship of the board is often the route to becoming AMA president, a high-profile job with little power, which entails making loads of speeches, making appointments to committees, eating lots of chicken dinners, and collecting about a $200,000-a-year stipend.

The Delegates Are Not Representative

The AMA makes much of its "democratic" House, but its delegates are not representative of the medical profession, as AMA research has shown. Delegate positions tend to go to older, more established physicians with the time and interest to devote to medical politics. But the views of such delegates may not be those of the broader physician population.

The typical delegate is an office-based private practitioner at a time when physicians increasingly are working for hospitals and health-maintenance organizations or in other nontraditional settings. The AMA has student, resident, and young physician sections and has spots on its board earmarked for students and residents. But, generally, younger physicians who are building practices simply are unable to get involved. As a result, the House of Delegates underrepresents today's younger, more ethnically and racially diverse group of physicians, and the greater number of female doctors.

Traditionally, minority groups within medicine have not felt welcome. The House of Delegates did not have its first woman delegate until 1915. Dr. Nancy W. Dickey was elected the first woman to be a full-fledged board member in 1989. For most of the AMA's history, blacks effectively were kept out of the organization. Because of their race they were barred from many county medical societies, and therefore from the national group. The first African-American delegate did not enter the House until 1949, and there have been few since. However, in 1993–94, the AMA Board's chairman is an African-American, Dr. Lonnie R. Bristow. He was the first African-American to be elected to the board in the AMA's history, and was named president-elect in June 1994.

Despite such changes, the House of Delegates remains an old boys' club. The average delegate is a white male, nearing senior citizen status at sixty-three, compared with the average physician, who is forty-five. AMA statistics show other contrasts: 19 percent of today's physicians are women vs. 7 percent of AMA delegates; just over 3 percent of American physicians are African-American vs. under 1 percent of delegates; and 21 percent of American physicians are foreign graduates, vs. 3.3 percent of AMA delegates.[3]

AMPAC: The Political Arm

Another important face of the AMA is AMPAC—American Medical Political Action Committee—the conduit through which the AMA collects and distributes money to politicians so it can have the access it needs to make its views known and sway votes. AMPAC operates officially as a separate organization, although there is overlap in doctors who move back and forth from board membership in both. Doctors oriented toward patient care or education traditionally have been distrustful of AMPAC, feeling it does not represent the best side of medicine. Yet, over the years, recent AMA leaders, including longtime chief executive Dr. James H. Sammons, moved to the top of the organization's hierarchy, having been active in AMPAC and its state affiliates.

AMPAC has won notoriety and fame as one of the biggest spenders on politics and as an innovator in new means of influencing politicians. The AMA and AMPAC always are at war with such public-interest groups as Common Cause and Public Citizen, which seek to reform campaign-finance laws to put stricter limits on monied interests. Common Cause president Fred Wertheimer describes the AMA and AMPAC as "arrogant."

AMPAC contributions provide a map for the issues that really matter to the AMA. Like all special-interest groups seeking favors, AMPAC channels funds to politicians in positions to advance its economic and "reform" agenda. Over the years AMPAC has rewarded members of Congress who voted for its favored legislation, and attempted to punish those who voted against it. And the AMA and AMPAC have declared innumerable wars against Congress when it was considering legislation that would curb physician pay or would affect their prerogatives.

But rarely, if ever, has AMPAC put its money on the line for public-health matters, such as gun control, tobacco, or abortion. Harvard medical student Joshua M. Sharfstein and his father, Dr. Steven S. Sharfstein, examined whether AMPAC contributed money to politicians who supported the AMA's stated positions on those three issues. The results, published in the January 6 *New England Journal of Medicine*, showed that AMPAC gave more money to representatives who opposed the AMA's public-health stands than it did to legislators who supported them. The AMA criticized the Sharfstein study as too "narrow."

MEDICINE'S PLUMMETING POLLS

In addition to the AMA's internal troubles, organized medicine is losing public confidence. A 1993 AMA-sponsored opinion survey reported new lows in the public perception of the image of the AMA and doctors in general.

Mrs. Clinton alluded to the bad news in her speech to the AMA. "Most doctors and other health-care professionals choose careers in health and medicine because they want to help people," she said. "But too often . . . that motive is clouded by perceptions that doctors aren't the same as they used to be, they are not doing what they used to do, they don't care like they once did."

Furthermore, people do not trust the leaders of medicine as they once did. In fact, polls show a dramatic drop in the proportion of people who said they had a great deal of confidence in medical leaders: from 73 percent of those surveyed in 1966 to 33 percent in 1986.[4] After Harvard professor Robert J. Blendon reported that stunning downturn, the AMA began asking people to rate the job the AMA is doing to help assure quality medical care. The first five years of the survey recorded a gradual decline in the AMA's combined good and excellent rating, from 59 percent to 51 percent, while its poor rating doubled to 10 percent. But in 1993 the proportion who thought the AMA was doing a good or excellent job plummeted to 43 percent, while those who thought it was doing a poor job held fast at 10 percent.[5]

Though most of the public probably would be hard-pressed to detail the AMA's activities, in this poll, the organization continued to lose ground in the public eye as a scientific and educational organization. From 1989 to 1993, the survey asked people to say how reliable they believe the AMA is as a source of information on health. More than half think the AMA is *somewhat* reliable—indicating more than a hint of doubt or skepticism about the AMA as the house of medical experts. More importantly, the AMA researchers found, the proportion of people surveyed who said they believed the AMA was a *very* reliable source of information on health dropped from 31 percent to 23 percent.

The Doctors' Image Is Declining

As the AMA's reputation has suffered, so has the image of physicians in general. The vast majority of people consistently give high marks to their own doctors, but they don't feel the same way about the medical profession. This finding is comparable to the way the public feels about politicians: they like their own representatives, but distrust Congress as a whole.

Most people agree that doctors stay up-to-date on advances in medicine and take a genuine interest in their patients. But the most recent results from AMA polls found than 71 percent think doctors keep their patients in the waiting room too long, about 60 percent think doctors do not involve patients enough in deciding on treatment, and 44 percent believe doctors act like they are better than other people. Those statistics are a far cry from the more positive picture painted in an AMA survey in 1956.[6] Back then, only 22 percent thought doctors kept them waiting too long, 19 percent thought doctors were not sufficiently frank with them in discussing their treatment, and just 9 percent said doctors "think he's better than other people."

More damning to the medical profession, however, is the growing belief that doctors are too interested in making money—a rise to 69 percent in 1993 from 60 percent in 1982. More than two-thirds of the people surveyed the year before said they think doctors' fees are too high.

But worst of all, the share of those who think people are beginning to lose faith in doctors—62 percent in 1982—hit an all-time high in 1993 at 70 percent.

Indeed, the image of the doctor in popular culture has changed dramatically in the past two generations. Science writer Natalie Angier noted the decline of doctors' images—"From Dr. Welby to Dr. Giggles, a Steep Slide," is how the headline writer put it—in an article about the treatment of doctors in movies and on television shows for the *New York Times* Sunday Arts and Leisure section. Dr. Welby was everyone's dream of a good doctor; Dr. Giggles was the star villain in a slasher movie. It is almost startling to see a rerun of Dr. Ben Casey on television simply because he seems so in control. Angier noted that today's TV doctors have more problems than their patients.[7]

Many commentators note that all authority figures fell in popularity during the anti-establishment decade of the 1960s and the antiheroic decade of the 1970s. Lawyers, judges, businessmen, and, of course, politicians and journalists, all saw their ratings sag. Blendon, considered the top expert on health-care polls, found that the leaders of medicine still ranked twice as high as leaders of other major institutions. But while the others have enjoyed an upswing in confidence, the trust in medical leaders has continued to decline.

There is much speculation about this. Hillary Clinton, in her pitch to the AMA for health-care reform, pointed out that the tremendous stress from the breakdown of the health-care system—and "because . . . we haven't taken responsibility for fixing it"—has added to the clouds hanging over doctors' heads. Others have pointed out that doctors' high income—on average $177,400 and rising—makes them easy targets for criticism by most wage earners, who on average make about a sixth as much as doctors do.[8] Some suggest that people put so much faith in medicine's ability to cure—reminiscent of religious faith in the Dark Ages—that a sharp disappointment results when it fails to fulfill the unrealistically high expectations.[9]

Blendon said the public generally has a lot of confidence in professions or institutions that show altruistic behavior, scientific competence, and a nonpolitical nature. If public confidence is based on those three factors, it is not surprising that the image of the AMA has sunk so low.

Looking After Doctors' Well-Being

Dr. Arnold S. Relman, the respected editor emeritus of the *New England Journal of Medicine,* sought to explain the public's sense of betrayal by the AMA in an interview published in the *AMA Journal:* "I think that the

AMA has the image of a trade organization. It represents what is best for the economic and political interests of its members, and the American public expects more than that from its doctors. Society subsidizes the education of our physicians and then it grants them the licensed monopoly to practice, assuring them authority and independence and power. This power is granted on the condition that physicians put their patients first—truly ahead of everything else."[10]

The AMA is well aware of its image problem, in part because of its polls and in part because of the prodding of people like Relman. Even its own editor, *JAMA's* George D. Lundberg, recognized the seriousness of the AMA's ailing reputation in 1985. He wrote an editorial following the release of an AMA poll showing the sharp decline of public trust of physicians and organized medicine. He outlined a series of steps to rehabilitate the image of medicine, including one point about appearances vs. reality. "We should spend less time and money on influencing laws and regulations and on formal public relations and should spend more time and money on making things right," he declared.[11]

Health-care reform offers the AMA that possibility, but so far the actions of the AMA appear once again to be focused on issues that primarily benefit doctors and the AMA: legal tort reform limiting a doctor's liability if he or she is sued for malpractice, an attack on a global budget and other fiscal devices that might limit doctors' pay, and relief from antitrust laws to strengthen the doctors' bargaining position over economic and other practice issues. To woo the AMA, Hillary Clinton offered to help doctors rebuild their image.

But the AMA so far has not taken her up on her offer. Instead, at their December 1993 meeting AMA delegates backed away from the Clintons and their own four-year-old plan. The AMA doctors simply could not stomach the idea of requiring employers to pay for the insurance of their workers. Many of them, after all, have offices that employ people. That means they, too, would have to pay for their employees' health insurance.

The AMA's switch brought a harsh rebuke from Hillary Clinton. She said, "Remember that the AMA institutionally opposed nearly every health-care reform we've ever been able to achieve." She downplayed the AMA's importance as a force in the health-care debate. Her husband shared her chagrin. The President said he was "real disappointed" at the AMA's action. Although both expressed hope that the AMA would return to the fold, and support their plan, they also looked to other doctors for support.[12] After all, the majority of the nation's physicians do not belong to the AMA.

Fighting "The Inevitable"

Stopping National Health Insurance at All Costs

Health care reform seems inevitable these days. Nearly everyone agrees that the time has come to mend the United States' patchwork system of health care. It appears to be out of control, as it races toward consuming 18 percent of national resources—more than $1 trillion a year—while it still does not cover at least 37 million Americans.[1] Since 1992, President Bill Clinton and his wife, Hillary Rodham Clinton, have raised expectations that they will succeed in overhauling the way we receive and pay for medical care.

This is not the first time reform has seemed inevitable. Five times previously liberal reformers believed they were on the brink of restructuring the delivery or financing of health care to make it more widely available and more affordable to greater numbers of people. But each time, they ran into a no-holds-barred battle with the forces of reaction led by the conservative leaders of the American Medical Association. The AMA won every battle but one, the passage of federal Medicare for the elderly.

With that one exception, the AMA has managed to stave off significant reform for most of the century. The AMA is responsible, in large part, for the way we get our health care today. And the health-care system bears its stamp: it is a system that has made American doctors the wealthiest in the world, but allows the health of Americans to lag behind those in many other industrialized countries.

The history of the AMA and the five previous battles reveal the AMA's true interests: the protection of doctors, their control of the system, and their earnings. It also reveals the AMA's tactics and strategies. The AMA has won by creating coalitions to directly defeat reform bills or by working with key lawmakers to stall legislation until the moment for change passes. Although the AMA's power has waned, it still looms as a key factor when lawmakers ponder whether reform is politically possible.

The AMA is now engaged in the sixth battle over health-care reform. Early on, the AMA set out to protect the existing system by promoting limited reform to avert a major restructuring or greater government involvement. And the AMA declared war on any proposals that borrowed from the Canadians' government-run "single-payer" health-care system.

The AMA has sought to refashion its image from an obstacle to a proponent of change. But, as in the past, it has evolved from acknowledging the need for reform to adopting a hard line against it. AMA leaders employ a sophisticated doublespeak, proclaiming "the status quo must go," while actually opposing fundamental structural change. They attack national systems in other countries by insisting on an "American" solution. And they resort to scare tactics, raising alarms of "rationing" as they did in the past with cries of "socialism."

The AMA has vowed to use every tactic and spend every dollar it can to protect what it deems as the best interests of patients and doctors during the national-health-care debate. Let the public beware: the AMA is playing for keeps, and it is working for doctors. When the battle is over, the AMA may be five out of six.

THE FIRST BATTLE

Many leaders of the AMA were among those who thought compulsory health insurance was inevitable in the years before 1920. At the time, the AMA was in its Progressive phase, fighting for federal regulation of food and drugs and a federal department of health run by a doctor, and the prospect did not alarm it. In fact, the AMA stopped just short of endorsing a model health-insurance bill in 1916. In a letter to the bill's authors, Dr. Frederick R. Green, secretary of the AMA's Council on Health and Public Instruction, wrote, "Your plans are so entirely in line with our own that I want to be of every possible assistance."[2]

The proposal was a cross between the German and English systems and was meant for the working class only. German chancellor Otto von Bismarck adopted the first national health program in 1883, mainly to buy workers' loyalty to the government in the face of a popular socialist movement. Versions of the program soon spread to most European nations. A form of it reached Great Britain in 1911, when Prime Minister Lloyd George established a government-run health system.

Reformers in the United States proposed a system that would help workers pay for doctors, hospitals, medicine, maternity benefits, and even funerals. Employers and employees each would kick in 40 percent of the cost, and the government would pick up the rest. It was "compulsory" because nearly all workers making under $1,200 a year would be required to participate. Middle- and upper-class people would continue to pay for their own care, which was then delivered primarily by family doctors.

But the AMA had its concerns, fearing that reformers might use insurance laws to change the traditional way that doctors practiced medicine. In this tradition, which the AMA had helped create, each doctor worked independently, charged patients a fee for each service rendered, expected patients to pay at the time of treatment, and provided free care to those whom doctors deemed worthy of charity. Some reformers said medical care could be delivered more efficiently if doctors instead worked in groups and were paid a fixed annual amount for each patient, with the payments spread among a pool of people through insurance or taxes. But the AMA adamantly opposed those changes because they would undermine physician control and limit their potential earnings.

To study the proposal—and protect the doctors' way of life—the AMA set up a Committee on Social Insurance, chaired by a prominent AMA member and insurance proponent, Dr. Alexander Lambert. He was the doctor of former President Teddy Roosevelt, a supporter of compulsory health insurance in his failed bid for president as the Progressive candidate. For his staff, Lambert hired the Progressives' insurance expert, Dr. Isaac M. Rubinow, a nonpracticing doctor, Russian immigrant, and socialist.

Lambert and Rubinow advanced three arguments for compulsory health insurance. First, it was good for the people. "No other social movement in modern economic development is so pregnant with benefit to the public," said an editorial in the *Journal of the American Medical Association*.[3] Most people simply did not have access to a doctor or medical care. An AMA official had earlier estimated that each year there were 600,000 deaths and 3 million illnesses at a cost of $1.5 billion in economic loss from preventable illness.[4] Second, it would boost doctors' incomes. *JAMA* reported that some British doctors saw their incomes double in poor industrial districts under national health insurance.[5] And finally, it was inevitable. If Great Britain had adopted it, the thinking went, surely the United States was not far behind.

To head off any major changes that might threaten doctors' incomes or autonomy, the AMA's policy-setting House of Delegates in 1917 laid down guidelines for health-insurance plans. The first insisted the insured have freedom to choose their own physician, which would help preserve independent practice. The second required payment of the physician in proportion to the amount of work done, which would protect the fee-for-service system. The third sought to relieve doctors from administrative work. And the last sought to ensure AMA influence by requiring M.D. representation on the program's oversight agencies.6

A Hostile Turnaround

But it was during 1917 that momentum for social change began to flag in the United States. Within the ranks of the AMA, a split over national health insurance grew. Generally, doctors at medical schools favored it, and practicing physicians—fearing it was a threat to their autonomy and incomes—opposed it. Meanwhile commercial insurance firms lobbied against a government plan and business fretted about the costs. Even the head of the American Federation of Labor opposed it because it took away an issue he could use to organize workers. Many special-interest groups lined up against it; few groups formed to support it.

When the United States entered the World War, an anti-German fever spread at the AMA and across the country. The AMA's president urged a witch-hunt for disloyal German doctors. Soon compulsory health insurance was tainted as "un-American" because of its origins in Germany. Following the Russian revolution, the AMA became caught up in the Red Scare sweeping the country. And some AMA leaders branded national health insurance as a detestable form of "socialism."

By 1920 the aura of inevitability surrounding compulsory health insurance had vanished. *JAMA* began publishing attacks on it, and the AMA's Dr. Green denied he had ever embraced it. States that had considered the model bill dropped it, and the concept was DOA at the AMA's annual meeting. The House of Delegates dissolved the Committee on Social Insurance and passed a resolution that stood for years as official policy: the AMA is opposed to any compulsory plan of health insurance run or regulated by any state or the federal government.

After the meeting, Lambert wrote to the reform group pushing health insurance, advising it to go forward without organized medicine. He told the reformers to offer physicians a fair proposition, and then hammer the inadequacy of the health-care system and the profession's refusal to improve it. "That will throw them on the defensive," he wrote. Meanwhile, Lambert was philosophical about the AMA's German-bashing and red-baiting. "I think that my profession will get over its present state of hysteria just as my ancestors got over the Salem witchcraft," he wrote. "They had it bad at that time, and the profession has 'got it bad' now."[7]

THE SECOND BATTLE

In simple, stark, and shocking terms, the AMA's key spokesman in 1932 described what he saw as the struggle over the future of medical care in the United States: "The alinement [sic] is clear—on one side the forces representing the great foundations, public health officialdom, social theory—even socialism and communism—inciting to revolution; on the other side, the organized profession . . . urging an orderly evolution . . ."[8]

A dozen years had passed since the AMA had turned against compulsory health insurance, and in that time, physicians had come into their own. By the 1930s physicians and the AMA had succeeded in shaping the health-care system so that doctors were the dominant force. But contrary to Lambert's prediction, the AMA had not gotten over its hysteria. It still had it bad.

The declaration of war came from the pen of Dr. Morris Fishbein, the glib, prolific, and omnipresent editor of the *AMA Journal.* For more than a quarter of a century Fishbein personified the AMA, his visibility spread through countless articles, columns, and books, and his voice well known from myriad speeches and radio broadcasts. He had earned an M.D., but he never practiced; he joined the staff of the *Journal of the American Medical Association* as an assistant editor in 1913 and rose to its editorship in 1924. He remained in that post until the AMA Board, long outshone by the editor, ousted him in a coup in 1949. Fishbein turned the journal into the AMA's meal ticket; he became the AMA's mouthpiece. A master of the well-turned phrase, Fishbein supplied physicians with verbal ammunition against any and all perceived enemies of organized medicine. And he decided that the Committee on the Costs of Medical Care was a threat to the AMA and to doctors.

Founded in 1927, the committee had forty-five members that included doctors—twenty-three had medical degrees—academics, social workers, insurance company executives, and others. Eight private foundations underwrote the committee's $1 million cost. The committee had made it a point to reach out to the AMA. Indeed, its chairman was

Dr. Ray Lyman Wilbur, a former AMA president and staunch Republican who served as Secretary of the Interior under Herbert Hoover.

Over five years, the committee produced the most comprehensive and detailed survey of health care in more than two dozen studies. It came up with the first estimate of national health expenditures: $3.66 billion, or 4 percent of the national income. A study found about 30 cents of every dollar spent on health care went to pay doctors. Another report said only half of lower-income families had received medical care, and the country needed a new, more efficient system to make sure they could.

The health-care system recommended by the majority of the committee relied on group practices—that is, several doctors working together collectively—based at hospitals. That would be a big change from the way medicine was practiced, with each doctor working alone, usually out of an office. To finance the care for most Americans, the majority recommended using insurance, taxes, or both. To pay for the poor, it said local governments should share the cost on a per capita or lump-sum basis. But the majority said doctors should be allowed to continue in the traditional fee-for-service practice. And while the majority backed voluntary insurance, it rejected compulsory insurance.

That should have made the doctors on the committee happy. But it didn't. In a sharply worded dissent, eight physicians declared the status quo was just fine. They rejected group practice as "mass production" medicine and insisted "the central place in medical practice" belonged to the independent, fee-for-service general practitioner. As for financing, the doctors attacked voluntary health insurance as a "bridge" to a compulsory system. Government's only role should be to care for the poor, they said, "with the ultimate object of relieving the medical profession of this burden."[9]

Fishbein immediately endorsed the dissenting doctors' view. His editorials contained some of his most acerbic attacks, such as calling group practices "medical soviets." Wilbur J. Cohen, an architect of Social Security and a key figure in health policy, said Fishbein launched the AMA's "devil theory of history" with his writings: liberals pushing national health insurance sought to persecute doctors, not bring care to unserved millions. Cohen added, "His use of that incendiary language set the tone of the discussions for years to come."[10]

Intimidating Roosevelt

By the mid-1930s the country was struggling with the Great Depression, and the nation's health-care problems appeared even starker than before. With upwards of 14 million workers suddenly unemployed, agitation for social legislation had regained credibility. The time seemed ripe for the passage for compulsory health insurance. The AMA feared Franklin D. Roosevelt would tack it on to his Social Security legislation.

In January 1935 a federal panel, appointed by Roosevelt, called for expanded public-health programs and nationwide preventive medicine. It also suggested the cost of health care be paid for with insurance. But the AMA intimidated Roosevelt. He did not recommend adoption of compulsory health insurance because he feared it would be used to block Social Security legislation and its retirement benefits for the elderly, regardless of income. The Social Security bill that came to Congress for consideration in 1935 mentioned health insurance in only one line, and that merely called for it to be studied. Yet even that line was deleted after the AMA sent telegrams protesting it.

The AMA did not take its victory for granted. In February 1935 it called a rare special session of its House of Delegates to reaffirm the guidelines placing doctors in control of all medical care and practice that they had established for any "social experiment in changing the nature of medical practice." And the AMA took its fight to every arena, and conducted surrogate battles through state and local medical societies.

AMA-affiliated medical societies launched a boycott against the Borden Milk Co. to get at the Milbank Fund, which the company funded and which advocated compulsory health insurance. The boycott worked. Milbank fired its director and muted its program on health.[11]

When federal employees organized the Group Health Association in Washington—creating what would now be called a health-maintenance organization—to provide medical care to government workers at a fixed fee per person, the local medical society and the AMA responded in 1937 by expelling the doctors and seeking to end their hospital privileges. The federal government successfully sued the AMA for antitrust. But more often such actions by AMA affiliates went unchallenged.[12]

And the AMA created its own "research" to knock other studies. For example, a government study found a large proportion of the population could not afford to pay for medical care and that the care given was inadequate. The AMA surveyed its medical-society affiliates, and, not surprisingly, found, "Fully 90 percent of all the sources consulted reported they knew of no significant number of persons needing and seeking medical care who were unable to obtain it." But as AMA historian James G. Burrow noted, despite such assurances, "an increasing percentage of the population became harder to convince."[13]

No New Deal on Health

In July 1938 health-reform advocates in the Roosevelt administration orchestrated a three-day National Health Conference in Washington, D.C., to sell a national health program. Studies presented there showed health-care needs had outgrown the health-care system—a third of the population received inadequate or no medical service, and an even larger segment suffered financially from illness. The conference recommended a program that the states would operate with federal subsidies. It called for expanded public-health services as well as maternal and child health services, through the Social Security system; expansion of hospital facilities; increased aid for those on relief or who had no money for health care; and a plan to compensate lost wages from a temporary or permanent disability. It also called for a comprehensive medical program financed by insurance, or taxes, or both.

Once again, a national health-insurance plan appeared to be inevitable. In a private meeting, AMA leaders offered the Roosevelt administration a deal: the AMA would support all of the other proposals if the Administration would drop compulsory health insurance. The Administration rejected the deal. When the AMA called another special session of its House of Delegates, it publicly adopted the terms of the spurned deal. To avoid national health insurance, the AMA was willing to make concessions.

But circumstances once again dissipated the aura of inevitability, rendering many of the AMA's concessions unnecessary. Roosevelt backed off from personally pushing the suggested reforms after a more conservative Congress was elected in 1938. The health-care bills introduced by New Deal legislators went nowhere. The entire movement ground to a halt soon after the United States entered World War II. The AMA stalled long enough so that changing politics and war again shoved social reform aside.14

THE THIRD BATTLE

The AMA went into shock in 1948. President Harry S Truman defied conventional wisdom and defeated the Republican presidential candidate, Thomas E. Dewey. Truman had made health care a major issue in his campaign, lashing out at the "well-organized medical lobby" and the "Republican 80th 'do-nothing' Congress." While Dewey sided with the Republicans on health care, Truman chided them for killing the national health plan he had supported when he became President following Roosevelt's death.15

The Democratic plan sought to create a national health system under Social Security that would cover everyone, regardless of income, and would be run by the federal government. It was the most far-reaching proposal ever offered, and it was the first to be backed by a president. When Truman triumphed—he also regained Democratic control of Congress—the election was deemed a mandate for his health-insurance plan.

A major change in the American health-care system again appeared to be inevitable. But this time the reform focused primarily on the financing of care. Unlike reformers of the Progressive era, Truman did not seek to reorganize the system by pushing doctors into group practice. Nor did he try to change fee-for-service payments. He wanted the federal government to finance the system so everyone, no matter how rich or poor, would have equal access to medical care. The United States was spending only four cents on the dollar for health care, and Truman declared, "We can afford to pay more than 4 percent."

Although the AMA was willing to endorse federal subsidies for hospital construction, public-health departments, and medical research, it continued to draw the line at a national health-insurance system. The AMA acted out of ideology: it and its members railed against the encroachments by the Big Government created under the New Deal and feared the rise of socialism, such as had happened in Great Britain after the war. But the AMA also sought to defend the autonomy and incomes of its members. After all, even if the government allowed doctors to continue to rule medical care, under a national system it could decide to change the way medicine was delivered or even set fees. And the AMA was wedded to the status quo.

Public sentiment, however, appeared to be running in favor of sweeping changes, according to various polls. For example, 52 percent of New Yorkers favored a compulsory system and 70 percent of Washington, D.C., residents backed Truman's plan. Even a poll taken by a physicians' group that the AMA set up to fight compulsory health insurance found that 55 percent of those surveyed favored a federal prepaid medical plan.16

In 1949 the AMA kicked off a counteroffensive. In an emergency session, it passed a special $25 assessment on its members to build a war chest. The assessment was controversial, especially among newspapers, whose editorial pages criticized it as unseemly. Even some doctors blanched at the thought of a political fund. But the AMA's members responded enthusiastically, sending in more than $2.2 million in the first year of the campaign.[17]

Meanwhile the AMA scrambled for an alternative to Truman's plan, and found it in an innovation in health-care financing it had once spurned—private health insurance. Over the years, *JAMA* editor Fishbein and other AMA spokesmen had sniped at all forms of insurance, suggesting they might interfere with the doctor-patient relationship. They said people should put money into savings accounts so they could pay for health care when the need arose. And they complained that too many people spent more money on movies and candy than on medical services. But faced with Truman's plan, the AMA began vigorously boosting what it called voluntary private health insurance.[18] For those who could not afford to buy insurance, the AMA unofficially backed the Republican plan of appropriating $200 million in federal funds to subsidize the purchase of private health insurance for the poor.

Five Million Bucks Stop Here

To sway public opinion, starting in 1949 the AMA launched one of the first nationwide political–public relations campaigns in U.S. history. The AMA hired the San Francisco–based husband-wife public relations team of Clem Whitaker and Leone Baxter, generally considered the first modern-day political consultants. They came to the AMA's attention by helping Earl Warren become Governor of California, and then, at the behest of the AMA-affiliated California Medical Association, running the campaign that defeated Warren's plan for a state-run health system. The AMA paid Whitaker and Baxter $100,000 a year until 1952, when they left to run the Eisenhower-Nixon presidential campaign. During its three-and-a-half-year run, the AMA's campaign cost nearly $5 million, an unprecedented sum.[19]

Whitaker and Baxter's National Education Campaign on National Health Insurance consisted of hundreds of pamphlets, leaflets, and radio and print ads. The duo created coalitions with civic and farm groups, veterans' and other conservative organizations, and businesses. They promoted an image to capture people's imagination: an 1891 painting by the British artist Sir Luke Fildes of an old-fashioned doctor watching over a sick child. They printed 65,000 copies of a poster of the painting—to be hung in physicians' offices—with the headline: KEEP POLITICS OUT OF THIS PICTURE! The poster went on to describe compulsory health insurance as "political medicine" that would create inferior medicine, red tape, and a heavy tax burden, and would bring "a politician between you and your doctor." And the AMA adopted a simple slogan: "The Voluntary Way Is the American Way."

The campaign also resorted to red-baiting, heating up the Red Scare already gripping the country as the hot war turned into the Cold War. The AMA asserted the U.S. system was the best in the world, and that its deficiencies were being greatly exaggerated. It charged Truman's program of "socialized medicine" would turn doctors into "slaves," and accused Truman aides of being "importers of alien philosophies."[20] An AMA president speaking on radio during peak listening time said, "American medicine has become the blazing focal point in a fundamental struggle which may determine whether America remains free or whether we are to become a socialist state."[21]

Within a year of the start of the intense, controversial campaign, Whitaker and Baxter had won over the public in the debate on Truman's plan. They had seized the initiative from Truman by redefining the issue in the popular imagination. No longer was it a question of greater health security, as Truman defined it. Now it was a battle over "socialized medicine." In 1950 the effort to enact a national health-insurance plan ground to a halt. Conservative Republicans won control of Congress, and with the start of the Korean War, Truman backed away from national health insurance. The AMA's stall had worked again.

THE FOURTH BATTLE

After the AMA defeated Truman's health-insurance plan, it faced few challenges during the 1950s. But the decade also brought about a shift in tactics by proponents of national health insurance: focusing on the elderly. Health needs and costs were greatest for those over sixty-five, and the number of older people has grown steadily with the rise in standard of living. But the system of private insurance that developed to finance medical care began to exclude the elderly as bad risks.[22]

The liberal-Democratic response was to seek to help the elderly by including hospital coverage in the benefits they received from Social Security. After all, senior citizens had a reasonable claim on assistance in the Social Security program, which they had helped finance. And by accepting Social Security, society had agreed that the elderly needed special help.

The AMA's leaders opposed any extensions of Social Security, primarily because it covered those who could afford to pay for their own medical costs, but also because they feared it would be an incremental step to a national health-insurance program for everyone, regardless of age or income. As it had in the past, the AMA insisted that the government should help only the poor. It also said that any national program to do even that should be run by private business or, failing that, state governments.

The war began in 1957, when an obscure Rhode Island congressman introduced a bill to cover hospital costs for the elderly under Social Security. The AMA reacted strongly and quickly—too much so, one of its lobbyists said years later in retrospect. For the next eight years, the AMA engaged in an expensive and intense battle with the AFL-CIO and other proponents of national health insurance. In its filings with the government, the AMA reported it spent about $1.6 million on lobbying, including $1 million in 1965 alone for an advertising blitz. Doctors complained they had to spend so much because of the concerted efforts of Big Labor. But during that period, the AFL-CIO reported spending a little more than half the AMA amount.[23]

In 1960 Massachusetts Democratic senator John F. Kennedy won a narrow victory over Republican vice president Richard M. Nixon. Enactment of a government-run health program for the elderly stood out as a priority on Kennedy's agenda. Once again, the AMA found itself on the defensive. And it again responded by seeking an alternative that did little to seriously change the status quo while protecting the dominance of doctors. First, the AMA gave its conditional backing to a law creating what was known as the Kerr-Mills program, in which the federal government provided matching grants to states to offer insurance assistance to the needy elderly. No one was particularly enthusiastic about Kerr-Mills, named for its sponsors Senator Robert Kerr (D-Okla.) and Representative Wilbur Mills (D-Ark.). But to the AMA, it was preferable to the legislation that would become Medicare.

The battle to influence the public became intense. The AMA started a mass-media campaign to counter materials being distributed by the labor-backed National Commission of Senior Citizens. Among its propaganda techniques, the AMA's red-baiting stood out. In the early 1960s, for example, an actor-cum-political spokesman, Ronald Reagan, cut a 33⅓ rpm record for the AMA's "Operation Coffee Cup." The AMA's Women's Auxiliary urged doctors' wives to hold coffees to play the recording, entitled "Ronald Reagan Speaks Out Against Socialized Medicine." Reagan warned listeners, "One of the traditional methods of imposing statism or socialism on a people has been by way of medicine." If Medicare passed, he said, "one of these days you and I are going to spend our sunset years telling our children and our children's children what it once was like in America when men were free."24

The AMA also battled Kennedy on his own turf, and in his favorite medium, television. In a nationally televised address from Madison Square Garden, where 20,000 elderly people cheered him on, Kennedy argued for the passage of legislation that would extend Social Security to cover hospital care of all the elderly. But Kennedy, a usually charismatic speaker, fell flat, delivering one of the worst addresses of his career.

After the crowd cleared out, Dr. Edward R. Annis, the AMA's most dynamic speaker, stood at the podium where Kennedy had been a few hours earlier. The AMA had rented the hall—and even paid extra to keep it from being cleaned—to film Annis delivering a rebuttal. In a speech that was nationally broadcast the next night in a time slot purchased by the AMA, Annis looked out over the empty seats and the pennants, paper cups, and flyers that littered the floor. He then gave a "hellfire and brimstone" speech staking out the AMA's unyielding opposition to Kennedy's plan. Annis warned viewers, "The public is in danger of being blitzed, brainwashed and bandwagoned. . . . "25

The Johnson Juggernaut

The AMA and its allies succeeded in stymieing Kennedy during his shortened term in office. But Kennedy's assassination, and the assumption of power by Lyndon B. Johnson, changed everything. A master politician, Johnson, more than Truman or Kennedy, knew how to whip Congress into line. And when Johnson campaigned for president in 1964, he promised he would make Medicare a top priority. He won in a landslide, and his coattails helped elect one of the most liberal, Democratic Congresses ever. On the first day of his new term, he kept his campaign promise by sending up Medicare as House Resolution No. 1. A national health-insurance program for the elderly appeared to be inevitable.

The AMA stood fast in its opposition to Medicare, and offered an alternative plan. In February 1965 Dr. Donovan Ward, the AMA's president, and three other AMA officials presented their objections and their plan in an executive hearing on Medicare at the invitation of the Ways and Means Committee. Mills, the committee's chairman, was a friend of the AMA who believed the financing of Social Security should not be tampered with.

"The American Medical Association opposes H.R. 1 as it opposed the same legislation which was rejected by the last two Congresses," Ward said. "It would represent a dangerous venture by the Federal Government in the field of health care. . . . Government regulation and control which would be established under this bill is not compatible with good medicine."[26]

The sponsors of Medicare had hoped to tiptoe around the AMA by simply excluding doctors from the legislation, making it a hospital-payment program only. But the AMA made hay of this fact. "We are opposed to offering false promises to the unfortunate who do need help. This bill would provide only a fraction of the care necessary in any serious illness, a fact which many of our aged do not realize," Ward said.[27]

The AMA proposed its alternative, Eldercare. For poor seniors only, the plan covered hospital and doctor bills. Meanwhile, an AMA ally, Representative Thomas W. Byrnes (R-Wis.), also jumped on the fact that Medicare covered only hospital care. He introduced a bill allowing the elderly to purchase private insurance to cover hospital and doctor bills in a federally administered program. It was also a voluntary program. General government revenues would pick up two thirds, and the elderly would pick up the other third through deductions from their pension checks.

Mills had put aside his reservations and signaled to the President that he would go along after Johnson's huge victory. To everyone's surprise, he sought a consensus by including a scrap from each major proposal into a whole new program, and in the process, creating an even more ambitious and far-reaching program than Medicare's sponsors had dared to propose. The result was referred to as a "three-layer cake." Medicare Part A, taken from H.R. 1, covered hospital costs. Medicare Part B, borrowed from Byrnes, covered doctor bills. And Medicaid, fashioned from the AMA, covered the poor. The President's point man on Medicare, Wilbur J. Cohen, crowed: "In effect, Mills had taken the AMA's ammunition, put it in the Republicans' guns, and blown both of them off the map."[28]

In a set of extraordinary circumstances, the AMA had lost. The AMA was at the peak of its power—seven of every ten doctors belonged to it, a higher percentage of doctors as members than ever before or since. In defeat, the AMA would never wield quite as much power. But it had learned about the value of money, the significance of working Congress, the importance of staking out a position. And after the AMA's leaders quelled a move by its members to boycott Medicare, it made sure doctors would benefit from the new national program. Johnson, like Truman, did not seek to reorganize health care, but simply to expand it. Medicare became a pipeline of money to hospitals and doctors.

THE FIFTH BATTLE

The AMA, still smarting from its defeat on Medicare, soon faced an even more daunting challenge. United Auto Workers president Walter P. Reuther renewed the campaign for national health insurance in a speech to the American Public Health Association in November 1968. He said the U.S. system was in a state of crisis, and announced a new Committee for National Health Insurance would push for a government-financed and -run program of universal health insurance. His call for reform opened a floodgate of proposals. Politicians from conservative Republican president Richard M. Nixon to liberal Democrat senator Edward M. Kennedy echoed his declaration that a crisis faced the U.S. health-care system. The rush to reform placed doctors and hospitals once again on the defensive.[29]

The AMA denied the system faced a crisis. It called the U.S. system the best in the world and insisted that many of the health problems cited by studies and experts were more likely the result of societal factors and economics than the absence of medical treatment. The few gaps in the system could be fixed, the AMA said, warning that frustration with rising costs should not automatically lead to the scrapping of the existing system.

To patch the cracks, the AMA offered a plan called Medicredit. It would have given everyone under sixty-five tax credits, graduated from 100 percent for those who pay no taxes to 10 percent for those at the upper bracket, to buy a private health-insurance plan. The AMA assigned its lobbyists to round up legislators to back the plan. Within a year the AMA published a list of ninety-five Medicredit sponsors in the House. Two thirds of them got contributions from the AMA's political-action committee for their campaign funds for the next election.[30]

According to an official AMA history, Medicredit's acknowledgment that the federal government has a legitimate role in the financing of health care was a sharp break from the AMA's past. But the history also admits, "No one in the AMA was so naive as to think that a Medicredit bill would pass." It was little more than a bid to gain a seat at the negotiating table.[31]

At that table were two key players, Kennedy and Nixon. Kennedy, who held the key chairmanship on the Labor and Public Welfare Subcommittee on Health, became labor's chief sponsor for national health legislation. Hints of presidential aspirations gave his position added strength. Nixon, a pragmatist, faced the problem of fashioning a conservative response in a liberal era.

Kennedy and Nixon agreed on fundamental problems: too many Americans did not have access to health care, and those who did were paying more but getting less for their health-care dollar. They expressed concerns about the skyrocketing costs of health care. The Department of Health, Education and Welfare, for example, showed that per capita health spending had more than doubled to $270 in 1969 from $128 in 1960.

But Kennedy and Nixon responded with very different plans, sparking a debate about the proper role of government in health care. Kennedy proposed the Health Security Act to create what is now called a tax-based "single-payer" system. It would wipe out private health-insurance companies and finance health care for everyone through Social Security. Nixon offered the National Health Insurance Partnership, a prototype of what today is "managed competition." It would preserve private health-insurance firms, require companies to offer insurance to employees, and restructure the delivery of care through prepaid group practices called health-maintenance organizations, or HMOs.[32]

In 1974 the timing seemed ripe. Both Nixon, to the dismay of most of his cabinet, and Kennedy, to the outrage of labor, moved toward compromise. They both sought to require employers to offer standard-benefit insurance plans to employees, make the people pay out of pocket, deductibles and copayments, and also require them to pay at least $1,000 before covering catastrophic care. Both also accepted the continued existence of insurance companies, although Nixon would have them sell policies while Kennedy would have them administer a federal system. Nixon would make participation by employees voluntary, and Kennedy would make it mandatory. Nixon also would decentralize the system by requiring states to administer it, while Kennedy would impose federal control.[33]

Although compromise seemed to be in the air, labor and the AMA blasted Kennedy's proposal. Labor abandoned Kennedy and stayed with the Health Security Act. The AMA reintroduced Medicredit and criticized both Kennedy's and Nixon's efforts to restructure American health care. The reform movement momentarily stalled with the start of impeachment proceedings against Nixon. After he resigned, the new President, Gerald R. Ford, started the ball rolling again, saying, "Why don't we write—and I ask this in the greatest spirit of cooperation—a good health bill on the statute books before Congress adjourns?"[34]

The Doctors' Dozen

Ways and Means chairman Mills took Ford's words to heart in August 1974. He whipped together a compromise plan in which employers and employees would have to participate in a national program financed through private insurance premiums; the poor, the self-employed, and others would be covered in a state-run alternative program funded by new general revenues, and catastrophic costs would be covered under a federal program funded by a 0.4 percent hike in employer payroll tax.

The committee became a magnet for lobbyists and PAC contributions from special interests with a stake in a national health-care system. The AMA tapped its wealthy members to raise ample funds for its political action committee, which gives money to the campaign funds of political candidates. In 1974 the AMA's PAC set aside $25,000 strictly for contributions to members of the Ways and Means Committee—a large sum in those days. In 1973 and 1974 the PAC contributed more than $1 million to 245 federal candidates—an even larger sum. Half of the candidates supported Medicredit and the other half were undeclared.[35]

When Mills met with members of the committee to seek support for his proposal, he found that what he once thought of as solid ground had turned to quicksand. No coalition could form a clear majority, with labor insisting on the single-payer plan and the AMA and other conservative groups backing tax credits. The committee first took a vote on the AMA's approach. It deadlocked at 12–12, with 7 Republicans and 5 southern Democrats voting for the AMA's Medicredit plan.

That twelve-member bloc determined the fate of the Mills proposal. The leader of the AMA's congressional sponsors and a key member of the Ways and Means committee, Representative Joel T. Broyhill (R-Va.), insisted that any health-care proposal had to win the support of the AMA-led medical profession. After the committee split on several votes, Mills realized that the twelve committee members wedded to the AMA plan held the key to any future compromise. On August 21, 1974, Mills gave up. "I think the members of the committee will agree with me that we've done everything we can to bring about a consensus," he said. "We don't have that consensus."[36]

The AMA and labor were pleased. The AMA had locked up enough votes to undermine the compromise. And labor had succeeded in delaying consideration of what it perceived as a weaker program. Labor looked to the 1974 elections, in which it predicted there would be a liberal landslide in Congress, giving it a better chance of getting its preferred program passed. They were right about the election: seventy-five new Democrats backing a labor-supported health plan won, and fifty-four of the legislators who had supported the AMA plan lost or retired, including Representative Broyhill.

After the election, AMA leaders feared that a national health-insurance plan looked even more likely to pass in 1975. Dr. Russell B. Roth, the AMA leader, shifted the AMA's position to accept what appeared to be the lesser of two evils. Rather than face a national healthcare system, Roth said requiring employers to offer medical coverage to workers "seems an acceptable alternative to our Medicredit approach."37 At the AMA's December meeting, its delegates reluctantly went along.38 Of the proposals on the table, the AMA's had changed the most.

Ironically, as 1975 opened, the future of a national health-care plan dimmed. Mills left Congress in disgrace after being caught in an escapade with an Argentine striptease artist, and Kennedy returned to labor's fold, again sponsoring the single-payer Health Security Act. Dealing with a worsening economy, Ford did not offer a health-care plan at all. Instead, he slapped a moratorium on any new federal programs that would create additional federal spending.

Meanwhile, unexpected roadblocks arose for the path for health legislation in Congress. In the post-Watergate atmosphere of reform, Congress changed its committee structure, triggering a dispute between Ways and Means and Energy and Commerce. The committee chairmen argued about which one would write the national health-insurance legislation. After they failed to resolved their differences, each committee held separate hearings and let the bill die. The moment had passed.39

The "Evils" of HMOs

The AMA also had to fight against attempts to restructure the way health care was delivered during the 1970s. Reformers again sought to create a more efficient system by pushing prepaid group practices, once again threatening the private independent fee-for-service practice. The AMA leaped to its protection and succeeded in slowing and limiting the change.40

The AMA had long opposed prepaid group practice, or what it called "the evils of contract practice." The AMA believed that doctors were exploited in systems that paid physicians a fixed fee for each patient, rather than a fee for each service. And the AMA's distrust remained despite the camouflage of a new name: health-maintenance organizations, or HMOs.

President Nixon introduced HMOs in his first plan for the healthcare system. Taking and recasting a liberal reform, Nixon proposed HMOs as a middle path between labor's centralized system and the fee-for-service system. Unlike a centralized system, HMOs would not require a new government bureaucracy. And at the same time, HMOs would reverse the "illogical incentive" of fee for service to reward doctors and hospitals for providing more services and to penalize them for returning patients to health.[41] Nixon called for planning grants and loan guarantees, hoping to increase the number of HMOs to 1,700 in 1976 from thirty in 1971.

Kennedy also favored the development of HMOs, and he proposed a more ambitious $5.1 billion aid package to rapidly expand the number of them. But the AMA and conservatives together beat back the program. Nixon scaled back his request, and the AMA, which accepted "limited, experimental" HMOs, urged defeat of Kennedy's proposal. What finally passed was an experimental pilot program for about 100 HMOs costing $325 million over five years. The AMA had succeeded in restraining the growth of HMOs, even if it could not stop them altogether. By 1978 just 168 HMOs were in operation, and only fifty-two met federal requirements—a far cry from Nixon's goal of 1,700.

The Last Gasp

National health insurance had one last gasp during the 1970s. Jimmy Carter's election to the presidency in 1976 seemed to brighten the prospects for national health insurance since he had campaigned for it to court labor's support. The aura of inevitability returned. Yet when Carter assumed office, he shifted gears and declared that health-care costs had to be slowed first. Instead of national health insurance, he proposed limiting hospital-cost increases to 9 percent in 1978 and increasingly smaller percentages until a new payment system was created.[42]

The AMA staked out its compromise position on reform. Among the key elements were standard benefits, an employer mandate to offer employees health insurance, a patient's freedom of choice of benefit plan and physician, subsidies for the poor to buy private insurance, and a pluralistic system of health-care delivery. The principles were contained in a bill before both houses of Congress.[43]

"We recognize that the present system is not perfect," Dr. William C. Felch, chairman of the AMA's Council on Legislation, told a government hearing on national health insurance. "But any modifications must be accomplished without radical restructure that would undermine or sacrifice the great strengths of our system which far outweigh any imperfections."[44]

By September 1979 no longer willing to wait for Carter, Kennedy introduced the Health Care for All Americans Act, which resembled his compromise plan. Developed by a labor coalition, the plan would insure everyone for basic medical services. It attempted to combine the benefits of competition with the controls of regulation. It set both national and state budgets for health-care spending, but allowed five consortia of insurance companies and providers to compete for business. But it was so complex that some joked it was a Rube Goldberg design.

Carter responded by introducing a more limited plan. It included only care for catastrophes, but required that everyone be covered. Among its equally confusing features were a requirement that employers offer their workers health insurance meeting federally established standards, and the merger of Medicare and Medicaid into one program called HealthCare. Carter also sought to use market competition in his plan by allowing private insurers to sell both employer and HealthCare plans.

Neither plan passed. The rivalry between Kennedy and Carter spilled into the Democratic primaries as both ran for President. Carter won the first round, promising "to kick Kennedy's ass," and then doing it. But Carter lost the second round, going down to defeat at the hands of the former AMA pitchman, Ronald Reagan. Under Reagan, national health insurance lay dormant. The AMA celebrated its survival of another bout of inevitability.

THE SIXTH BATTLE

In January 1989 a proposal for a government-run system of national health insurance appeared for the first time since the 1970s. National health insurance was a dead issue during the Reagan years, but with the start of the new Bush Administration a small but growing group of liberal doctors sought to revive it. In its opening shot, the 1,500-member Physicians for a National Health Program declared: "Our health-care system is failing. Tens of millions of people are uninsured, costs are skyrocketing, and the bureaucracy is expanding. . . . It is time for basic change in American medicine."[45]

Every authority on the nation's health was struck by the same paradox: costs for care continued to soar, accounting for 12 percent and more of the gross national product, while at the same time the number of people without health insurance was some 37 million and increasing. The growing problems of cost and access led to the creation of a host of committees—including a business-labor commission headed nominally by three former presidents, and a bipartisan congressional committee—to figure out how to fix a system that appeared to be badly broken.

The liberal doctors behind the national health-insurance proposal thought their timing was right. The paradox facing the United States does not exist in other Western industrialized countries because they have national health-care systems. Only the United States and South Africa do not. Americans were becoming more disenchanted with the U.S. system. Perhaps it was time for the government to step in, as it had in Canada. In Canada the federal and provincial governments collect taxes to finance health care, eliminating the need for private insurance companies, and negotiate budgets for spending on health care directly with doctors.

In March 1989 a widely quoted poll sponsored by a pharmaceutical firm found that 60 percent of U.S. citizens said they preferred the Canadian health-care system over the one in the United States.[46] The liberal doctors' proposal for a single-payer program similar to Canada's was published in the New England Journal of Medicine, accompanied by an editorial declaring: "Universal Health Insurance: Its Time Has Come."[47]

The conservative doctors at the American Medical Association viewed the turn of events with alarm. Already, the AMA was in a fierce battle with Congress over a plan, borrowed from the Canadian system, to limit the growth of physician pay under Medicare. Now a proposal to adopt the entire structure of the Canadian system was gaining ground. In June, when delegates met for the AMA's annual meeting, they kicked off a counteroffensive.

They endorsed a new AMA Board report that echoed Dr. Morris Fishbein's assessment of half a century earlier: "It is not an overstatement to emphasize that American medicine is at a crossroads, with one road leading to government controls, rationing of care, and other objectionable results inherent in a nationalized system, and the other leading to a strengthened U.S. system preserving all of the advantages that mark the American system as being the best in the world."[48]

The AMA's Reacts

The AMA adopted its well-worn strategy of fighting major change to the health system, which organized medicine had spent millions of dollars and mighty effort to help shape. The AMA delegates, who regularly renew their opposition to "socialism," passed a resolution directing AMA staff to run a public-relations campaign attacking the flaws in the Canadian system.[49] They also endorsed the board's campaign— "Strengthening the U.S. Health Care System"—and authorized a budget of up to $2.5 million for a campaign to run at least through 1990. Dr. James H. Sammons, the AMA's top executive, said, "I wouldn't argue with anybody who says that $2.5 [million] is just a beginning."[50]

Dr. James S. Todd, then the AMA's second-in-command, replied to the *New England Journal*'s editorial, claiming, "It's Time for Universal Access, Not Universal Insurance." He compared the prospects of a government-run health program to the hapless Post Office, and questioned the "siren song of foreign programs."[51]

As in the past, the AMA sought to identify alternatives to a major restructuring of the system. To patch the system's cracks, the AMA turned to its past policies. The keystone was requiring employers to offer workers a standard health-insurance package, an idea the AMA had adopted in the 1970s. To cover the uninsured, the AMA called for expanding the coverage of the Medicaid program through national minimum standards and a plan to develop state risk pools for the uninsured and medically uninsurable. The AMA developed those proposals after unemployment and loss of insurance soared in the recession of 1982. Since the 1930s, the AMA had urged the government to pay for the health care of the poor.

The AMA still considered health care a privilege, not a right. In an attempt to make points with the public, and to soften this position, the AMA's leaders announced with great fanfare that the delegates would be voting on a patients' Bill of Rights at its December 1989 meeting in Honolulu. But to the leaders' embarrassment, the delegates balked and failed to ratify the Bill of Rights.[52] However, the delegates finally passed a version of the Bill of Rights, which said patients have a right to "the availability of care," after a lengthy debate at their June 1990 meeting.[53]

The delegates did agree with the leadership on one major issue. They recommended that the counteroffensive against a Canadian-style system be repackaged and promoted, "so that in future debates physicians will be able to present and identify with a positive and proactive health-care program."[54]

The "New" AMA's "New" Plan

In February 1990 Dr. James H. Sammons abruptly resigned as AMA executive vice president in the wake of a scandal, and Dr. James S. Todd took his place. Todd immediately went to work fashioning a "new AMA" that was less confrontational, more willing to compromise, and eager to end the AMA's isolation from other groups. One of the first incarnations of this "new AMA" was the renaming of its battle plan as "Health Access America."

The AMA held a press conference in Washington on March 7, 1990, to unveil the sixteen-point plan. "It's a double package, something we can take to Congress and the American people," said president Dr. Alan R.

Nelson. He added the AMA's real purpose: "We've got to put a merciful end to all those preposterous discussions about a national health system such as England's or a national health-insurance system like Canada's."[55]

If the AMA wanted a place at the negotiating table over the future of American health care, it had to offer a plan. Other proposals had begun appearing almost monthly. In January 1989 the National Leadership Commission on Health Reform suggested in broad outlines a system relying on employer-provided health insurance. In August 1989 the American Academy of Pediatrics released its plan for universal health care. In September 1989 the AFL-CIO announced it was resuming its drive for a national health plan, although it would not push any one specific plan, and the American Academy of Family Physicians and the American Society of Internal Medicine had released their plans. Just days before the AMA's announcement, the bipartisan Pepper Committee created by Congress approved a recommendation for requiring employers to either provide insurance to workers or pay into a government-run pool, commonly known as a "play-or-pay" plan.

Not surprisingly, the ideas contained in Health Access America tilted toward the interests of physicians. By requiring employers to cover workers and a broad expansion of Medicaid, the plan made sure doctors would be paid for their work. By opposing total reliance on HMOs or budget caps to control costs, it sought to avoid reductions in physician pay. And by insisting on changing laws to make it harder for patients to sue doctors accused of malpractice, it sought to remove a nagging form of physician accountability. The plan also would strengthen the AMA by making it the negotiator between doctors and the government.

Not all doctors bought the AMA line. The American College of Physicians, the country's largest specialty group, representing 77,000 internal medicine specialists, demonstrated a breach in the AMA's vision of physician unity. Dr. John R. Ball, ACP executive vice president, said his group had quit the AMA's sessions on reform. "The ACP attempted to get the AMA to speak more bluntly of the physician's responsibility," Ball said, but there was no "substantial discussion" of the M.D.'s role in assuring the quality of care or containing costs. Another ACP official derided the AMA's plan as a "Band-Aid solution."[56]

Influencing the Inevitable

Throughout 1991 the AMA tried to position itself as a proponent of change, not an obstacle. Todd met with old AMA enemies and surprised them by his conciliatory approach and a demeanor far less arrogant than that of Sammons. The AMA president, in a rare occurrence, met with the president of the AFL-CIO. They agreed that Medicaid should be expanded and that an employer-based approach appeared more politically feasible than a single-payer plan.

But the AMA continued warring on the Canadian system. In April it released a poll that it said showed most Americans wanted only a repair job, not a replacement, of the health-care system. The leading expert on health-care polls, Dr. Robert Blendon of Harvard, said the AMA's survey stacked the deck by asking leading questions. He also said the AMA poll was contradicted by eight other polls that found that more than 60 percent of Americans wanted a national health-insurance plan.[57]

In May 1991 the AMA sought to solidify its new image. In special-theme issues *JAMA* published thirteen different health-care-reform plans, and the AMA's nine specialty journals ran another fifty-two articles on reform and the uninsured. Dr. George D. Lundberg, editor in chief of the AMA's journals, editorialized that it was no longer acceptable for so many people to be uninsured. He said the system had to change: "An aura of inevitability is upon us."[58]

Todd proclaimed that the AMA was forging the beginnings of a national consensus on health care. "We want to talk to people and not reject anything out of hand. Changes are inevitable, and it is never wise to oppose the inevitable. Our goal is to achieve a position where we can influence legislation and proposals early in their development," he said.[59]

The AMA's push fanned the flames of political change, and John Sununu, George Bush's chief of staff, saw health care as little more than a Democratic campaign issue for the presidential election in 1992. Sununu called AMA's leaders on the carpet for their agitation for health reform. But the AMA did not back down, and it proved right about the voters' interest in health care. Harris Wofford, an underdog Democratic candidate for an open senate seat in Pennsylvania, pounded away at the need for reform and won. (The AMA's political action committee, of course, contributed to the campaign of his Republican opponent.)[60]

By 1992 the concern over the ailing health-care system had reached epidemic proportions, and nearly every expert and interest group, and most politicians, offered a cure. A week before the first presidential primary, even President Bush presented a plan. Lundberg, in the second *JAMA* dedicated to reform, counted fifty-seven national and state legislative proposals. He urged AMA members to continue to push for reform, despite unavoidable trade-offs.

As if to goad doctors into getting on board with the AMA's strategy, Lundberg wrote an editorial titled "The Aura of Inevitability Intensifies." In it, like Fishbein before him, Lundberg exploited the fears of the AMA doctors: "If business continues as usual without major change [in the health-care system], I predict a meltdown by 1996. At that point, in a worst-case scenario, the Congress would panic and nationalize the entire health-care industry; they can do that." And, to scare his physician-readers even more, he said doctors would be "conscripted as government employees."[61]

Meanwhile the AMA's chief executive continued to mend fences by appearing before the Group Health Association of America, the country's largest HMO organization, and burying the hatchet. "While the AMA has long recognized the existence of HMOs, we have been slow in recognizing and accepting the benefits of HMOs," Todd said.[62]

But while Todd was carrying olive branches to former foes, the American College of Physicians released its own version of health-care reform, which was far different from the AMA's. "Health care is a fundamental right, not an economic privilege," ACP chief executive Ball said. Added ACP president Dr. Willis C. Maddrey, "With this proposal, our physicians acknowledge that the health-care system is so broken that something much greater than incremental reform must be done to fix it."

In its plan, the ACP was inviting the government to take a greater role in health care. The ACP called for a national budget to limit health-care costs; the AMA had always said this would cause rationing of care.[63] At its December 1992 meeting, the AMA rejected a national budget and stuck with letting "the market" control costs. The ACP, in an unusual move, took a shot at the AMA, saying it was disappointed. "Health-care reform begins with cost control, and cost control begins with the commitment to living under a budget," Ball said.[64] AMA delegates declared the ACP shot "inaccurate, unprofessional, and insulting."[65]

But the signs were clear. Unlike in the five previous battles over health-care reform, the AMA could not keep the House of Medicine together. Not only had the ACP gone its own way, but the American Academy of Family Physicians and the American Academy of Pediatrics appeared to be at odds with the AMA.

Preparing for the Inevitable

The election of Bill Clinton put the first Democrat in the White House in a dozen years and gave the country the first president in nearly a generation who had campaigned for health-care reform. He emphasized how serious he was by putting his political career on the line by appointing his wife, Hillary Rodham Clinton, to head the task force that would create his reform proposal. He promised to unveil a proposal in 100 days after his inauguration, but missed his deadline by months.

Lundberg, in an editorial, declared, "The Aura of Inevitability Becomes Incarnate."[66] As in the past, the AMA gradually moved from a conciliatory stance toward the Clintons to a harder line against true reform. In the early stages of the process, the AMA sought to follow the strategy Todd had earlier described: it would not oppose inevitable change, but it would do everything it could to shape the proposals being developed by the new Administration. To do this, the AMA dipped into its ample financial reserves to run $3 million worth of advertising in major national newspapers and magazines as part of its $10 million, four-year Health Access America campaign. And the AMA's political action committee spent $6.3 million in the 1991–92 election cycle, more than other health groups or special interest of any kind.[67]

But much to the AMA's chagrin, Mrs. Clinton did not include the AMA or any other special-interest group among the 538 members of her Health Care Task Force. And the AMA publicly whined about being kept from the table. And for the first months of the Clinton administration, the AMA and the Clintons publicly tested each other. Mrs. Clinton hinted that certain special-interest groups were greedy, and the AMA reacted with offense. The AMA accused the Clintons of locking out doctors, and the Clintons assured the country that doctors were involved.

To greet Clinton's proposal, the AMA planned a three-pronged attack. First it would deploy its lobbyists in its $8.7 million Washington operation to buttonhole politicians to explain the AMA's angle on the plan. Within a week of the announcement, the AMA would mail its analysis to the nation's 718,000 doctors and medical students and to the media. And the AMA told its members to urge their patients to contact their representatives.

The AMA had fought fiercely in the past, and Todd pledged to do no less during his watch: "We will mount the most vigorous congressional effort in our history, fighting for what is best for patients and physicians alike."[68]

The AMA showed it could mobilize doctors by staging a "lobbying day" in Washington in March 1993. Hundreds of members went to Capitol Hill to meet with their representatives, and the AMA invited politicians to speak to an audience of doctors. Responding were all the major health-care players, from Vice President Al Gore to Representative Fortney "Pete" Stark (D-Calif.), the frequent AMA antagonist and chairman of the Ways and Means Committee health panel.

The AMA sent representatives to meet with the Health Care Task Force several times, and just before Clinton abandoned his reform-plan deadline, Todd wrote a boastful note to AMA's trustees: "It would appear that the President may need us more than we need him to get his health-system reform plan through the Congress. The negotiating leverage should be ours."[69]

In June, Mrs. Clinton addressed the AMA at its annual meeting, and she pressed every button she could to evoke an emotional response among doctors to win them over to her side. She praised them, and promised change in malpractice laws and federal clinic regulations. As a high-ranking AMA official said after her speech, "I couldn't have written it better myself."

When Clinton's rough draft was leaked in September, a diplomatic James Todd said he was "cautiously optimistic," and AMA public-relations people smiled and said that the AMA was happy with about 80 percent of the plan. The AMA had won a key battle when Clinton rejected a single-payer plan as an option. Instead he offered a vaguely defined program called "managed competition," which borrows many ideas of the old Nixon plan. Clinton proposed to build on the existing employer-based health-insurance system, emphasizing giant HMOs that compete with each other as well as continuing to offer traditional fee-for-service medicine at higher prices. But issues dear to the AMA's heart remained unresolved: whether there would be malpractice reform, health-spending caps, and cuts in physician pay under Medicare.

The AMA's conciliatory tone abruptly changed following Clinton's September 22 televised address to Congress on his health plan. In its $700,000 mailing on September 24 to all the nation's doctors and medical students, the AMA rolled out its artillery and blasted away. The language of the package, actually an appeal for an AMA battle fund, left little doubt about where the AMA stood: "We have serious reservations about the President's proposal. . . . We are troubled by the degree of centralized regulation. . . . We are also deeply concerned that the means to finance reform are unclear."

The AMA's rejection of key provisions of the Clinton plan stood out by the way the package described the opposition. The AMA "unequivocally" and "staunchly" opposes a national health-spending budget and a national board that would set the budget. It "strongly opposes" a single-payer health system. And it "is adamantly opposed" to restrictions on fee-for-service practice.

The cooperative and conciliatory AMA had given way to the confrontational AMA. The AMA appeared to be following its old path, switching into high gear to battle in Congress what it could not change in conference with the Clinton administration. As much as the AMA has claimed it has transformed into a friendlier, more flexible "new" AMA, as Clinton's campaign for health reform began in fall 1993, it sounded like the "old" AMA of hardball politics.

The delegates at the AMA's December 1993 meeting further eroded the image of a "new" AMA. Leading the charge back to the past was Dr. Edward R. Annis, who was the AMA's chief spokesman in its battle against Medicare three decades earlier. "The AMA is going hand-in-hand with the Clinton Administration," Annis said in his first speech to the House since he was AMA president in 1963–64. "The Administration is determined to dictate and control the way American medicine is practiced."[70]

His rhetoric led conservative delegates to attempt to rescind AMA support of employer mandates, the foundation of the AMA's Health Access America plan. But AMA leaders, fearing the political fallout from such a move, worked out a compromise. The resolution, which the House adopted, says the AMA supports one of three options: 1) requiring employers to pay for their workers' health insurance, 2) requiring each individual to buy health insurance, or 3) a combination of the two. In one vote, the delegates had nearly severed one of the few links between the AMA plan and Clinton's proposal.

The partially successful assault on the AMA's own policy by a bloc of conservative members showed again how out of touch delegates are with the mainstream of physicians. The AMA released a poll it had commissioned showing that 70 percent of U.S. doctors support an employer mandate. Dr. Robert Graham, chief executive of the American Academy of Family Physicians, attended the meeting as a delegate. He said, "The AMA leadership really believes reform is important, but the rank and file [delegates] would kill it without qualm."[71]

A week after the AMA meeting, Clinton hosted a pep rally in the Old Executive Office Building next to the White House. There representatives from ten doctors' organizations expressed their support for Clinton's health-care plan. "The presence of these physicians here debunks the notion that the plan we have presented is some sort of big-government bureaucratic plan that erodes the doctor-patient relationship," Clinton said.

In February 1994 the AMA suffered another body blow at the hands of the independent American College of Surgeons. Dr. David D. Murray, chairman of the ACS Board of Regents, representing 55,000 members, told the House Committee on Education and Labor that it would support a single-payer, Canadian-style system because it provided "the best assurances that patients would be able to seek care from any doctor of their choice . . . can probably be made more simple and more workable administratively."[72]

Support by such a prominent group for an idea that the AMA long had tarred as no less than un-American heartened the many single-payer supporters in Congress while it upset the self-styled reformers at the AMA. Dr. Robert E. McAfee, the AMA's president-elect and a surgeon himself, expressed astonishment at the surgeons' position. He warned that a single-payer system would take "medical decisions out of the hands of doctors and their patients and [give] that power to faceless government bureaucrats and bottom-line-oriented MBAs." He said single-payer medicine would result in rationing of care and in new technology not being made available.[73] It was the sort of propaganda against "socialized medicine" that made the AMA famous.

The stands by the surgeons and the others—representing more than 350,000 physicians, far more than the AMA's membership—again demonstrated that if there is one Voice of Medicine, it was not the AMA. As the director of the Washington office of the American Academy of Family Physicians put it: "The AMA doesn't speak for the entire medical community."[74]

CHAPTER 3

License to Make Money
Turning Medicare into a Cash Cow

IN THE CENTURY-LONG struggle over national health insurance, Medicare is the only major political battle that the AMA lost. But now doctors are hooked on Medicare, the federal program that helps 35 million elderly and disabled people pay their hospital and doctor bills. That's because even in defeat, the AMA won a victory for doctors. The price the AMA demanded for not boycotting Medicare was the government's agreement to allow doctors to set their own fees. Critics refer to this arrangement as the federal government's "open checkbook."

Soon after the enactment of Medicare in 1965, the AMA's opposition turned into an obsession with keeping the checkbook open. That is not surprising. Medicare transformed the way medical care is delivered and paid for, and with private insurance is the driving force in the health-care system today. Medicare also has changed the way doctors practice medicine. About a third of a doctor's earnings, on average, come from Medicare. Even though many doctors complain that Medicare pays too little, it has helped make many doctors wealthy.

But the personal financial gains that doctors have made through Medicare have come at the expense of the very people who are supposed to be helped by the federal health program: the elderly. Senior citizens' share of hospital and doctor bills have risen so much that they are spending as much out-of-pocket on health care now as they did before Medicare. And as any worker can tell from looking at the Medicare deductions and taxes from his paycheck, the burden on taxpayers continues to grow.

For the past three decades, the AMA has battled to protect doctors' earnings under Medicare in the face of government attempts to curb the skyrocketing costs. Each time Congress has considered measures to slow Medicare expenses, and specifically to rein in doctors' pay, the AMA has gone to war. Physician income is the AMA's bottom line. And its obsession with Medicare illustrates how the AMA is not that different from a plumbers' union. As Princeton economist Uwe E. Reinhardt, one of the leading experts on physician pay, puts it, "The AMA is a trade union. I know they hate the word 'trade union,' but I mean let's face it, that's what they are. And the overwhelming preoccupation is the professional freedom and the economic achievement of their members."[1]

The AMA has been largely successful in its goal. Total earnings of U.S. physicians make them the envy of doctors around the world. During the 1980s, professionals such as lawyers and accountants also saw their incomes rise rapidly. Yet as one study of doctors' incomes concluded, "Physicians remain the most highly compensated professionals, and their absolute income gain in the 1980s exceeded that of any other profession."[2]

RAGS TO RICHES

Doctors were not always as wealthy or influential as they are today. Most doctors fell into the lower end of the middle class when the AMA was founded in 1847. A few doctors rose to wealth and prominence, but most were simply not rich. In the 1850s, for example, a Massachusetts doctor earned an average of $600 per year, while a typical annual budget for a family of five in New York was about $540, according to Paul Starr, who traced the rise of the medical profession in *The Social Transformation of American Medicine*.[3] He cited an article from that era complaining that medicine was "the most despised of all the professions." When a young man chose to become a doctor, the article said, "the feeling among the majority of his cultivated friends is that he has thrown himself away."

Fifty years later, doctors had made gains but still weren't rich. A doctor's yearly income was in the range of the $1,000 made by federal employees and the $759 made by ministers, and about double the $540 made by the average worker. But by the 1920s, doctors' earnings were rising much faster than the cost of living, and a 1928 AMA survey found doctors' average annual income was $6,354. During the Depression, doctors, like everyone else, saw their incomes drop. But the gap between doctors and most workers continued to widen: doctors on average made about $4,000, four times as much as the $990 average earned by all workers.

The long, slow road to prosperity closely followed the medical profession's success in persuading society to give it a licensed monopoly. For most of America's history, doctors and their fees were either regulated or subject to truly competitive markets. When America was a colony, governors played a major role in setting doctor fees. After the United States won independence, states continued licensing doctors. In the 1830s and 1840s, states repealed licensing laws. That unleashed the competitive market. Soon just about anyone could declare himself a doctor, and many people did. These "irregular" practitioners created fierce competition for the "regular" doctors, who followed a style of practice they said was based on science. For most of the 1800s, the regulars had too many competitors and too few paying patients.[4]

A year after the state of New York repealed its physician licensing law, the regulars founded the AMA, primarily to upgrade medical-education standards, but also to improve the image, status, and incomes of doctors. In the AMA's first Code of Ethics, one section called for the posting of fee bills listing the range of fees for particular services to discourage price-cutting among physicians. Another section warned wealthy physicians not to give free advice to affluent patients because that made it harder for poorer doctors to collect from their rich patients. The Code did little to reduce competition.[5]

The AMA took other steps to advance the interests of doctors. It campaigned against the irregulars, calling them quacks; it fought against hospitals and dispensaries for the poor, which it accused of stealing paying patients, and it lobbied for licensing laws and improved educational standards. By the 1870s states began reestablishing physician licensing laws, but it wasn't until after the turn of the century that the AMA's drive for education reform was successful. The AMA played a major role in setting the rules for admittance to medical school, education and training, licensing, and even hospital privileges. The number of medical schools dramatically shrank. Fewer schools meant fewer graduates. That meant fewer competitors. And doctor incomes began to rise.[6]

Ensuring Doctors' Pay

When the Great Depression hit in the 1930s, it became clear that many people could not afford to pay their doctor bills. An answer to that problem was private health insurance, which the AMA reluctantly accepted only after making sure doctors remained in control. In fact, it was doctors associated with the California Medical Association, an AMA affiliate, who created the first Blue Shield plan in the late 1930s as an alternative to a state-run health insurance program. Other doctor-controlled private insurance Blue Shield plans soon followed in other states. The plans created an important precedent by allowing doctors to set their fees. The plans could limit their payments to doctors, but allowed doctors to bill patients for the difference between the plans' payments and the doctors' usual fees. Doctors called this practice "balance billing"; critics tarred it "extra billing."

After World War II, the private health-insurance industry boomed, aided partially by government intervention. To control postwar inflation, the government froze wages but allowed companies to compensate employees with health benefits and exempted those benefits from taxes. As a result, most contracts between management and labor unions included company payment for workers' health insurance. The increased demand for medical care coincided with a shortage of physicians. Not surprisingly, doctors' incomes began to rise, at a rate of 5.9 percent a year, twice the consumer price index.[7] By 1965 doctors' average annual earnings hit nearly $30,000, about five times the median average income.[8]

MAKING MEDICARE PAY

Since the 1920s the AMA has balked at the prospect of the government running a national health program. Its leaders worried that the government would try to tell doctors how to do their jobs and feared it would set physicians' fees. At the heart of the AMA's battle against "socialized medicine" was its determination to protect the independence and economic standing of doctors.[9]

Bitterness and anger characterized the AMA's eight-year war beginning in 1957 against health-care legislation that ultimately became Medicare. The AMA refused to accept the need for it, even though studies showed that senior citizens were increasingly having a hard time paying for health care and an even more difficult time finding health insurance. Medicare was designed to make sure the elderly would continue to have access to health care at an affordable price.

On July 29, 1965, the day after Congress enacted Medicare and the day before Johnson signed the bill into law, the President met with eleven AMA leaders at the White House. Many doctors talked openly about boycotting Medicare. One right-wing doctors' group loudly urged physicians to shut down the new program. Without the doctors' cooperation, Medicare would flop, Johnson and his staff knew. The President wasn't about to let that happen.

Johnson used all his wiles to impress and ingratiate himself with the AMA doctors. He relied on his folksiness, his presence, and a ten-point memo written by his health aide, Wilbur J. Cohen, to placate the doctors. He promised no government interference in physicians' practices, and invited the AMA to help write Medicare's rules. And he opened the government checkbook. Medicare would become a conduit for cash to doctors and hospitals.

Johnson allowed doctors to set their own fees under Medicare. The plan would pay "reasonable charges" based on what doctors customarily charged and what the prevailing charges were in the area; and charges would be updated each year. But no one had determined what was a customary and prevailing rate, leaving doctors free to create the baseline for future increases. And they did that by hiking their fees. As a result of the higher fees and the increased number of patients in the first year of Medicare in 1966, the average physician's earnings rose 11 percent to its highest level ever, $32,170.[10]

Representative Wilbur Mills (D-Ark.), the House Ways and Means Committee chairman who fashioned Medicare, also gave doctors a financial bone. Retired AMA lobbyist James W. Foristel recalled, "Right after Representative Mills gave in to President Johnson on Medicare, he called in eight AMA trustees to give them the bad news. 'Here's what I can do for you,' Wilbur said. 'I'll write into the law a provision that will allow physicians to direct bill for their services, rather than being forced to accept the Medicare payment as payment in full.'"[11]

That provision borrowed the practice of physician extra billing from the doctor-controlled Blue Shield plans. And it meant doctors could choose to be paid by the government directly—called "taking assignment"—or to collect from the patient, who would then seek reimbursement from the government. If doctors took assignment and billed the government, they knew the government would pay, but they had to accept the government-established "reasonable charge" as full payment. If doctors billed the patient, they depended on the patient's ability to pay, but could charge more than the government would pay.

Doctors said they sought the privilege of extra billing because they thought the government should be in the business only of helping seniors who could not pay their bills. Repeatedly, the AMA sought to include a "means test" in federal health insurance to determine whether a person needed the help in the first place. The AMA maintained it was the right of the elderly to pay their doctors as much money as they wanted, and extra billing allowed this right to be exercised.

But Medicare did not give the elderly a free ride. They had to pay the first $50 and 20 percent of the rest. If their doctors billed the government, that was all they paid. If the doctors billed the patient, the sky was the limit on what the patient might have to pay.

After meeting with Johnson, the AMA's leaders took the golden bait and urged their members to comply with the law. In October 1965 the AMA held an emergency meeting. Its members were hostile to Medicare and cool to their own leaders. By the end of the two-day meeting, however, the AMA membership decided to go along with Medicare. It slowly dawned on them that Medicare may be government-run, bureaucratic, and even a tad socialistic, but it was an unparalleled opportunity.

The next summer, the AMA held its annual convention just days before the official start of Medicare on July 1, 1966. The House of Delegates passed a notable resolution: it recommended AMA members to bill Medicare patients, not the government—freeing doctors to charge whatever the traffic would bear.[12]

Unreasonable Costs and Charges

In February 1970 the Senate Finance Committee released a stunning report, which opened: "The Medicare and Medicaid programs are in serious financial trouble."[13] Medicare had started just four years earlier, the report said, but the cost of paying hospitals and physicians had soared beyond expectations and belief. Already Congress had to increase Medicare taxes 25 percent to meet skyrocketing hospital costs. And the government had to hike the premium paid by senior citizens 33 percent to cover the rapidly rising doctors' bills.

The report blasted the way the government set physicians' "reasonable charges" under Medicare. The law said charges should not be higher than what local insurance companies paid. But that was what was happening, according to the report's survey of eight common procedures performed on the elderly in 1968. A comparison of the maximum Blue Shield payments for the procedures with the average Medicare charges produced astonishing differences. In Illinois, for example, the most the Blue Shield plan would pay for cataract surgery was $165; Medicare paid on the average $444, nearly three times as much. In Florida, Blue Shield paid at most $117 for a hernia operation, for which Medicare paid an average of $255, more than twice as much. And in Texas, Blue Shield's top payment for a gallbladder operation was $95, while Medicare's average payout was $303, triple the amount.

"No one can say for certain how much money has been overpaid as a result of the failure to apply the statutory limitation on 'reasonable charges,'" the report said. But it added, "It is safe to say Medicare has spent many hundreds of millions of dollars more than otherwise would have been required."

Overpaying for Medicare

Worse, the report disclosed that in 1968 the government paid more than $25,000 in Medicare reimbursements to at least 4,300 individual practitioners and 900 physician groups. And Medicare payments exceeded $100,000 to at least 68 solo practitioners. The staff examined the records and created profiles on the doctors who were raking in the most. "Hundreds of the payment profiles indicate that the physician involved might be abusing the program," the report charged. "For example, we found many general practitioners each paid $15,000, $20,000, or more for laboratory services. We found large payments being made for what appear to be inordinate numbers of injections. In many cases we found what is apparently overvisiting and gang-visiting of patients in hospitals and nursing homes."

The report described this practice: "A physician may see as many as 30, 40, and 50 patients a day in the same facility—regardless of whether the visit is medically necessary or whether any service is furnished. The physician in many cases charges his full fee for each patient, billing Medicare for as much as $300 or $400 for one sweep through a nursing home."

In a congressional hearing on the report, AMA president Dr. Gerald D. Dorman showed a film to legislators to display physician involvement in Medicaid and Medicare. The film followed one doctor working in a poor Chicago neighborhood and another one in a rural Kentucky county. The country doctor said he kept his clinic open twenty-four hours a day, 365 days a year. He said every day he saw more than 100 patients, and sometimes as many as 200. After the film, Senator Russell B. Long (D-La.), who had originally opposed Medicare, spoke.

"May I just make one comment on that film? I think that the kind of thing we just saw in Kentucky is a disgrace," Long said. "Based on the figures he gave, these people are getting about three minutes attention each. I don't think anybody, I don't care if he's Louis Pasteur, can give anybody much treatment if he is only giving them three minutes attention." He added, "We are willing to pay for the care patients are getting. We are not willing to pay for the care patients are not getting. We don't feel we ought to have to pay for a half hour's attention when the patient only got three minutes' attention."

One of Medicare's original sponsors, Senator Clinton P. Anderson (D-N.M.), told the AMA officials: "The key to solving these problems is the physician. He is the common element of control in all aspects of health care. He literally and figuratively has his finger on the pulse of these areas of difficulty and their potential solution."14

APPLYING THE BRAKES

In the decade that followed the hearing, three different presidents tried a mix of refinements, fee freezes, peer-review systems, and complicated regulatory schemes to curb costs, all to no avail. The AMA managed to defend the basic way Medicare paid doctors—a fee for each service, updating what the doctor customarily charged or what the prevailing rate was in the area. For most of the 1970s the government continued to pump money to hospitals and doctors to fulfill its primary goal: to help people get health care, not to control costs.

That all changed with the 1980 election of Ronald Reagan, a conservative Republican who had opposed Medicare in the 1960s. Previously presidents had placed health concerns above costs concerns in their approach to Medicare. Reagan reversed the order. Ironically, organized medicine had hailed Reagan as its champion during his campaign for President. But the AMA leaders' joy turned to apprehension as his budget-cutters began wielding an ax.

For the first time in its history, Medicare became a target for budget cuts. The AMA and other health-care providers found themselves facing an unexpected united front: Reagan's ideologically conservative budget officials teamed up with the liberal-Democratic legislators who controlled the tax-writing Ways and Means subcommittee on health. The White House wanted to cut the budget, and Congress wanted to protect the elderly. That left hospitals and doctors targets for budget savings.

The budget-cutters first took on hospitals, responsible for nearly two-thirds of Medicare costs. When Medicare was first enacted, the government paid hospitals their costs and an added amount to allow the hospitals to expand their facilities to meet the increased number of patients. President Jimmy Carter had sought to impose a cap on hospital costs, but hospital and AMA lobbyists persuaded Congress to block his initiative. By 1980 Medicare costs had soared.

To nearly everyone's surprise, a major overhaul of Medicare hospital payment sped through Congress and the bureaucracy in a matter of months, not years. The new system was called Diagnosis Related

Groups, or more commonly DRGs, which set standardized reimbursements to hospitals based on the diagnosis regardless of actual cost. The idea was to give hospitals an incentive to monitor costs. It went into effect in September 1983.

Next came the doctors' turn under the knife. Most people believed their fees were too high, particularly for the elderly and disabled covered by Medicare. In 1983, according to a report in the *New England Journal of Medicine*, 80 percent of doctor bills exceeded Medicare's "reasonable" rates. That resulted in the elderly paying $2.5 billion extra for physician services. Indeed, the elderly were being hit hard, the report said: Medicare beneficiaries paid more than half of physician charges through premiums, additional insurance, deductibles, and extra billing.[15]

But revamping Medicare payments to doctors did not come as easily as it did for hospitals. A struggle ensued between 1983 and 1989. Nearly all of the AMA's long-held and treasured notions about how doctors make a living were questioned. The AMA became obsessed with Medicare during the 1980s, as shown by its record of its official communications with the federal government. During the 1981–82 session of Congress, about a quarter of the AMA's communications dealt with Medicare. By the 1989–90 session, more than one-half did.[16]

FIGHTING THE FREEZE

The AMA often attempts to preempt or prevent government action by recommending a voluntary approach be taken by doctors. In 1983 the organization could feel the hot breath of government panting down doctors' necks. Government experts were projecting that rising hospital and doctor bills would bankrupt Medicare in a decade. As a way of getting those costs under control, Congress began eyeing doctor bills paid by Medicare.

On the eve of an AMA conference in February 1984 that would discuss the future of Medicare among other things, Dr. James H. Sammons, the AMA's chief executive, returned *USA Today* reporter Steven Findlay's call. Findlay later recalled he asked what the AMA was prepared to do. Sammons "blurted out" that the AMA would call on physicians to voluntarily freeze their fees for six months or a year. He assured Findlay that the Board of Trustees would approve of the plan. "It's time we [doctors] helped get the economy of the country back on its feet," he told Findlay.[17]

On the day the interview appeared on the front page of *USA Today*, the board met and, true to Sammons' prediction, approved the call for a one-year voluntary freeze. The AMA's PR apparatus hastily arranged a press conference for the rest of the news media. In a few hours the board members put the best face they could on the new policy.

"It is a sincere attempt on the part of the AMA to participate in the solution rather than contribute to the rapid escalation of the cost of health care in our country," said Dr. Frank J. Jirka, Jr., the AMA's president and one of the few Democrats ever to make it to the top in the conservative doctors' group. "We felt that at this particular time in history, when we have some really depressed conditions in this country, that it is incumbent on us as physicians to reduce some of these rising costs." The board chairman, Dr. John J. Coury, predicted that most physicians would comply with the AMA call. "I'm not a gambler," he said, "but I'm willing to bet that 85 percent to 90 percent of the physicians of this country will participate."[18]

Critics of the AMA and physicians in general took a different view. They all noted that the timing of the call for a freeze coincided with a movement in Congress to tighten the regulations on how Medicare would pay for physician fees. Members of Congress were discussing, among other things, a bill that would end extra billing by requiring "mandatory assignment." That is, the bill would make doctors accept the government's reimbursement as full payment for treating Medicare payments. AMA officials reviled this notion as "public-utility regulation of medicine" and predicted that as many as 60 percent of the doctors accepting assignment voluntarily would drop out. That would force many Medicare patients to find new doctors and could cripple the whole system.

Another suggestion was to apply the new payment system developed for hospitals to doctors—in other words, create Diagnosis Related Groups (DRGs) that would carry a price tag that the government would pay up front. That way, if doctors could do it for less, they made a bigger profit. The AMA rejected this notion as too complicated and unworkable. It pointed out that the listing for medical procedures contained at least 7,000 different codes, making it nearly impossible to create usable DRG categories. And a third way was a government-imposed freeze on the fees doctors could charge for treating Medicare patients. Reagan had told the AMA he would seek a fee freeze the year before, when he addressed the AMA's annual meeting.[19] The AMA opposed any mandatory government policy.

Among the skeptics of the AMA's voluntary fee freeze was House Ways and Means chairman Dan Rostenkowski (D-Ill.), who was pushing legislation creating mandatory assignment. He said the AMA's call for a voluntary fee freeze showed that the "AMA agrees that doctors are charging Medicare patients too much." He added that Congress had squeezed hospitals and hit beneficiaries with Medicare cuts, and it was now time to reject the notion that "it is not all right to restrict doctors' fees."[20] Representative Andrew Jacobs, Jr., (D-Ind.), chairman of Ways and Means Subcommittee on Health, derided the AMA's fee freeze, calling it a "New Year's resolution" that doctors would not follow. He earned the lasting enmity of the AMA by pushing for mandatory assignment and a government-imposed freeze.[21]

War Threatened

Sammons warned the Reagan administration and Congress if they continued to push mandatory assignment they would have a war on their hands. Doctors revived talk from the 1960s about boycotting Medicare, leaving seniors and the disabled stranded. The AMA had flooded the halls of Congress with doctors. In April 1984, on a voice vote, Congress backed away from mandatory assignment for doctors under Medicare. *American Medical News* noted the defeat of mandatory assignment and patted the AMA, its owner, on the back for its call for a voluntary fee freeze.[22]

But the Administration and Congress were determined to find savings in Medicare doctor fees. And two months later, in June, Congress enacted a fifteen-month freeze on Medicare doctor fees. The mandatory fee freeze made doctors accept reimbursement from the government at the rate they charged in July 1983. Congress also added inducements to doctors to accept assignment of Medicare fees as a "participating physician." The incentives included an earlier end to the fee freeze and a form of free doctor advertising through a "participating-physicians" directory the government would distribute to the public. The law also authorized fines or a suspension from Medicare for "nonparticipating physicians" with a pattern of increasing charges to Medicare patients during the freeze. Doctors had until October 1, 1983, to decide if they would participate.

In September, Department of Health and Human Services secretary Margaret M. Heckler, Senator Robert Dole (R-Kan.), Representative Jacobs, and Cyril Brickfield, of the American Association for Retired Persons, held a press conference to promote the new wrinkles in Medicare physician payment. They wanted to call the problem to the attention of the more than 30 million elderly and disabled citizens covered by Medicare. Dole hailed the AMA, which, he said, could have been "a key potential roadblock" to the Medicare reforms. Jacobs later recalled he was stunned by the praise heaped on the AMA by Dole, Brickfield, and Heckler. The AMA already had announced it was planning to file a suit to block the freeze.23

When the AMA disagrees with the government, it frequently goes to court. A week after the press conference, the AMA sued the Department of Health and Human Services, charging that the government-imposed fee freeze was unconstitutional because it violated the equal protection clauses in the Fifth and Fourteenth amendments. The lawsuit complained doctors were the only professionals whose fees were frozen to reduce the federal budget deficit. It argued that the freeze denied senior citizens the right to select their own doctors because it prevented them from paying the higher fees doctors charged non-Medicare patients. The suit also sought a delay in the program's October 1 start because doctors did not get fee information as early as promised, making it difficult for them to decide whether to become "participating physicians."

"As part of their lawsuit," Jacobs recalled later, "they had to file against HHS secretary Margaret Heckler. She lived in Boston and worked in Washington. Should they file it in Washington? Did they file it in Boston? No, they filed it in Indianapolis. They went directly to my mother's doctor and asked him to be one of the plaintiffs."24

On April 18, 1985, a federal judge dismissed the lawsuit, ruling that the AMA lacked standing to bring the issue to court because no patients had been denied care as a result of the freeze. Backed by the courts, Congress extended the freeze to May 1986 for participating physicians and through the end of 1986 for nonparticipating physicians.

Pump Up the Volume

The AMA, acting as the self-proclaimed leader of medicine, claimed a big victory in holding the line on Medicare costs. And lots of rhetoric was exchanged, but in the end it was shown that the freeze did not help consumers. In fact, doctors found a way to outfox freezes implemented by the AMA as well as by the government.

The AMA estimated that 73 percent of the physicians chose to comply with its voluntary fee freeze. It said the average doctor's fees rose 5.5 percent, higher than the overall rate of inflation of 3.7 percent but the lowest fee increase since the last government-imposed freeze on fees in the early 1970s. As a result, the AMA declared its year-long freeze a success.25

Others were less laudatory. Government economist Daniel Ginsburg said, "The fee freeze definitely inhibited price movement. But obviously not all doctors felt obliged to go along with it." And some were plain critical. Charles Inlander, executive director of the consumer group the People's Medical Society, said, "The fact is that doctors' fees are rising at a 66 percent higher rate than inflation. That to me is not a great victory of consumerism in this country. It shows that the medical profession has a long way to go to bring their prices into the reality of the American economy."[26]

Research later showed decisively that neither the AMA's nor the government's fee freeze had worked. One study examined Medicare spending on doctors in four states between 1983 and 1986. It found, "By 1986, Medicare and its beneficiaries were spending 29.5 percent more for physician services than three years before. This amounted to a $132 increase [per beneficiary], up from $450 annually in 1983 to $582 in 1986."[27]

Why had the fee freeze failed? Simply, doctors did not want a pay cut, and they found a way to actually increase their pay by increasing the number of services they provided their patients. The study concluded, however, "a real possibility" existed that doctors had responded to the freeze just by increasing the number of services per patient. More services meant more bills. More bills meant more Medicare spending. And that meant the freeze did not cut into doctors' incomes.

Not all physicians had pumped up the volume, the study found. Medicare spending increased disproportionately for surgery, radiology, and special diagnostic tests, which together accounted for two-thirds of the expenditure growth. Those services tended to be initiated by physicians rather than patients, countering the argument that patients demanded more services.

The authors drove home their conclusion by pointing out that patients would not likely know how to determine whether it was appropriate to undergo X rays and specialized tests, such as echocardiography and cardiac monitoring. And, the study said, "It is also noteworthy that increased surgical volume was observed frequently among those procedures that are considered 'overpaid' relative to the physician effort involved in performing them."

PRESERVING FEE-FOR-SERVICE MEDICINE

During the mid-1980s the AMA had to make a choice about how it wanted doctors to be paid. Medicare was under siege and on the brink of bankruptcy. The AMA found itself fighting a two-front war: protecting

Medicare from budget cuts and protecting doctors' pay from layers of regulations and restrictions. It also was struggling with an image problem, as more and more people viewed doctors as greedy and avaricious. AMA public-relations specialist Toba Cohen told *The Wall Street Journal* in 1986, "If I could knock 'avarice' off the phrase 'greed and avarice,' that's probably doing what I was hired to do."[28]

Meanwhile, nearly everyone agreed, the inflationary system of paying doctors under Medicare, which had made many a physician prosperous, had to go. The old method of customary, prevailing, and reasonable fees was no longer customary, prevailing, or reasonable. The system, critics said, encouraged the growth of doctor charges and the volume of services. It also sent the wrong signals to doctors in their decisions on where to locate and what to specialize in. The system, which was based on a series of updates of what doctors had charged in the past, favored surgeons and specialists and slighted family doctors and pediatricians. It also tended to favor the time a doctor spent conducting a procedure and worked against the time a doctor spent with patients. And it was so complex, layered by the government with regulations and modifications, that it confused patients and doctors alike.[29]

Even top AMA officials conceded that the way doctors were paid under Medicare had to change. But the alternatives being bandied about in Washington did not look promising to the AMA. All of them rejected the AMA's preferred basis of payment: a fee for each service. Liberal Democrats, such as Senator Edward M. Kennedy, continued to suggest imposing the DRG payment system on doctors. Conservative Republicans, led by the Reagan administration, still favored a type of payment known as capitation. Under it, Medicare would pay doctors a yearly lump sum for each patient, rather than a fee for each service. This system is widely used in health-maintenance organizations. The AMA criticized that method for using the profit motive to discourage proper treatment. Capitation also resembled the contract practice the AMA had damned as unethical.

Given the alternatives, the AMA opted for a fee schedule, which some of its affiliate state medical societies had used before Medicare. The schedule would be based on a scale that placed "relative values" for each service performed. For example, it would assign one value to an office visit, and then rank that in relation to, say, a surgical procedure. The ranking was supposed to be "budget neutral"; that is, it would not be used to cut the amount of money the government set aside for Medicare. And, most importantly, it would preserve the AMA's preferred method of fee-for-service payments.

The other incentive for the AMA to opt for a fee schedule was that it would also probably make the payment system more rational by basing it on the effort, training, skill, and time it actually took a physician to do his or her job rather than relying on the fees he or she had always charged. This in theory would increase payments to family physicians and pediatricians—the lowest-paid doctors—and lower the payments to surgeons and other specialists—who were the highest paid.

PAY ON A NEW SCALE

In 1986 Congress created a thirteen-member Physician Payment Review Commission to advise lawmakers on how to reform the way Medicare pays doctors. The first thing it did was reject DRGs and capitation as the only payment methods for physicians. Instead, it endorsed the idea of creating a fee schedule. The schedule would be based on the amount of resources a doctor spent in effort and time to complete a procedure. Then the scale would rank the procedures relative to each other. Hence the schedule took on the unwieldy name, Resource-Based Relative Value Scale, which was shortened to RB-RVS.[30]

To create this device, the commission contracted with Harvard sociologist William C. Hsiao. Hsiao in turn subcontracted with the AMA to use its "masterfile," the nation's most complete list of doctors, and other expertise. The AMA originally sought the contract, but the Justice Department nixed its bid, noting possible antitrust problems. As a doctors' organization, the AMA had potential conflicts of interest in creating a Medicare physician fee schedule, the government lawyers warned. Two years and $2.5 million later, Hsiao unveiled the first model RB-RVS. He published the version initially in the *New England Journal of Medicine* on September 29, 1988, and a month later in the *Journal of the American Medical Association*.[31]

The long-awaited study got a chilly reception. Dr. James S. Todd, the AMA's second-in-command, expressed the AMA's ambivalent view in an editorial. The scale, he conceded, "provided an acceptable alternative to such dubious schemes as diagnostic related groups for physicians and mandatory capitation." But now the AMA had to evaluate the scale's true impact, whether it could be "translated into the cold, hard realities of Medicare policy."[32]

Hsiao was undaunted. "The RB-RVS could provide a fair and equitable approach to compensating physicians for the services they provide," he wrote in *JAMA*. "We believe that RB-RVS could also enhance cost-effective medical care and ameliorate the manpower shortage in some primary-care specialties."[33] Hsiao also said at a press conference,

"The playing field is tilted against office and hospital visits and time spent with patients—not just for internists and family physicians but across all specialties. Physicians are much more generously rewarded for diagnostic tests and surgery."[34]

The Physician Payment Review Commission struggled with many issues raised by a national fee schedule, including such fine points as whether allowances should be made for the differences in the cost of living found, say, in Los Angeles vs. Paris, Texas. About a year and a half into the commission's deliberations, Representative Fortney "Pete" Stark (D-Calif.) and Representative Willis D. Gradison, Jr. (R-Ohio), of the Ways and Means health panel, sent a letter complimenting the commission for its work on geographic variations, but asked how the schedule would hold down the Medicare costs for doctors' services.

"That put a much more difficult issue on our agenda," recalled commission member Thomas E. Reardon, a doctor from Portland and an AMA Board member. "We began to look at ways to do that. And that is when ETs came up."[35]

Lowering the Volume

The Physician Payment Review Commission had a problem. It had embraced fee-for-service as a basis for paying doctors in its new fee schedule. But, as medical economists had long pointed out, fee-for-service encouraged doctors to perform more services. And studies showed that doctors, when confronted with the Medicare fee freeze, had responded by simply requiring more patient visits and ordering more clinical tests. In other words, they increased the volume of service to make up for lost income. The commission began studying ways to encourage doctors to perform only appropriate services, to cut out unnecessary and marginal procedures.

The AMA offered its suggestions: change the laws to 1) make medical malpractice lawsuits harder to file and the awards to victims smaller, 2) begin studies of what it called practice parameters (guidelines for treatment), and 3) free doctors from antitrust laws. The AMA insists that fear of malpractice lawsuits leads many doctors to practice "defensive medicine," that is, to conduct tests of marginal value simply to avoid being sued. The AMA also pushed studies of practice parameters to create guidelines on appropriate treatments and care.

The commission acknowledged these problems, but it instead looked north and east for a way to control costs. It examined the way doctors were paid in British Columbia and Quebec as well as in Germany, which in 1985 had undergone a major reform. The commission came away with a budgetary device known as "expenditure targets."[36] The targets were quickly dubbed ETs in a nod to the popular movie *E.T.*, about an extraterrestrial alien who comes to earth and befriends a little boy.

ETs were designed as a carrot-and-stick for doctors. Each year the government would set targets as a goal for the increase in Medicare payments to doctors. If the growth of doctors' expenses stayed under the targets, the government would reward physicians by setting higher targets the next year. But if the doctors' expenses exceeded the targets, the government would lower the next years' targets to recoup the excess.

Another problem for the new fee schedule arose. If doctors thought the Medicare fees were not high enough, they could simply pass on the additional cost to their patients through extra billing. The representatives of senior-citizen groups on the commission especially worried about this problem. But commission members representing doctors argued that doctors needed the ability to bill beyond Medicare's set fees, which they said were too low. The commission heatedly debated whether the fee schedule should simply ban extra billing.

At the end of the debate, the commission settled on a reform package that was described as a "three-legged stool." One leg created a new, fairer fee schedule for doctors, the RB-RVS. A second leg protected seniors by putting a cap on the extra amount a doctor could charge them. And the third leg was ETs, which sought to bring skyrocketing doctor costs back to earth.[37]

Medicine's Schism

The commission's proposal posed a great challenge to the AMA. At its interim meeting in Dallas in December 1988, the AMA and about two dozen specialty societies debated Hsiao's fee schedule. Because the schedule rated the value of different work, it pitted specialist against generalist, surgeon against family practitioner, doctor against doctor. But the AMA managed to keep all the participants together, stressing the need for doctors to speak with one voice in the process of reforming Medicare. Members of the Physician Payment Review Commission all complimented the AMA's diplomatic abilities in keeping medicine together. Reardon played a key role in persuading the AMA and the specialty societies to compromise. By the end of the meeting, organized medicine supported the use of a relative value scale—with refinements, of course—but rejected proposals to limit extra billing and to impose ETs.[38]

One major specialty association, however, boycotted the AMA meeting. The American College of Surgeons had from the start opposed the AMA's decision to support the switch from historical-based charges (usual, customary, and prevailing) to a resource-based relative value scale. The reason was clear: surgeons stood to lose the most from any fee schedule derived from such a scale.

On February 7, 1989, the American College of Surgeons held a rare Washington press conference to announce its proposals for physician-payment reform. The statement, read by Dr. Paul Ebert, the College's director, did not make front-page news in the general press, but it shook the House of Medicine: "At the heart of our new comprehensive plan is a public commitment from the American College of Surgeons, the surgical specialty societies, and their more than 85,000 members, to work directly with Congress . . . to reach an agreement on a broad range of physician-payment goals that can be implemented in an orderly manner." Key among its proposals was an acceptance of ETs as long as Congress set up a specific target for surgeons, separate from the target for other physicians.

In other words the surgeons had broken with the rest of organized medicine to cut a separate deal with Congress. "Those of us in surgery believe that it is impossible to effectively and efficiently address the volume issue across the entire spectrum of medical services," Ebert said. The college instead proposed having its own ETs in "an attempt to address the issue of increased volume of services exclusively within the scope of surgical specialty."[39]

The defection of the surgeons was a big blow to the AMA. The College of Surgeons had undermined the AMA's position that physicians and specialty groups were unified in opposing ETs. An AMA official lamented, "The surgeons made ETs a viable legislative and political issue." It also gave Representative Stark the upper hand in the debate, allowing him to use the "divide and conquer" approach to dealing with medicine.[40]

THE SHOWDOWN

In March 1989 Stark launched a series of hearings on the "three-legged" payment reform devised by the Physician Payment Review Commission. Stark, chairman of the health subcommittee of the budget-conscious, tax-writing House Ways and Means Committee, made his goal clear at the outset: "The fundamental problem is that Medicare gives doctors a blank check. The more services they provide, the more they earn whether or not the services are needed. Payment reform must correct this perverse incentive."

The government blank check had to stretch further every year, Stark complained. In 1989 Medicare spending on doctor services soared 16 percent, far above the rate of inflation. In the previous five years, Medicare spending on doctor services alone more than doubled to $28 billion. "We cannot continue to pass these cost increases on to the elderly for their 25 percent [share of the tab] or to the taxpayers at large for the approximately 75 percent they are paying," Stark said.[41]

The increasing financial burden on the elderly, one of the nation's largest voting blocs, particularly worried Congress. The premiums seniors paid to cover their share of Medicare's doctor services had nearly doubled in five years, and in the previous decade their out-of-pocket costs had nearly tripled. Seniors were paying 15 percent of their income for medical care, the same that they paid when Medicare began in 1966.[42]

Why were Medicare payments to doctors going up so quickly? Inflation, expensive new technologies, and an aging population figured in. But studies also traced a major cause right back to the doctors. They were increasing the volume of their services to patients: more office visits, more diagnostic tests, more surgical procedures, and, of course, more bills. Dr. Phillip R. Lee, of the Physician Payment Review Commission, testified, "Some studies suggest in some areas as many as 20 to 30 percent of the procedures performed are either unnecessary or of marginal benefit. If we could eliminate or reduce those, we could save all the money we need to finance Medicare and still have some left for other things that need to be done."[43]

The AMA's vice-chairman, Dr. Joseph T. Painter, assured Stark that the AMA supported one leg of the stool: the creation of a new fee schedule. But the AMA vigorously objected to the other two legs: the limit on doctors' extra billing of patients and the spending goals of ETs. Painter focused the AMA's attack on ETs, which Lee's commission had designed specifically as an incentive to discourage unnecessary procedures. Painter said ETs "may appear to be a painless way to hold down expenditures, but it must be recognized for what it is, an implicit system to ration care."

"Why is it rationing?" challenged Stark. "All we are suggesting is that you go back at the end of the year among yourselves and say, 'Guys, we spent too much.' It doesn't have to be rationing. You all would say that when you don't get as much money as you want, but you could also reduce your fees, couldn't you, and come to the target? That doesn't have to deny quality service. [But] that is the AMA's position: if we don't get what we want, we won't treat people."[44]

On June 14 Stark's subcommittee approved the package in an 8–3 vote. It contained the fee schedule, with the the automatic ETs and limits to extra billing intact. The Bush administration signed on, seeking a way to control Medicare costs. In fact, the top Bush health adviser, William L. Roper, insisted on ETs. He much preferred paying doctors a set fee per patient as a way of cutting the Medicare budget, and initially he was lukewarm to a fee schedule. ETs made the fee schedule acceptable.[45]

The War on ETs

But the AMA mounted an effort to keep the government checkbook open, even if it came at the expense of Medicare patients and taxpayers. In a blunt, angry speech before the AMA's annual meeting on June 19, 1989, organized medicine's top doctor, Dr. James H. Sammons, declared war on ETs, growling, "It's rationing, no matter what the hell they say."[46] ETs were one of the AMA's worst nightmares. When the AMA fought Medicare in the 1960s, it warned that medical service would depend on government budgets, not patients' needs, under "socialized medicine." Twenty-five years later, no AMA leader would publicly brand ETs socialism. But in his speech—and his last crusade as the AMA's chief— Sammons resurrected bitter memories of the battle over Medicare by calling ETs "the biggest challenge facing the AMA since 1964."[47]

To wage the war, Sammons activated the same kind of political and public-relations machine that the AMA had used to successfully fight proposals for national health care since the end of World War II. Sammons unleashed the AMA's lobbyists in Washington and revved up the PR apparatus in Chicago. He urged state and local medical societies to join the battle and encouraged members to contact their representatives and senators. The AMA set up a telephone at its annual meeting so doctors could call their representatives in Washington. And the AMA's newspaper ran a front-page appeal to doctors to contact their congressmen.[48]

In Washington the AMA's lobbyists orchestrated more than a dozen floor speeches by House members assailing ETs.[49] Top AMA leaders visited the White House to press their case with President Bush. Within six weeks of Sammons' declaration, the AMA had sent three letters to every member of Congress and several more to members of key House and Senate committees. More noticeably, the AMA took out a full-page ad in major newspapers aimed at Congress. The ad showed a picture of an elderly woman and in large type asked: "How Do You Tell Someone on Medicare She's an 'Expenditure Target'?"[50]

The ad campaign created a storm of complaints. Labor unions and seniors' groups blistered the AMA for conducting "a slick and dishonest media campaign to protect their control of Medicare's golden goose, while pretending to be acting for older Americans who are in fact being squeezed by skyrocketing doctor charges."[51] Gradison, the ranking Republican on Stark's subcommittee, angrily attacked the ads as "heavy-handed" and a "scare tactic" aimed at the elderly.[52] Health and Human Services secretary Louis Sullivan, an AMA member, called the ads "misleading" and a "deception on the American public." Sullivan threw the Bush administration's support behind ETs.[53]

On June 28, 1989, the full Ways and Means Committee, after two days of closed-door meetings, also approved the package, and carved out a separate target for the surgeons. The AMA had few friends among the committee's members. Indeed, Stark was the AMA's worst enemy. And the ranking minority member, Gradison, declined to take any political action committee contributions, closing an avenue for AMA influence. After the vote, the AMA issued a statement criticizing the closed-door meetings and accusing the committee of attempting to leave the "dirty work" of rationing care in the hands of doctors.[54]

The reform package still faced a rough road. First it had to pass the health subcommittee of Representative Henry A. Waxman (D-Calif.) and then the full committee on Energy and Commerce in the House. Then it had to go through the Medicare subcommittee of Senator Jay Rockefeller (D-W.Va.) and the full Finance Committee in the Senate. Finally, it had to pass the full House and Senate. The AMA's prospects for knocking off ETs along the way looked good. The AMA had many more friends on the Energy and Commerce and Senate Finance committees than it had on the Ways and Means Committee.

On June 29 Waxman's health subcommittee passed a version of the reform package—but, as the AMA had hoped, it had dropped ETs. Two weeks later, the full Energy and Commerce Committee approved the "two-legged" stool. Coincidentally, the AMA had honored Waxman as its legislator of the year and gave him $5,000 in contributions in 1989.[55] But Waxman carefully distanced himself from the AMA's lobbying campaign against ETs, telling Congressional Quarterly, "I hold my point of view in spite of their ad campaign, not because of it."[56]

By the fall, the reform package had moved to the Senate Finance Subcommittee on Medicare, headed by Rockefeller. The senators had two versions of the legislation to consider: Stark's bill with the ETs and

Waxman's without ETs. Rockefeller, and the subcommittee's ranking Republican, Senator Dave Durenberger of Minnesota, proved to be determined to pass the reform package. The AMA pinned its hopes on its long relationship with Durenberger, and did all it could to establish one with Rockefeller.

When Durenberger went through a particularly tough election in 1988 because he faced charges of ethics violations, the AMA's political action committee came to his aid, contributing $9,800 directly to his campaign and spending another $134,527 independently to campaign for him.[57] The AMA also focused much energy on Rockefeller. Sammons recounts how he paid several visits to Rockefeller and even chased him to an underground shuttle to the Capitol, trying to persuade him to junk ETs.[58] And although the AMA's PAC had supported Rockefeller's opponent in his last election, it gave Rockefeller two $1,000 contributions in 1989 and another $5,000 in 1990 for his reelection campaign.[59]

Rockefeller and Durenberger worked with the AMA to find an alternative to ETs. Bush, they felt certain, would not sign a reform package into law without some way to control the volume of physician services. And they knew Stark would not give up ETs very easily, either. Finally, the two senators came up with a compromise—MVPS, which stood for Medicare Volume Performance Standards. The AMA signed on after Rockefeller agreed to ensure that the new standard would require action by Congress, would only be advisory, and would include a role for the AMA.

The *Congressional Quarterly* noted, "The AMA had succeeded in making 'expenditure target' a dirty word. Rockefeller went so far as to disavow a committee briefing paper that used the name. 'We do not have expenditure targets,' he insisted. 'We have volume performance standards, and I insist that the words be changed.' "

Over five days, Rockefeller led the drive to get Congress to pass Medicare physician-payment reform in 1989. Other legislators, including powerful congressional leaders, even told him to drop the entire reform package. But he pushed on, often working late into the night to hammer it out. Finally, in a late-night conference in November, ETs died. Rising from the ashes were the MVPS, toughened to include a default mechanism that would set the standards if Congress failed to act. MVPS did just about everything ETs did, said the Physician Payment Review Commission staff, and though more flexible had the same overall effect. Many in Washington, and even other doctors' groups, saw MVPS as little more than a face-saving deal for the AMA. But Sammons claimed victory: "We are pleased the expenditure target proposal has been soundly rejected."[60]

Dr. Phillip Lee, the payment-review-commission chairman, said, "I think the AMA clearly has got to say they defeated expenditure targets, and that's fine with me. But I think the volume performance standard gives the clear message to doctors that we must do something about the volume of unnecessary services now being provided." He added, "The fundamental problem of the American system is that we gave an open checkbook to hospitals and physicians. Now we are trying to close that checkbook."[61]

The federal government has begun phasing in Medicare physician-payment reforms, which will not be completely in place until 1996. But early reports indicate the reforms have begun to work, although the AMA has described the government's handling of the MVPS a disaster. Extra billing has dropped dramatically, with fewer than a tenth of all doctor bills under Medicare seeking additional payment from patients.[62] And the growth in doctors' Medicare expenses have come in lower than the government-set targets.[63]

Charging More, Making More

Even if the AMA was not entirely successful in its battles over Medicare-payment reform, it served a useful purpose for physicians. It bought them time to make a bundle of money. While the AMA and Congress argued over the best way to reform physician pay, doctors were busy making up for any sacrifices they may have made under the government-imposed Medicare fee freeze by upping their fees faster than the rate of inflation. Not surprisingly, their incomes also outraced inflation during this time of playing catch-up.

In 1987 and 1988, AMA surveys found, doctors' average incomes rose twice as fast as inflation. During the three years of the Medicare fee freeze from 1983 to 1986, average net physician income rose to $119,500, an increase of $15,000. In 1987 average income jumped to $132,300, nearly matching the increase of the three previous years.

By 1990 doctors' average net income before taxes had risen to $164,300, nearly twice what it was a decade before. Or, viewed another way, three-quarters of the doctors made more than $90,000, and half of them made more than $130,000. In 1992, the AMA reported, the average doctor's income was $177,400, with surgeons making an average of $244,600, internists $159,300, and family physicians at the bottom, making $111,800.

The AMA acknowledges that doctors make much more than other people, but it notes doctors require years of training, have specialized skills, and make life-and-death judgments. Doctors graduate with huge debts and start careers later in life. Most doctors work long hours and face great stress. The AMA also pointed out that in real dollars, adjusted for inflation, doctor incomes dipped slightly from 1989 to 1991.

Those arguments offer little comfort to most working people, who make nowhere near the earnings of doctors but who must bear the brunt of the cost of the nation's health care. From 1982 to 1990, the average earnings for full-time employees grew from about $18,500 to $25,900, a raise of 4.3 percent a year. During the same time, doctors' average income rose from $98,000 to $164,000, or 6.6 percent a year. At the start of the 1980s, a doctor earned about five times as much as the average worker. By the end of the decade, a physician made six times as much.[64]

Deep Pockets
Buying Time and Clout
in Washington

THE AMERICAN MEDICAL Associa-
tion may not win every political battle in Washington, but more often
than not it gets its way. That's because politicians have learned that when
the AMA talks, it pays to listen. The AMA represents the country's
wealthiest profession, and it is not shy about using money to gain access
to lawmakers. Few other special interests have invested as much money in
politics, or have the resources to do so, as the AMA.

In the past two decades, the AMA easily has spent more than $100
million of its own money to influence public policy by lobbying through
its Washington office and providing "political education" to its members.[1] In fact, about a quarter of each AMA member's dues—$420 each
year for full-fledged members—goes directly to finance lobbying alone.
In addition, the AMA's political funding arm, the American Medical
Political Action Committee (AMPAC), raised and distributed another
$34 million to political activities and congressional campaigns across
the country.[2]

AMPAC best illustrates the AMA's ability and willingness to use
money to make friends in Washington. In nearly every election since
1972, when the government began keeping records of political donations, AMPAC has been at or near the top of the list of special interests
that contribute to candidates' campaign funds. In fact, AMPAC ranks
second out of more than 4,000 PACs in making direct contributions to
federal candidates in the past two decades. And AMPAC—whose sponsor has 270,000 members—has donated much more than the PACs

sponsored by larger, well-known special-interest groups: a fifth more than the United Auto Workers (1.4 million members); 50 percent more than the National Education Association (2 million); and three times as much as the National Rifle Association (2.5 million).

Not surprisingly, the AMA has become a fixture in Washington as the rich, powerful, and politically sophisticated Doctors Lobby. It is so entrenched that it has special ties to the Federal Election Commission, the only federal agency created to monitor and regulate political action committees. A former top AMPAC executive is one of six commissioners on the FEC. And when the cramped agency decided to move, the commissioner helped select an AMA-owned building as the new site.

As the jockeying for position at the negotiating table for the health-care reform of the 1990s began, the number of health-related lobbies has rapidly multiplied. Increasingly, the AMA appears to be one voice of many. But to retain its disproportionate clout, the AMA has reached into its deep pockets and again has outspent them all. The AMA and AMPAC have written checks at one time to the campaign chests of nearly every representative and senator in the current Congress, which will decide the future of the health-care system. As in the past, the AMA will seek to protect doctors and scuttle major reform by persuading lawmakers to delay, dilute, or delete legislation it doesn't like. The AMA is banking that its investment in this Congress—a total of $11.4 million—will pay off.

Birth of a New Political Machine

At one time the AMA had scant power and little influence over lawmakers. From its founding in 1847 until the early part of this century it was a weak organization, with no full-time staff, a meager budget, and little prestige. Created as an educational and scientific association dedicated to improving the status and image of doctors, it began laying groundwork for the future by pushing for state licensing of doctors and waging war on abortion.

At the turn of the century, the AMA restructured itself into a stronger organization and at the same time created a lobbying arm, the Committee on Medical Legislation. The three-member committee set up the AMA's first political machine: a network of doctors across the country who volunteered to contact their state and federal legislators to press the profession's interests "by any honorable means."[3] Special interests certainly plied candidates with money—most money came from Wall Street and Big Business—but they didn't have to report it. The AMA then most likely was too poor, and perhaps too idealistic, to spread much money around.

The AMA's political strength grew over time, and the AMA became, like most special interests, adept at blocking change it did not like. With the onset of the Depression and the New Deal, the AMA continued its lobbying and propaganda campaigns, putting its prestige on the line against the liberalism of the times. But the AMA's clash with reformers gave it a reputation as a powerful trade group rather than the AMA's self-image of a high-minded educational and scientific organization.

The AMA's first foray into establishing a separate political fund came at the end of the Depression, when the doctors of the AMA sensed their power had slipped. To avoid a clash with the IRS over the AMA's tax-exempt status, a past AMA president and other members founded the National Physicians' Committee for the Extension of Medical Service. The committee was endorsed by the AMA's House of Delegates, and 90 percent of its funds were donated by pharmaceutical companies. But in 1948 it closed down after embarrassing the AMA with an anti-Semitic letter addressing "fellow Christians" and an ill-advised contest for editorial cartoonists seeking to ridicule national health insurance. In its nine years of existence, the committee spent about $1 million on ads, pamphlets, radio, and other propaganda.[4]

Big Money

The AMA solidified its reputation as a big-money lobby after World War II, outspending even the AFL-CIO's $835,000 unsuccessful advertising campaign against the Taft-Hartley Act in 1947.[5] To fight President Harry S Truman's plan for a government-run and tax-financed health-care system, AMA leaders assessed their members $25 each. With that money, the AMA reported it spent $1.5 million in 1949. And over three and a half years, the AMA spent nearly $5 million for its campaign. In today's dollars, that would equal nearly $30 million.[6]

The AMA also spent money liberally to influence congressional races. In 1950 it organized a massive $3.1 million advertising campaign, tying into business ads, against liberals and for conservatives during a two-week stretch just before the election. Meanwhile doctors from state medical societies set up "healing arts committees," patterned after union committees on political education, to beat liberal Democrats. In two cases the doctors' victories came back to haunt them. Florida doctors helped fund a successful drive to defeat Senator Claude D. Pepper. He returned to Congress in 1962 when he won a seat in the House, where he focused on liberal health initiatives until his death in 1989. Wisconsin doctors defeated Representative Andrew Beimiller, who joined the AFL-CIO and became a key leader in labor's fight for national health insurance and Medicare.[7]

But the AMA did buy itself some time. After watching the AMA's expensive campaign against Truman, Dwight D. Eisenhower welcomed not only the support of the AMA but also hired its PR firm, Whitaker and Baxter, for his successful presidential bid. According to author Richard Harris, Eisenhower made a deal with the AMA. His Administration would oppose national health insurance if the AMA would back a new Department of Health, Education and Welfare. The AMA had blocked similar departments in the past because it wanted a separate health department headed by a doctor. Eisenhower tapped Oveta Culp Hobby to head HEW, and she announced she would run it as an "AMA Administration."[8] National health insurance lay dormant in the 1950s.

Off the Charts

The AMA, like other special interests, was well aware that in Washington perception of power is as important as real power. Since money is power, big spenders are seen as powerful. When Congress after the war passed a law requiring special interests to register and report how much they spent on direct lobbying, many groups refused to file, or if they did, underreported expenses. The AMA filed its reports under protest, and one year itemized spending in a blinding eight-page report of single-spaced type without breaks. *Congressional Quarterly,* which annually publishes lobby spending, noted, "This method of reporting is unique with the AMA." But the AMA reported a large enough sum each year to become a fixture on the *CQ* list.[9]

The AMA, like other special interests, used the list as needed. When it did not wish to be seen as a big spender, it changed its reporting procedures to lower the amount. For example, in 1954 the AMA said it spent $39,120 on direct lobbying, but its audited financial statement showed it spent $210,700 on its Washington office.[10] When the AMA wanted to impress friends and foes with its economic power, it filed more complete reports.

CQ each year published a list of the top lobby spending, and the AMA reported the three highest annual lobbying expenses recorded, each of them coming in at more than $1 million. The AMA reported spending the two highest yearly amounts in 1949 ($1.5 million) and 1950 ($1.3 million) on its successful campaign against Truman. And it spent the third-highest amount in 1965, $1.1 million, on its unsuccessful fight against Medicare.[11]

PAC ATTACK

In 1960 the razor-thin victory of John F. Kennedy over Richard M. Nixon again jarred AMA officials into action. The AMA's archenemies— liberals and labor unions—backed Kennedy, who as a senator had pushed for Medicare. Just four months after he took office, the AMA created the American Medical Political Action Committee, or AMPAC. Through AMPAC, the AMA could collect money from members and others to make contributions to House and Senate candidates who agreed with the agenda of the M.D.s.[12]

It was a gutsy move. No trade or business group had set up a national PAC before. The field belonged to labor. During World War II, the Congress of Industrial Organizations created the first PAC. When it merged with the American Federation of Labor in 1955, the new AFL-CIO started several national Committees on Political Education. The next year the COPEs spent $2.1 million on candidates.[13] AMA Board members and staff took note, and pondered the idea of starting their own PAC. At least eight state medical societies had set up PACs, but AMA officials hesitated.

Most of them feared the reaction of the Justice Department and the IRS. The AMA's tax-exempt status could be jeopardized, they said, since law bars not-for-profit organizations from making political contributions. They also worried about being accused of violating the Federal Corrupt Practices Act. And they simply did not trust the federal government, with which they had clashed so long.

So the AMA took special pains to set up a separate organization, settling AMPAC into a building three blocks away from AMA headquarters. The board's final vote also hinged on the reaction of the Justice Department. When it did not react, the board officially launched AMPAC. The new PAC immediately began soliciting AMA members, their spouses, and their friends to join. In keeping with the AMA's hostility to government oversight, AMPAC set sustaining membership dues at $99, because contributions of $100 or more had to be reported. In its first year, AMPAC raised about $200,000 from more than 13,000 members.[14]

But for a real boost, AMPAC secretly turned to the Pharmaceutical Manufacturers' Association, a trade group for drug companies. The AMA-PMA connection was strong. The two groups often joined forces to lobby Congress, and the AMA's general counsel became the PMA's executive director. Seventeen of the nation's biggest drug firms gave nearly $1 million to AMPAC in its first three years, according to internal AMA documents that were leaked years later. AMPAC could not use the money for campaign contributions, but it could use it to set up its offices and pay administrative costs, as well as to solicit funds it could give to candidates' political funds.[15]

In its first two elections, AMPAC funneled support to conservatives on the powerful House Ways and Means Committee, the tax-writing body that considers bills on national health insurance. In its first outing, AMPAC claimed that 70 percent of the candidates it backed won. In the 1962 and 1964 elections, AMPAC spent about $700,000. Although it was too little and too late to stop Medicare, it helped the AMA shape the program to benefit doctors.

AMPAC Flexes Its Muscles

The enactment of Medicare in 1965 demolished the AMA's image as an invincible lobby and demoralized AMA members. Soon the aftershocks of defeat shook the AMA. Labor and liberal Democrats announced a drive to pass a universal national-health-care system, and AMA membership began declining rapidly. The AMA needed a victory badly to prove both to the outside world and to its own members that it remained an organization to be reckoned with.

The opportunity came along in 1969 with the opening of a position in the new Nixon White House of the top health official, the Assistant Secretary for Health at the Department of Health, Education and Welfare. The new HEW Secretary, Robert Finch, had made up his mind by the time Richard M. Nixon was inaugurated to push for the director of Massachusetts General Hospital in Boston, Dr. John H. Knowles. But Finch soon found his choice was far too liberal and too antagonistic for the AMA to survive.[16]

For five months Finch urged Nixon and his top aides to appoint Knowles to the post. But the AMA had turned to its friends in Congress to lobby against the liberal Boston physician, who was associated with hospitals more than with doctors. AMA officials did not like Knowles, and they had other candidates in mind, including the nephew of the AMA's president.

The AMA had a powerful ally, Senator Everett Dirksen (R-Ill.), working behind the scenes. But Finch, a close Nixon friend, appeared to win and in June sent a letter to the White House nominating Knowles. At the last minute the AMA's case was bolstered by the top GOP fund-raisers in the Senate and House. Press reports say Senator John Tower of Texas visited the White House and said, "There are a lot of well-qualified men for this job. There's no reason to alienate a large group of contributors." The contributors he referred to were the doctors at AMPAC, which gave some $682,000 to the campaigns of Republicans and conservative Democrats in the 1968 election.

Nixon pulled the plug on Knowles. Knowles blamed the AMA and AMPAC, which he said were his only opponents. Newpaper editorials thundered about the power of the AMA and the influence of AMPAC's contributions on politicians, especially Dirksen. True to the secretive politics of the day, the AMA denied it had opposed Knowles. Years later, the AMA acknowledged its opposition, and one official said the Knowles affair was important in reestablishing the clout of the AMA.

AMPAC had been key to bolstering the image of AMA power following Medicare, but AMPAC took steps to consolidate its position, and by the end of the 1960s the AMPAC crowd had taken over the AMA. Soon after its founding, AMPAC became the breeding ground for future AMA leaders, who before had come from more scientific or educational backgrounds. The AMA's chief executive then, Dr. F. J. L. Blasingame, distrusted AMPAC and was well aware of its threat to what he labeled the "scientific-educational" AMA. Blasingame described the new breed spawned by AMPAC: "What you had now were people interested in political action, people who liked that kind of life. It was a tougher crowd. More aggressive." By 1968 Blasingame was openly challenging the AMPAC crowd and the AMPAC crowd was fighting back. In the end, the AMPAC faction won by electing its candidates to the AMA board of trustees, reorganizing the board, and setting up a showdown with Blasingame. The board asked for Blasingame's resignation. He refused. So the board fired him.[17]

The complete takeover came six years later. In the most controversial election in AMA history, the board picked Dr. James H. Sammons to be the AMA's chief executive. Sammons had risen rapidly through the ranks, making stops as chairman of the Texas Medical Political Action Committee and AMPAC before becoming the AMA's board chairman. Sammons' mentor was a former AMPAC chairman, Dr. John Kernodle (who was forced to resign because of an unrelated bank-fraud conviction) and his righthand man was Joe D. Miller, AMPAC's first director. When Sammons took over and found the AMA finances deep in the red, one of the first things he did was to shrink the number of the AMA's scientific councils.

AMPAC Rising

During the 1970s, AMPAC quickly moved up among the ranks of all PACs to dominate the field. In its first decade of existence, AMPAC spent far less than the labor unions. But in its second decade, it caught up and passed them. The progression came election by election. In the 1972 two-year election cycle, AMPAC trailed only the AFL-CIO and the United Auto Workers in political contributions. In the 1974 elections, AMPAC moved up a place to become second only to the AFL-CIO. By 1976 AMPAC had risen to the top, becoming only the second PAC to contribute more than $1 million to federal candidates in an election cycle. AMPAC contributions have never dipped below the $1 million level since.[18]

More and more the AMA focused on the "socioeconomic," which was the buzz word then for politics, and less and less did it concern itself with educational and scientific efforts. Although the AMA spent just a fifth of its budget on its political efforts in 1971, a top AMA official noted "the ballgame for medicine will be won or lost in the socioeconomic area."[19]

The 1970s also ushered in an era of campaign-finance reform. A congressional flap in the 1960s and the Watergate scandal pushed Congress into enacting the most sweeping campaign reforms ever. The laws legitimized political action committees set up by special interests such as labor unions, corporations, and trade associations. But the laws also required them to disclose how they spent their money: PACs were required to file finance reports ten times during each two-year election cycle.

But AMPAC wasn't satisfied with filing only ten reports. In 1972 FEC records show AMPAC filed dozens more reports than most other PACs. And in 1973 and 1974, an AMPAC bulletin noted, AMPAC filed 130 times, many times amending earlier reports. This defeated the purpose of the law, which was to make it easier for citizens and voters to see who was contributing money to candidates. But when asked directly, AMPAC officials, unlike those for other PACs, refused to say which candidates it was supporting or even how many contributing members it had. AMPAC's chairman said, "We have conscientiously and explicitly followed the letter and intent of the law in reporting our contributions."[20]

AMPAC had created a complicated arrangement with the fifty-two PACs of state and territorial medical societies. They conducted joint fund-raising campaigns and shared information about candidates. They shifted funds back and forth, filing amendments and other documents with the FEC when they did. AMPAC officials claimed the final decisions on which candidates to support came from the state PACs. And when it came time to contribute, AMPAC would usually send a check to a local doctor who was the politician's key contact. A letter accompanying the check would point out that AMPAC was giving the money at the request of local doctors. Sometimes a state PAC would add a check of its own.[21]

AMPAC insisted that it and the state PACs were completely separate entities. And it emphatically stated that the AMA had nothing to do with AMPAC. The AMA took reporters to task for writing that the AMA had contributed to political candidates. The AMA, officials said, has never spent a penny on a political campaign. AMPAC, they said, does that.

But that assertion was undermined when someone dubbed "Sore Throat" in the 1970s leaked several confidential AMA memos to the press. One series of memos described how drug companies had contributed $851,000 to AMPAC in its first three years, a secret until then. Another package of a dozen memos described how AMA lobbyists requested AMPAC contributions for specific candidates, and AMPAC usually complied. For example, lobbyists asked AMPAC to give to a reception for Mendel J. Davis (D-S.C.), because "Mendel has introduced every bill we have provided." And the lobbyists asked AMPAC to make up for its "mistakes" by giving a donation to a particular candidate: "We opposed [him] in the primary. This might be a vehicle for patching that up."[22]

The published reports caught the interest of the Federal Election Commission, the agency set up by Congress to make campaign-finance records public and to investigate violations of campaign laws. The press widely reported that the AMA was being investigated for possibly violating prohibitions against nonprofit organizations making campaign contributions.[23] But the FEC backed off after a review of the law. It never determined if the charges were true. Its letter to the AMA explained why: even if it was true that the AMA was directing AMPAC's campaign contributions, it was not a violation of federal law.[24]

A Pack of PACs

At the end of 1974, when Congress passed its sweeping campaign reforms, AMPAC officials assessed the impact, and, with political astuteness, decided the "reform" was good for them. The AMPAC bulletin noted, "Many of the authors of this law were in favor of reducing the influence of special-interest groups. However . . . they, in fact, increased the importance of special-interest giving." The law put a limit on spending for congressional races (later thrown out by the courts), and allowed PACs to give up to $5,000 per election (which the courts upheld). The bulletin noted that if AMPAC and a state PAC each contributed $5,000 to a candidate for the primary and another $5,000 for the general election, they could give $20,000. That, it said, is "a fairly substantial portion of a candidate's budget," giving medicine "a more effective role" in campaigns.[25]

In May 1976 Congress added amendments to the campaign act, including a "non-proliferation" clause to bar groups from using affiliates to exceed contribution limits. But that did not stop AMPAC and the state medical PACs. In September 1976 the reform group Common Cause released a study that showed that AMPAC and its state affiliates had contributed more than the legal limit of $5,000 each in contributions to twenty-one congressional candidates. Aggravating the situation was the fact that AMPAC and its affiliates, with a couple of months to go before the election, had contributed nearly $1 million, more than any other PAC.

A week later, Common Cause filed what it called the first major complaint against a PAC under the federal campaign-reform law. It wanted AMPAC stopped immediately. "It is patently unfair to allow the American Medical Association to play by its own set of rules in the 1976 elections while others are complying with the letter and spirit of the new campaign finance law," said Common Cause's vice president then, Fred Wertheimer.[26]

One of the candidates named by Common Cause returned $1,000 of the $6,000 contributed by AMPAC and a state PAC. And AMPAC filed its next financial report to the FEC under protest, blaming the FEC for not making Common Cause keep its complaint confidential. A few days later, AMPAC filed a formal complaint with the FEC, accusing Common Cause of violating the campaign law for publicizing its complaint. Ironically, AMPAC's executive director went public with his complaint that Common Cause might have broken the law in going public with its complaint. But the FEC quickly cleared Common Cause.[27]

The FEC, however, also did not stop AMPAC and the state medical PACs from continuing their excessive joint contributions. In June 1978 Common Cause again filed a complaint with the FEC, this time disclosing that AMPAC and affiliate contributions were over the limit to forty-five candidates. The FEC staff investigated the complaint, compiled information from the state PACs, and took depositions from AMA leaders. The doctors' responses were nothing less than hostile, FEC documents show. In October 1979 the FEC's general counsel found it was likely AMPAC and at least four state medical PACs had violated the campaign law's limits. Facing lengthy litigation, AMPAC and its affiliates entered into a consent agreement with the FEC, stating they would no longer exceed the limit of $5,000 per election to a candidate.[28]

Combating Carter

Having beaten back national health insurance in the early 1970s, the AMA now faced a different kind of threat: medical-care cost containment. The federal government's aim had shifted from simply ensuring universal access to reining in the skyrocketing costs of health care, particularly under Medicare and Medicaid. To that end, President Jimmy Carter proposed a cost-containment program that would cap hospital expenditures. But the AMA knew from experience that after hospitals, doctors would be next.

HEW secretary Joseph Califano claimed Carter's cost-containment plan would save the country some $50 billion over the next five years, but Carter and Califano found themselves stymied by the AMA and its allies, the American Hospital Association and the Federation of American Hospitals. Carter's frustration at being blocked spilled over at a town meeting in Spokane. "I know that doctors care very seriously about their patients," Carter said. "But when you get doctors organized into the American Medical Association their interest is to protect the interest not of patients, but of doctors. And they've been the major obstacle to progress in our country in having a better health care system in years gone by."[29]

At the suggestion of a powerful conservative Democrat, the AMA, AHA, and FAH created an alternative plan to Carter's proposal. It was called, fittingly, the Voluntary Effort, and relied on the providers to hold down costs. A substitute amendment, creating a national commission to study and monitor hospital costs, was introduced to replace Carter's plan. And the showdown came on November 15, 1979: the House approved the substitute amendment 234–166, scuttling Carter's bill.[30]

Califano cited the "effective and well-bankrolled lobbying" of the AMA and its allies as he spread the blame around for the defeat.[31] The late PAC opponent Philip Stern took a look at the vote and AMPAC contributions and wrote, "Did AMA campaign contributions affect that vote? Again, the figures suggest that they did."[32] A Common Cause study found that AMPAC had contributed nearly four times more to the legislators who voted to kill Carter's bill than to those who supported it. Common Cause's Fred Wertheimer said, "The American Medical Association has played the central role in the determination of our nation's health policies, and political contributions are the primary source of its power."[33]

Correlation studies like the one done by Common Cause are controversial. Many political consultants, legislators, and academics doubt their validity. PAC officials and some politicians also bristle at the idea that PAC giving is simply a form of bribery—honest graft. One FEC commissioner captured this skepticism well: "Saying 'PAC money buys votes' is the equivalent of looking at the obituary page and concluding that people die in alphabetical order."[34]

But the AMA's response to the study was a nondenial denial. AMPAC's chairman called it misleading and scolded Common Cause for attributing the contributions to the AMA instead of AMPAC, according to the AMA's newspaper. And AMA executive vice president James H. Sammons said Congress voted against Carter's bill because it was so poorly drawn. Neither specifically nor directly denied the charges Common Cause had leveled.[35] And three years later an AMA political official who looked back on the defeat of hospital-cost containment as a big achievement credited "4 A's": "We had allies, an alternative, arguments, and AMPAC."[36]

One academic who liked PACs found convincing evidence that AMPAC had rewarded and punished candidates in the next election in 1980 using the cost-containment vote as a "litmus test." Based on roll votes and 1980 contributions, he found that AMPAC gave its supporters an average of about $2,500, and opponents about $340. The study controlled for the liberal or conservative ideology of the candidate, and found that even liberals who supported the AMA position were rewarded: AMPAC gave them three times as much as it contributed to conservatives who opposed the AMA. The study concluded: "The fact that one specific roll call affected contributions in this case is quite clear."[37]

Big Daddy

At the start of the 1970s, the AMA appeared to be a struggling has-been—weakened by defeat, red ink, and uncertainty. By the end of the decade, the AMA had turned itself around, becoming a financially sound and politically vigorous contender. It had emerged victorious over the reformers pushing national health insurance and cost-containment schemes. And AMPAC had become the dominant PAC in the business. As Wertheimer put it in 1979: "The AMA is the 'Big Daddy' of the American PAC movement. It has made little secret of its willingness to use political money to influence public policy."[38]

No other PAC contributed as much money to congressional candidates as AMPAC did during the 1970s, FEC records show. In the five elections from 1972 through 1980, AMPAC contributed $5.5 million, or an average of about $10,300 for each of the 435 seats in the House and

100 seats in the Senate. The second-largest contribution total in that period was $4.7 million by the United Auto Workers. AMPAC spent another $2.1 million on administrative expenses and the political education of physicians—it held workshops where politicians and party officials spoke to doctors, produced pamphlets and videotapes about the political process and the AMA's aims, and even encouraged doctors to run for office.

AMPAC insisted it was bipartisan, giving money to both Democrats and Republicans. Indeed, during the Carter years, AMPAC made about as many contributions to Democrats as it did to Republicans. But the amount of the contributions made AMPAC a virtual arm of the Republican Party. Of AMPAC's nearly $3 million in contributions in the 1978 and 1980 elections, $2.1 million, or 70 percent, went to Republican candidates.

This partisanship spilled over to the presidential race. AMPAC's policy was to give money only to congressional and senatorial candidates, not to presidential candidates. But five former AMA presidents helped establish a separate committee, "Physicians for Reagan-Bush." To underscore the AMA leadership's de facto endorsement of the conservative Republican Ronald Reagan, the committee paid for a full-page ad in the AMA's newspaper. The ad was so unusual and unprecedented that the newspaper ran an editorial in the same issue defending the practice.[39]

AMPAC's support of Republicans paid off after Reagan won the election. The new President appointed Lee Ann Elliott as one of the six commissioners of the Federal Election Commission. Elliott, a conservative Republican active in Illinois politics, had the backing of both the Republican and Democratic senators from Illinois. Since 1979 she had worked as a political consultant. But it was Elliott's earlier job history that mattered: from 1951 to 1962 she worked for the AMA in its law division, and from 1962 to 1979 she served as assistant, and later associate, executive director of AMPAC.

For AMPAC there were few greater signs of power. To have a former official, its number-two executive, appointed to the sole regulatory agency for PACs was a coup. Earlier appointments also had partisan backgrounds; Big Labor had had its share of appointments. By design Congress gave the FEC a partisan balance: three commissions were Democrats and three were Republicans. But a majority of four had to approve before the FEC could act.

During the 1970s the FEC had looked into two major complaints about AMPAC, and since it was the nation's largest PAC, it was likely the FEC would get more complaints about it. But Elliott dismissed potential conflicts of interest in her written response to Senate Rules Committee questions before it unanimously approved her appointment. She disclosed she would receive a monthly AMA pension for the rest of her life, but she described what she would do if she faced any potential conflict of interest: "I would recuse myself from decisions where there was a direct conflict or the appearance of conflict based on the facts of the particular case."[40]

The AMA was at the peak of its power in the post-Medicare era. One survey of 135 health care organizations ranked it as the most influential organization in health policy during the 1970s.[41] And it sought to reinforce its presence in Washington by buying three parcels in the capital. It paid $675,000 for a town house—Needham House—where visiting AMA officials could stay. It spent $13.3 million for the old Potomac Electric Power Co. headquarters as investment property. And it bought a piece of property for $3 million at 1101 Vermont Street NW.

That parcel became the site of the AMA's official presence in Washington: a new twelve-story building that it constructed at a cost of $12.5 million to serve as headquarters for its Washington office and its political action committee. The AMA and AMPAC moved into the top two stories; the lower floors were leased to other medical-specialty societies. Sammons said the building showed lawmakers that the AMA was here to stay.

PAC AND PROUD

Success with lobbying and PAC contributions in the 1970s encouraged the AMA to become more aggressive and more open about its political nature. In 1981, following two studies and a bit of soul-searching, the AMA board presented its delegates a report explaining the new "functional profile" of the AMA. Identified as the primary goal of the AMA was representation of doctors.[42] Second to that came scientific information. Over the next few years the AMA put its new profile into action, and the balance of the budget gradually shifted from science to representation. The AMA's shift—foretold by Dr. F. J. L. Blasingame in 1968 when he was ousted by the AMPAC crowd—had become official policy.

Meanwhile the political AMA took a higher profile. In 1982 the AMA officially opened its new Washington office—named the American Medical Association building, complete with a multimillion-dollar art collection. That same year, nearly all of the members of the AMA's policy-setting House of Delegates joined AMPAC as sustaining members, the highest-dues-paying category. AMPAC officials even publicly spoke about their strategies and named the candidates they hoped would win. The FEC's efficient operation made such disclosure a must.

Besides, it was the decade of PACs. The amount of money PACs spent on elections soared as FEC and Supreme Court rulings unleashed corporations, which for decades were barred from contributing to federal candidates. Now they could set up their own PACs, and between 1975 and 1980 the number of corporate PACs exploded from 139 to 1,106, the FEC said. Now PACs were the allies of conservatives, unlike before, when labor PACs fueled the races of liberals. When Congress failed to pass public financing of congressional races in 1980, many speculated that Republicans might win enough seats in 1982 to control the House for the first time in decades.

With the ascendancy of PACs, AMPAC was no longer shy about its methods or its wealth. AMPAC defended the PAC movement, and bashed Common Cause and other critics, in a book it copublished in 1981. Its officials boasted about using such sophisticated political techniques as selected precinct polling for candidates, which AMPAC originated in the 1960s. And it proudly told of pioneering the use of two major loopholes in the campaign-finance laws that allowed it to get around the $5,000 per election limit on contributions to candidates' campaign funds.

One involved polling. Under an obscure provision of the campaign law, AMPAC has to report only a fraction of the cost of a poll it conducts for a candidate by withholding the results for two weeks or more. In 1982, the first year AMPAC reported using this loophole, it said it paid $10,000 each for home district surveys for thirty-six candidates, an expense that is twice the contribution limit of $5,000 per election. But because AMPAC held the results for sixty days for most of the candidates, it had to report only as little as 5 percent of the poll's actual cost as its in-kind contribution to the candidate.[43] FEC records show AMPAC reported only $91,070 for such in-kind contributions in the 1982 elections, even though AMPAC officials admitted they had spent at least four times as much money for the surveys.

Another innovation involved what are known as independent expenditures. In 1976 the Supreme Court ruled on a lawsuit charging that the limits on campaign contributions set by federal election laws violate First Amendment rights to free speech. The Court ruled that the limits could stand for direct contributions to a campaign, but that contributors could spend as much as they wanted to independently of the campaign.

This meant contributors, such as AMPAC, had to abide by the $5,000 limit for direct contributions to a candidate's campaign fund. But the contributor, on its own, could spend unlimited amounts of money promoting a candidate as long as the contributor acted completely separately and independently of that candidate and his or her campaign. So a contributor could spend thousands of dollars to run television advertising for a candidate as long as the contributor had no contact whatsoever with the candidate. Similarly, a contributor could spend thousands for advertising against a candidate as long as the contributor had no contact with the candidates running against the targeted politician.[44]

AMPAC made its first independent expenditures in the election that followed the Supreme Court ruling, spending about $58,000 on magazine advertisements for selected candidates and buying campaign buttons in ten congressional districts. And in the 1980 elections, AMPAC spent about $180,000 for television spots for seven candidates and direct mail for another seven. All but one of them won. In the 1982 elections, AMPAC increased its independent expenditure again, spending more than $220,000 on 21 candidates, FEC records show.

The Turnaround

Given the shift in the mood of the country from liberal to conservative, the 1980s should have been a replay of the 1950s for the AMA. Without the threat of national health insurance, and the Reagan administration's loosening of the restraints on capitalists, the AMA should have enjoyed the same prosperity and peace as it did under Eisenhower. But instead it faced a series of crises, some brought on by outside forces, others brought on by itself. The first test of power involved the Federal Trade Commission. Ruling on a lawsuit by the AMA, the Supreme Court upheld the FTC's jurisdiction over doctors and other professionals. Having lost its court battle, the AMA turned to Congress to pass a law exempting professions from FTC regulation.[45]

At first it appeared that the sophisticated lobbying of the AMA would work. The AMA and its allies had successfully tapped into the antiregulation fever that swept much of Washington and the country during the Carter years. The FTC was even described as "a rogue agency gone insane." Representative Thomas Luken (D-Ohio), the key sponsor of the exemption, said, "I don't want the FTC to practice its brand of quackery in regulating medicine."

But the tide began to turn against the AMA when unlikely partners joined together to oppose the exemption. Already, the AMA had battled against the consumer activists, who argued from a liberal point of view that doctors and other professionals needed to be regulated. But then the Reagan-appointed FTC chairman opposed the exemption on ideological grounds. Without regulation, he reasoned, the free market cannot work in health care.

Meanwhile the consumer activists discovered and publicized the link between AMPAC campaign contributions and the congressional sponsors of the legislation exempting professionals. The news media picked up on the link—at a time when PAC spending was controversial, it seemed to establish that special interests indeed do try to buy votes. AMPAC's strength as a big contributor was being turned against it and into a weakness.

Michael Pertschuk, the FTC chairman under Carter and among those opposing the AMA, later wrote in *Giant Killers* how the Naderite group Congress Watch issued a series of studies and press releases about the link. The first study and release, in March, said the PACs of the AMA, the American Dental Association, and a third health group, the American Optometric Association, had contributed $863,810 from 1979 to 1981 to 157 House and Senate sponsors of the exemption. The second one, in June, reported that the PAC contributions now topped $1 million, as 186 of the 192 cosponsors received an average of $6,145. The third study focused on the AMA.

The AMA and AMPAC officials derided the connection between exemption sponsors and campaign contributions as "total nonsense" and "baloney." And the AMA prevailed in the House, when it voted to exempt the professions—by seven votes. Later, political scientist Kirk Brown studied the vote and the contributions and concluded: "Since only seven votes would have had to be changed for the professionals' exemption to have been defeated in the House, it is not difficult to conclude that AMA's and ADA's campaign contributions of over $1.5 million to House members during the 1982 election provided the margin of victory."[46]

But a few days later, feeling the pressure of negative publicity, the Senate spiked it, with fifty-seven senators voting against it. The AMA and AMPAC had lost both the exemption and a chunk of their reputation for political effectiveness. Their success in raising and contributing campaign funds had been turned against them. It would be a tactic thrown up against them again, and AMPAC's reputation as a big spender began working as much against the AMA's goals as it did for them.

The FEC's Landlord

Thousands of reporters and consumer activists have walked through the front doors of the old PEPCO building at 999 E Street NW in Washington to use the well-lighted first-floor public-document room of the Federal Election Commission. There, they examine the campaign-finance reports that detail the millions of dollars that PACs and individuals spend to influence Congress. But what they don't know is that the

American Medical Association—whose PAC is considered the Godfather of PACs—is the FEC's landlord.[47]

The FEC lease illustrates just how entrenched the AMA is in the nation's capital. Not only does the AMA have one of the biggest-spending PACs in the country, but it also owns the building that houses the only federal agency charged with monitoring PACs and campaign contributions. It is part of the quiet but effective power of the AMA that it has never publicized the arrangement with the FEC. True power rarely advertises itself.

The AMA paid a 33 percent markup when it purchased the PEPCO building in July 1981 for $13.3 million from a partnership that had just bought it in January. The D.C. real estate market was hot, and the AMA was gambling that the value of the building would continue to escalate: it was next to the block that investors planned to turn into a new Federal Triangle office complex, around the corner from the historic Ford Theater, and across the street from the FBI's new headquarters.

The University of the District of Columbia occupied the building, a nine-story masonry structure built in 1931 as the headquarters of the Potomac Electric Co. But the AMA announced it would not renew the university's lease when it expired in 1982. Instead, it would renovate the building and seek new tenants.

Meanwhile, the FEC in 1983 began contemplating a move from its cramped quarters at 1325 K Street NW, in Franklin Square North. Its lease was up in 1985, and for advice it contacted the General Services Administration, the federal agency that handles real estate for the government. The GSA hired a consulting firm to review the FEC's needs, and the firm reported that its office was not only inadequate, but that it was unsafe—the thirteen-story building had no sprinklers and only two fire escapes, prompting the FEC to consider buying emergency rope ladders.

On March 1, 1984, the FEC commissioners voted 6–0 to relocate. Lee Ann Elliott, at the time the FEC chairman and head of the FEC's site-search committee, initiated the lengthy bureaucratic process for a relocation by making a formal request to the GSA. By May the FEC had drawn up forty-three pages of specifications for the new space, including a preference for its location: four blocks from a Metro stop, five blocks from Franklin Square, and within an area in Northwest Washington. In September the GSA advertised for bids.

By the end of the month, GSA had received at least three bids. FEC staff director John C. Surina wrote a memo saying the GSA was, "contrary to normal procedures," inviting the FEC's search committee and consultant to tour the sites to speed up the process.[48] In an interview later, however, William B. Jenkins, at the time overseeing the relocation as director of the GSA real estate division for the Washington, D.C., area, said there was nothing unusual about the tour. Commissioners Elliott and Joan D. Aikens, along with three staffers and a consultant, visited the three original and a last-minute fourth site.

After the tour, the AMA-owned PEPCO building stood out as the favorite of the FEC staff and search committee. The other sites had major flaws, the committee decided. On March 1, 1985, a year to the day after they voted to relocate, the commissioners voted 6–0 to move into the PEPCO building. In July the GSA signed a ten-year lease, with a starting base annual rent of $1.68 million. In a letter to Jenkins, Surina wrote, "In all likelihood, 999 E Street will be the permanent home of the agency."49

FEC and GSA officials describe the FEC's selection of an AMA-owned building as a coincidence in an otherwise routine process. Elliott, in an interview, said she had no contact with the AMA during the search, and didn't learn that it owned the building until July or August 1985, after the lease was signed. She said her reaction upon learning about it was: "How about that." She added, "I didn't pay much attention to that after that. It didn't matter to me."

Surina said he and the staff also did not learn about the AMA's ownership until after the lease was signed. He stressed that the FEC was one step removed from the process. The GSA acted as the agent for the FEC, he said. Had the FEC been directly handling its own lease search, it may not have selected a building owned by the sponsor of one of the country's largest PACs, Surina said. Referring to the appearance left by the arrangement, he said, "It might have been a factor had we been our own agent."

The purchase, renovation, and leasing of the old PEPCO building turned out to be one of the AMA's better investments. The AMA added to its building's profitability with another highly successful attraction: a trendy Hard Rock Cafe. The AMA also leased space to the Bureau of Public Debt, a part of the Treasury Department that manages financial transactions related to the federal debt. Together the FEC and the Bureau pay more than $3 million in rent to the AMA each year.

Meanwhile, the AMA was weighing the future of its new Washington headquarters at 1101 Vermont Avenue NW. The D.C. real estate market was still hot, and foreign investors were buying up "trophy" properties at unbelievably high prices. A Japanese real estate firm made a $35 million offer to the AMA for its D.C. headquarters, which would give the AMA a $17 million profit. The deal would allow the AMA to keep its name on the building's façade, and the lobbyists and PAC staff to work out of its top floors. So, three years after its great fanfare about erecting a building to establish a permanent presence in Washington, the AMA sold it to the highest bidder.

Playing Hardball

AMPAC celebrated its twenty-fifth anniversary in 1986 by breaking its own record by spending $5.4 million during the two-year election cycle, almost $2 million more than it had for the previous election, which also had been a record-breaker. But AMPAC was not satisfied with simply spreading money around to help incumbents, as it normally did. This time, said AMPAC's tough-talking chairman, Dr. Thomas R. Berglund, AMPAC would play hardball.[50]

Of the four health subcommittees in Congress, the one that matters the most is part of the powerful, tax-writing Ways and Means Committee in the House. When the AMA first set up AMPAC, it channeled much of its money into the conservatives on that panel. It was the Ways and Means Committee of Representative Wilbur Mills (D-Ark.) who created Medicare and tried but failed to craft a compromise national health insurance system in 1974. In 1978 it was the Ways and Means health subcommittee chairman who suggested to hospitals and the AMA that they come up with a voluntary alternative to Carter's plan.

When the iconoclastic Representative Andrew Jacobs (D-Ind.) became chairman of the Ways and Means health panel in 1982, the AMA figured out quickly he was no friend of theirs. During the four years he ran the powerful panel, Jacobs managed to infuriate the AMA. He pushed a fee freeze and a limited-payment plan for doctors under Medicare. The thin-skinned AMA doctors also objected to his glibness. He publicly joked about AMPAC's attempt to give him a campaign contribution after he beat the candidate AMPAC had supported. And, noting that the AMA was lobbying against his Medicare bill while seniors were pushing for it, Jacobs told House members, "Vote for the canes, not for the stethoscopes."

Meanwhile, in 1985, during the shifting in committee posts that comes after elections, Representative Fortney "Pete" Stark (D-Calif.) took over the chairmanship of the Ways and Means health panel from Jacobs. A liberal Democrat and former banker, Stark had showed no interest in Medicare or health-system matters before. But he quickly took to the subject and immediately employed his sharp tongue to infuriate the AMA. He routinely called doctors "rich," "reactionary," and "greedy." But all seem to agree it was one comment that ticked off the AMA the most: Stark referred to AMA members as "troglodytes." That is, cavemen.

For the AMA and AMPAC, playing hardball meant launching the

most expensive and controversial "shadow campaign," or use of independent expenditures, ever conducted in a congressional race. In July
1986 the first vestiges of AMPAC's "shadow campaign" in Stark's East Bay
district showed up: a series of twenty-nine billboards promoting the
Republican challenger. AMPAC had found its champion in David M.
Williams, the fifty-year-old owner of a package engineering firm.
Williams was a political neophyte, but AMPAC officials had decided he
was their man.

Stark quickly made AMPAC the issue in his campaign. After the billboards started showing up, he again called doctors "greedy" and said
they had targeted him for defeat because "they've never met anybody before who wasn't scared of them." As election day neared, Stark's attacks
on the AMA and its PAC dominated the race. Williams, his opponent,
complained, "This campaign has come down to Stark calling the AMA
greedy cavemen, and the AMA putting up signs for me."

The Williams campaign itself was woefully underfunded. The California Republican state party gave it nothing, and the National Republican Congressional Committee contributed a total of $16.86. Williams
loaned $14,000 of his own money to his campaign. He said he would ac-
cept no PAC funds and would return checks from corporations. His fund
raised a total of $63,000. Yet more than half of that came from contribu-
tors responding to an AMPAC solicitation sent to its 57,000 members, a
practice known as bundling.

AMPAC spent four times as much on its shadow campaign as Williams did. Before it was over, AMPAC eventually sank $252,199 into
billboards, benchmark surveys, tracking polls, radio ads, direct mail,
flyers, opposition research, and consultants. But even though Stark
was a former board member of the anti-PAC Common Cause, he had
become a seven-term congressman in part by accepting PAC money. In
the 1986 election he raised $566,000 and spent most of it countering
AMPAC.

Meanwhile, in Indianapolis Jacobs noticed similar footprints left by
AMPAC. There, AMPAC found its challenger in James P. Eynon, a forty-
year-old real estate manager. Also a political newcomer, Eynon at least
had the savvy to raise more than $500,000 in campaign funds. AMPAC
gave $6,000 to Eynon's treasury and independently spent another
$315,838 on a media blitz, polls, and consultants. The amount AMPAC
spent on the shadow campaign against Jacobs set a record for independent expenditures in a single race. And the combined resources of
AMPAC and Eynon outspent Jacobs by a margin of 20 to 1. Jacobs raised
$52,000 and spent about $40,500. But Jacobs, too, had made the AMA

and AMPAC the major campaign issue. Eynon later complained, "The AMA entry was the major focus of the race."

In the end, AMPAC's highly visible spending backfired. Stark won with 70 percent of the vote, Jacobs with 58 percent. AMPAC had spent $1.5 million independently on fourteen races in the 1986 elections, and came up with an even split, winning seven and losing seven. Again, AMPAC's strength of having nearly unlimited funds had been turned back on it, handing the AMA a defeat instead of a victory.

Stark Reaction

But the AMA lost more than its bet on the election. It had enraged one of the most powerful members in Congress who would be in charge of issues crucial to AMA members, notably Medicare and physician payment. As Stark fought back, the AMA's attempts to intimidate him, or even send a warning to marginal candidates, loomed larger and larger as a miscalculation.

Stark immediately filed a complaint with the FEC, charging that AMPAC and the Williams campaign had been in contact, and that AMPAC's shadow campaign was therefore not based on independent spending. And he went on the attack against FEC commissioner Lee Ann Elliott, urging her to remove herself from the proceedings on his complaint because of her long history with the AMA. Stark pointed out she still received an annual pension from the AMA.

But after getting clearance from the FEC's attorneys, Elliott rejected Stark's request. The FEC staff reviewed Stark's complaint and recommended that some charges be investigated. But the matter required an FEC vote. The commissioners split the vote: three Democrats voted to investigate, three Republicans voted to drop it. The FEC requires four votes to take action. The AMA was off the hook.

By now Stark was so angry that he sued the FEC and Elliott, but the judge dismissed the case. Stark even showed up at Elliott's confirmation hearing in 1987 for a second six-year appointment to argue that she be denied a return to the FEC. He said she had a conflict of interest. She denied it. The Senate subcommittee approved her reappointment.

The AMA had made an irritant into an enemy. And he was a powerful enemy. Since the 1986 election, Stark has helped write and shape landmark Medicare bills and other legislation that was crucial to the AMA. To help him understand the effects of proposals being considered, he invited experts and those affected to testify before his subcommittee—except, that is, the AMA.

Too Much Money

University of Southern California professor Herbert E. Alexander, who has studied PACs for longer than any other political scientist, has a theory about why AMPAC pursued its disastrous policy on independent expenditures in 1986. "First, they wanted to scare some people who were not favorable to their viewpoint," he said. But it had so much money in its treasury, it had to do something with it.

"AMPAC has had so much money that it has a hard time distributing it," he said. "In dealing with Congress, for example, you'll find that if you look at the figures through the FEC and other ways, every two years they give to several hundred candidates. . . . They make contributions very liberally. Part of the reason is that they are flooded with money." He added, "They can't stand to have a cash balance at the end of an election year. They have to spend it, because if they don't they can't go so readily back to their members to ask for more."[51]

In 1988 AMPAC's membership fell off for the first time in many years. And the political action committee's new chairman, Dr. Joseph Hatch, the brother of conservative Utah Republican senator Orrin G. Hatch, announced that AMPAC no longer would go tilting against the windmills of secure legislators, even if they were hostile to the AMA. AMPAC was drawing in its claws. For the 1988 elections, AMPAC slightly increased direct contributions to candidates, but cut nearly in half the amount it spent on shadow campaigns, though it still made the second largest direct contributions to candidates of any of the nation's PACs. But the AMA went back to its policy of supporting friendly incumbents.

Its huge reserves of cash turned AMPAC into a cash-rich gambler looking for close exciting races on which to bet. In some cases the AMA poured money into obscure House districts simply because there was a contest with an open seat—a rarity in Congress, where most politicians have a lock on their jobs.

For example, AMPAC in 1988 spent $131,560 in independent expenditures to help elect Democrat Bill Sarpalius, a public-school teacher and agricultural consultant, to Congress from the 13th District of Texas. Sarpalius, a conservative who had served for eight years in the thirty-one-member state Senate, hails from Amarillo, in the Texas Panhandle. No expert on health, his real interest lies in agriculture, a mainstay of his district.

Phil Duncan, Sarpalius' chief of staff, offered an explanation for the AMA's large outlay: it was an open seat, and Sarpalius was "a proven quantity." Duncan explained, "He has always received significant contributions from the AMA, going back to his Texas state senate days. He had been a friend in the Texas state Legislature. He's someone who's voted very conservatively on issues that mattered to docs."

Duncan, who worked for former House Majority Leader Jim Wright for eight years, added that AMA lobbyists are among the most effective. "They have built up a lot of goodwill with this sort of thing," he said of AMPAC's independent expenditures, adding that AMPAC should help AMA lobbyists during the battle over health-care reform. "They are at least going to get a hearing in a lot of offices."[52]

UPPING THE ANTE

The AMA and AMPAC are no longer the lone Voice of Medicine in Washington. As the pressures for health-care reform began building during the 1980s, the number of competing specialty medical associations and health-related organizations proliferated. Two of the AMA's main rivals for influence in Washington, the primarily clinical and educational American College of Surgeons and the American College of Physicians, opened offices in Washington, though neither set up a political action committee.

Yet there was an explosion of health PACs plying Congress with money. The number zoomed from around 65 in 1980 to more than 150 a decade later. And although AMPAC kept upping the ante in its spending and contributions each election cycle, it found that it accounted for a smaller share of the political-health dollar. In 1980 AMPAC contributions represented more than 43 percent of all health PAC contributions. A decade later its share had dropped by half, to 22 percent.[53]

But the AMA insists it still has clout in Washington with policymakers, and has cited a survey of 152 senior congressional staff people that rated the AMA as one of the top five most effective lobbying groups in the country. In his last address as the AMA's top executive, Sammons defended the AMA he had built and its power: "We're still the Big Dog on the policy block."

Indeed, the AMA is still the biggest. The FEC ranked AMPAC as the biggest-spending PAC in the 1992 election cycle, with $6.3 million in expenditures. Common Cause called AMPAC the largest contributor to campaigns of all health PACs for handing out $12.6 million to both winning and losing candidates from January 1, 1983, through May 31, 1993.[54] The next-largest contributor donated half the amount given by the AMA.

As large as those figures may appear, they actually understate the investment the AMA and AMPAC has made in the current Congress, the one that will decide the future of health-care reform. Special interests such as the AMA have several ways to funnel money to politicians. The three best-known are 1) direct contributions to campaign funds, 2) through the old system, since modified, of honoraria, in which a group could give a fee to a politician for making a speech or dropping by for a visit, and 3) independent expenditures.

Over the past twenty years, the AMA and its PAC have used all three routes to channel funds to politicians, creating an enormous financial stake in Congress. Adding together the money the AMA and AMPAC have spent from 1975 through 1994 on the current representatives and senators shows the Doctors' Lobby has an investment in the 104th Congress worth $11.3 million, or about $24,000 for each of the 464 members who took AMA money.

That amount is down slightly from the $11.4 million invested in the last Congress, largely because some of the most senior members of the House and Senate either stepped down or were defeated in the Republican onslaught in the November 1994 election. Among the best known were Speaker of the House Tom Foley (D-Wash.), House Ways and Means Committee Chairman Dan Rostenkowski (D-Ill.), and Senator Dave Durenberger (R-Minn.) Even Representative Bill Sarpalius (D-Tex.), who ranked fifth with $162,560 of AMA money in 1992, lost his election to a Republican.

The AMA did not bankroll the new Republican members; it stuck to its pro-incumbent policy. But that does not mean the AMA has not laid the groundwork for influence with the new majority party. Indeed, for the first time in years, the AMA's investment in Republicans in Congress is greater than it is in Democrats. The analysis shows that the AMA and its PAC have invested $6.6 million in 241 Republicans, compared with $4.6 million in 223 Democrats.

And the Republicans' Top Gun has long been a favorite of the AMA. House Speaker Newt Gingrich (R-Ga.) ranks 12th overall in total AMA and AMPAC spending. But if only direct contributions are counted he ranks number one.

AMPAC's biggest overall investment, $328,085, remains in Representative Vic Fazio (D-Calif.), the chairman of the fund-raising Democratic Congressional Campaign Committee. It committed $255,085 to a shadow campaign in the 1992 election to help Fazio squeak by with 52 percent of the vote. (Fazio chaired Hillary Rodham Clinton's massive health-care task force.) In the 1994 election year, AMPAC gave Fazio the maximum, $10,000.

AMPAC's second largest investment, $248,108, is in Senator Bob Packwood (R-Ore.). It independently spent $227,808 in 1992 on television ads, polling, and other assistance to help Pakcwood, who was accused of sexually harrassing several former female staff members. Packwood has long been influential on health issues, and sits on the Senate Finance Committee.

The others, in whom AMPAC has invested more than $100,000, are Representative Scott McInnis (R-Colo.), $204,909, Senator Phil Gramm (R-Tex.), who is gearing up for a presidential campaign, $167,463; Representative David E. Skaggs (D-Colo.), $150,530; Representative James V. Hansen (R-Utah), $135,359, Representative Mike Parker (D-Miss.), $127,851; Representative Gary A. Franks (R-Conn.), $111,454, and Senator Tim Johnson (D-S.D.), $108,659.[55]

The analysis also shows that the AMA or AMPAC has handed a check at some time to 87 percent of the 535 representatives or senators on Capitol Hill. About three-quarters of those who have not gotten checks either won office for the first time in 1994 or do not take PAC contributions. That leaves just a handful of politicians—such as Senator Edward M. Kennedy (D-Mass.)—who are just too liberal or antagonistic for AMPAC to donate money to them.

The AMA has even reached out to its nemesis, Pete Stark. In 1992 it invited him to Chicago to appear on a panel about the future of health care. It also gave him an in-kind contribution of a dated poll recorded at $2,000 but worth much more, and a direct contribution of $4,000. Stark said, "I'll take money from anyone." The AMA also paid the way for one of Stark's health-panel aides to a luxurious resort to discuss health-care reform.[56] In 1994, AMPAC again gave to Stark, cutting three checks for a total of $7,500. But the last check, for $4,000, got lost in the mail. An aide to Stark said, "We hope that they'll give it to us again for the next election."

Buffeted by change and uncertainty, the AMA continues to hone itself as a sharp political tool for physicians' interests. In 1994 it increased the portion of its members' dues devoted to lobbying from one-fourth to one-third. And it continues to raise and spend some of its largest sums through AMPAC, which had about $830,000 in cash on hand at the end of 1994. Money may not buy votes or sway legislators, but it certainly can buy access to them. And as long as politicians need money, the AMA will have a potent voice.

CHAPTER 5

Principles for Profits
Keeping Medicine's Business Ethic Alive

THE DOCTOR-PATIENT relationship is almost sacred in American medicine. And there is a good reason for it. Without a patient's trust, a doctor can do little good in diagnosing an illness and prescribing a treatment. A physician can hold the trust of a patient as long as he believes that the physician is putting him first, ahead of interests in personal or professional gain.

The American Medical Association reveres the doctor-patient relationship and claims that the AMA Principles of Ethics uphold that trust. The essence of professionalism in medicine, the AMA says, is the importance of physicians always placing patients first. The AMA, in fact, calls itself a professional association, dedicated to the health of America, and tries to distinguish itself from a trade group primarily interested in the narrow economic or political interests.

But the AMA has always had a difficult time representing both its ideals and its members. The history of the AMA shows that when its ideals clash with its members' political and economic interests, the ideals often lose. The founders of the AMA tried to paint a bright line separating the profession of medicine from the business of medicine. And during the 1950s the AMA's more high-minded members attempted to highlight that line.

In showdowns over several highly publicized physician financial conflicts of interest in the 1950s and 1960s, and again in the 1980s and

1990s, the AMA's members put their personal interests ahead of ethical concerns—and their patients. Even when the leadership and the Judicial Council attempted to steer the association toward a higher ethical plane, its members reversed course.

CREATING A CODE OF ETHICS

From its origins, the American Medical Association attempted to establish a code of ethics to prevent doctors from putting their financial gain ahead of the interests of their patients. When the AMA was started in 1847, its founders wanted to make clear that physicians were professionals, not businessmen. This was no easy task. Unlike now, most states then did not license doctors. With no legal distinction between a snake-oil salesman and a doctor, it is not surprising that the public had a low regard for physicians as a group. To improve their image, the AMA doctors sought to distance themselves from other healers by adopting key distinctions of the traditional European "learned professions" of law, divinity, and medicine: a code of ethics.

The professions adopted such codes because they are in a position to exploit the people they are supposed to help. A doctor has skills that are difficult for non-physicians to readily evaluate. A doctor controls the path of the patient's treatment, and it is crucial that the patient trust the doctor for treatment to be effective. More importantly, patients—ill and often scared—are at their most vulnerable when they see physicians.

The AMA's first Code of Ethics contains the essence of codes going back to the beginning of medicine: physicians should put patients first. Or, as the AMA Code put it, physicians had to have "a sense of ethical obligations rising superior . . . to considerations of personal advancement." The code rejected the business practices of many doctors at the time. It declared that advertising by doctors was "highly reprehensible" and "derogatory to the dignity of the profession." And it sought to limit doctors' incomes basically to fees for the services they provided. The code barred doctors from profiting from patents on surgical instruments and medicine.[1]

In 1903 the AMA replaced the Code of Ethics with the Principles of Ethics. The organization changed the name from "Code" to "Principles" to emphasize that ethics are not enforceable laws or a penal code, but standards of conduct. The 1903 Principles echoed many of the words and sentiments of the 1847 Code, but broke the Code's image as an almost sacred icon.

Bodies for Sale

Among the issues addressed by the 1903 Principles was a nettlesome practice among doctors: fee-splitting. Fee-splitting did not begin until the 1890s and did not become widespread until the 1900s. This practice involved a kickback paid by a doctor—often a surgeon—to another doctor—frequently a general practitioner—for referring patients.[2] At first the AMA's House of Delegates did not entirely ban fee-splitting. Instead, it voted to kick out only those members proven guilty of fee-splitting "without the full knowledge of the patient." In other words, it was okay for a surgeon to give a kickback to a referring doctor as long as the doctor told the patient about it.[3]

In 1912 the House of Delegates reaffirmed its prohibition of "secret fee-splitting." A report explained the motivations behind the practice: surgeons' incomes had soared while general practitioners' earnings remained static. Meanwhile, the delegates added a ban on doctors accepting commissions or rebates from instrument manufacturers or medical-supply houses. This practice appeared to border on bribery since the doctors' decisions to recommend a particular brand of glasses or drug was influenced by a manufacturer's payment of money.

In 1913 surgeons organized themselves into the American College of Surgeons, a group of physicians independent of the AMA. The surgeons attempted to stamp out fee-splitting—after all, it was not in their economic interest to pay kickbacks. Members of the ACS had to sign an oath vowing to shun "dishonest money-seeking" and to "refuse utterly all secret money trades with consultants and practitioners."[4]

Finally, in 1929, the House of Delegates equated fee-splitting with commissions, and deemed both unethical. Doctors, however, continued to engage in the condemned practice. In the early 1950s the ACS conducted a crusade against fee-splitting. Dr. Paul Hawley, an ACS director, made headlines and outraged the AMA in an interview with *U.S. News & World Report*. He said fee-splitting was rampant among doctors and led to "ghost" surgery—that is, procedures in which patients were not informed about or were misled about the identity of the operating surgeon—and unnecessary procedures. Meanwhile, Dr. Loyal Davis, another prominent ACS member and stepfather of future First Lady Nancy Davis Reagan, also publicly condemned fee-splitting.[5]

AMA delegates responded to Hawley's highly publicized interview by introducing nearly a dozen resolutions condemning his remarks as damaging to the profession. Some of the resolutions even suggested censorship. The Chicago Medical Society attempted to discipline him for speaking out against fee-splitting without the medical society's permission. The practice never disappeared, but the AMA succeeded in lowering its high profile. The AMA in 1954 adopted a resolution calling for "a moratorium from the constant discussion of 'principles' about fees."

THE TEMPTATIONS OF WEALTH

After World War II the world of medicine underwent a major transformation, tempting doctors with new ways to make money off their patients. New technology advanced medicine, making it more effective in treating illness. New drugs came on the market in rapid succession. Federal money financed the construction of newer, better hospitals. And the explosion of private health insurance among workers through union contracts or in individual purchases pumped money into the health-care system. In the post-war era, medicine prospered.

Doctors prospered as well. With the influx of money and patients, there simply were not enough doctors to go around, so it was relatively easy for them to build practices. Doctors' lucrative practices gave them money to invest, and they began eyeing side medical businesses. These entrepreneurs sought the blessing of the Judicial Council, which serves as the AMA's "Supreme Court," and that set off an internal battle within the AMA over the ethics of making money.

The entrepreneurial doctors pushed for a fundamental change in the AMA's Principles of Ethics. But they met stiff resistance from the more conservative M.D.s on the Judicial Council. The question was whether doctors could engage in side businesses as a way to make money from their patients. The outcome of the battle would shape the direction of medicine and the AMA for decades.

In 1947, noting the dozens of proposals from entrepreneurial doctors, the Judicial Council reported with a weariness of voice: "It should be well known by this time that the traditional interpretation of the Principles of Medical Ethics . . . is that the doctor may receive no profit whatever from his patient other than payment for rendered medical services."[6]

In 1949 the Judicial Council persuaded the AMA's House to make the traditional interpretation explicit in the Principles. The new section stated: "An ethical physician does not engage in barter or trade in the appliances, devices or remedies prescribed for patients, but limits sources of his professional income to professional services rendered the patient."[7]

However, this was not a universally popular move. Dr. Allen T. Stewart of Texas assailed the "restrictive infringement" of the revised ethics, and asserted that the federal government was using the revision as "an entering wedge" to deprive doctors of their constitutional rights to engage in private enterprise. Stewart sought to loosen the restrictions at the AMA's next meeting in 1950, but failed.[8]

The arguments over physicians' side businesses surfaced in the popular press, tarnishing the image of M.D.s. Dr. Edwin B. Dunphy, the chairman of the AMA's section on ophthalmology, tackled this image problem in his annual address in June 1952. He noted that many politicians and citizens attacked the AMA as a group of "greedy" doctors, and warned, "The medical profession is not a luxury business but a profession dedicated to rendering service to humanity. Reward or financial gain is a subordinate consideration. Physicians should never lose sight of this principle. If they do, the medical profession will certainly be government regulated eventually and with public approval."[9]

The Lure of Drugs

Of the growing number of opportunities for doctor investments, pharmacies and pharmaceutical companies proved to be among the most profitable and tempting. A watershed battle within the AMA was fought over the ethics of these investments. Pharmacies seemed a logical extension of the services offered by doctors and group practices. Doctors knew something about the drugs they prescribed. And many group practices, patterned after the well-known Mayo Clinic, already offered a range of doctors and services, such as blood tests and X rays.

Retail drugstores and pharmaceutical manufacturers were enjoying a postwar boom. The sales at retail drugstores grew steadily, and rose to a record $4.5 billion in the mid-1950s.[10] In 1954 the Judicial Council urged the House to ban physician ownership of drugstores, or doctor dispensing of drugs, unless no other drugstore was available. The House complied. Under the revision, doctors who wished to own a pharmacy, or dispense drugs or other devices such as glasses, had to get a waiver from the local medical society stating no other adequate suppliers existed nearby. Even then, doctors were required to make the drugs or devices available "without profit."[11]

The revision created an uproar. Angry delegates came to the AMA's annual meeting in June 1955, determined to force a showdown. The fight pitted entrepreneurial doctors against the high-minded Judicial Council. The entrepreneurs launched ten resolutions proposing the repeal or at least the loosening of the Principles. One resolution claimed the physicians' right to dispense drugs to their patients dated back to Hippocrates; another traced it to Socrates. Others asserted physicians had a constitutional right to make money. Another said the revision indicated AMA leaders lacked faith in the medical profession's integrity while denying doctors "the right to a fair and reasonable profit in the providing of remedies to the patient."

The entrepreneurs won. A committee fashioned a compromise, which the House adopted. The new principle said: "It is not unethical for a physician to prescribe or supply drugs, remedies, or appliances as long as there is no exploitation of the patient."[12]

Selling the Birthright

The House action overturned an ethical precept long held by the Judicial Council. The council had always insisted that doctors should not even be in a position to financially exploit their patients by making money on the drugs or devices they prescribed. But now the House had set a different standard. The new standard distinguished the opportunity to exploit from the act of exploitation itself.

The rebuff of a key ethical precept deeply disturbed the chairman of the Judicial Council, Dr. Homer L. Pearson. In an anguished report Pearson accused the delegates of selling out the AMA's ethics for personal financial gain. Turning to the Bible, Pearson recalled the story of Esau, who sold his birthright for a bowl of pottage. In Pearson's sermon, doctors became Esau, the AMA's Principles of Ethics became their birthright, and financial temptations became the pottage. He wrote, "Birthrights are very hard to come by, but their selling price is sometimes very cheap—sometimes the price of meatless stew."[13]

Meanwhile, in 1957, the House of Delegates adopted a new, streamlined version of the Principles of Ethics. The House reduced its principles to ten sections, with much of the flowery language excised. The first section said service to humanity is the "principal objective of the medical profession," but no longer stated that reward or financial gain was subordinate. Instead, the Principles encouraged doctors to "merit the confidence of patients."

Another section seemed to limit the source of physician income. It said: "In the practice of medicine a physician should limit the source of his professional income to medical services actually rendered by him, or under his supervision, to his patients." But the Principles now included a loophole: "Drugs, remedies or appliances may be dispensed or supplied by the physician provided it is in the best interests of the patients."[14]

Income Over Image

The Judicial Council did not rest in its struggle with the physician-entrepreneurs. In 1961 Dr. George Woodhouse, the new chairman of the Judicial Council, picked up where Pearson had left off. The council conducted a year-long study of the pharmacy-ownership issue, and issued its report to the AMA's interim meeting in November 1962. The report took the hard line, proposing again a ban on doctors' making money off their patients by selling drugs or devices. It also branded as unethical doctor ownership of drug-repackaging companies—businesses that took drugs, put them in new packages under a brand name, and then sold them—and controlling interest in pharmaceutical companies. The council's report stated bluntly: "These practices are contrary to the best interest of the public and the medical profession. Any arrangement by which the physician profits from the remedy he prescribes or supplies is unethical."[15]

But the report was met with hostility at an AMA hearing. Speaking against the proposal were many physicians who owned drugstores or drug firms, ophthalmologists, and the association that represented clinic managers and owners, many of whom also owned pharmacies.

Only three physicians spoke in favor of the proposal. James H. Sammons, a Texas delegate and future AMA chief executive, was one of them. He was particularly vexed about the image of doctors, given the impending fight with the Kennedy administration over its proposal for Medicare. The Texas Medical Association deemed physician ownership of drugstores and pharmaceutical companies unethical, in part because of the temptations inherent in the arrangements. In speeches on the issue, Sammons stressed that he did not seek to limit physician income, "for most assuredly we do not want to do that." Instead, the issue was about the AMA's image.

"We feel very strongly that physician ownership of drugstores is adversely affecting medicine in the public eye. It is difficult, if not impossible, to discuss intelligently and convincingly the problems of the socialization and governmentalization of medicine with a patient who knows that the doctor or doctors in town own the drugstores from which he or they are buying their medications. This in the public eye becomes unequivocally greed of the worst sort," Sammons said in a 1962 speech.[16]

But the reference committee did not heed the warnings of Woodhouse or Sammons. Instead, it seized on a procedural issue—the Judicial Council had not published its report in the *AMA Journal* early enough—and killed the proposal. The council did not again attempt to restore the 1954 Principles, or anything similar, until 1991.

NEW TIMES, NEW PRINCIPLES

On July 22, 1980, the House of Delegates adopted a new looser and simpler version of the Principles of Ethics after little debate. The new Principles had been crafted and sold over a three-year period by a committee led by Dr. James S. Todd, the New Jersey surgeon who would a decade later become head of the AMA. In reality, the AMA had no choice but to change the code. Legally, its back was to the wall for two reasons.

First, chiropractors had filed a barrage of lawsuits against the AMA, accusing it of conspiring to prevent them from practicing medicine. In the lawsuits a key exhibit was the AMA's Principles, which said a physician shouldn't voluntarily associate with anyone whose approach was not based on science. The lawsuits said the AMA used this language to bar chiropractors from getting physician referrals and hospital privileges.

And the Federal Trade Commission also dogged the AMA. The FTC accused the AMA of restraining free trade by banning physician advertising and interfering with certain types of medical practice, such as health-maintenance organizations. After the FTC made its ruling, the AMA sued. Eventually, the U.S. Supreme Court, in a 4–4 vote in 1982, upheld the FTC. The FTC also cited the AMA's Principles as key evidence.

As a result, the 1980 version of the Principles surgically removed the offending sections and replaced them with more amenable language. The AMA dropped the ban on associating with unscientific healers and its limits on types of medical practice. The AMA also clipped language banning physician advertising. AMA lawyers stressed the revision in the legal battles with the chiropractors and the FTC. Todd denied the revision was simply a reaction to the lawsuits facing the AMA, though he acknowledged the association needed to meet certain legal requirements.[17]

But the AMA's leaders understood the potential danger of the changes facing the AMA. Among them was Dr. James Sammons, who in 1974 became the AMA's chief executive. At the 1980 meeting at which the House adopted the new Principles, Sammons said, "What worries me is a growing threat to professionalism itself." He said one problem with professionalism was that it had no single agreed-upon definition, but he listed three elements: ethical standards, competence, and the scientific method. "When you consider what has emerged from both the legislative and executive branches of government in recent times," he said, "you can see clear threats to all three of those elements that characterize a profession."[18]

The Corporate Challenge

Ironically, as the 1980s developed, the greatest danger to professionalism came not from government but from the private sector as corporations and even doctors themselves became entrepreneurs out to make a buck on technology that became a driving force in medicine. The Reagan administration aided and abetted the capitalistic spirit—pushing marketplace competition as the new path for medicine. Under this approach, doctors become health-care providers, and patients customers.

Dr. Arnold S. Relman, the editor of the *New England Journal of Medicine*, took note of the trend and reacted with alarm. He staked out his position against the growth of commercialism in medicine in an editorial, "The New Medical-Industrial Complex." He decried the rise of the for-profit businesses in a field that in recent history had been primarily not-for-profit. Relman urged the AMA to take the lead. The AMA must keep doctors on the straight and narrow path of professionalism, no matter what the pressures might be, Relman said.

He wrote, "If the AMA took a strong stand against any financial interest of physicians in health-care businesses, it might risk an anti-trust suit. . . . Yet, I believe that the risk to the reputation and self-esteem of the profession will be much greater if organized medicine fails to act decisively in separating physicians from the commercial exploitation of health care. . . . A refusal to confront this issue undermines the moral position of the profession and weakens the authority with which it can claim to speak for the public interest."[19]

Relman recalled in an interview years later that after his editorial ran he had gotten no direct response from the AMA. But as he continued his crusade he began to annoy the AMA. "Many of the editorials that I wrote were critical of the policies that were being supported by organized medicine," he said. "I heard indirectly from many sources that there was unhappiness in the AMA."

The AMA Way

The AMA again was confronted with an explosion of technology that created many tempting, lucrative investment opportunities for doctors.

And it continued to face the question that had been so nettlesome in the 1950s: should doctors be allowed to make a profit off their patients through side businesses that supplied or provided the cure or therapy the doctors recommended?

For its answer, the AMA resorted to its ambivalent past. At the interim meeting in December 1984, the House adopted conflict-of-interest guidelines proposed by the Council on Ethical and Judicial Affairs.[20] Over the next two years, the report would be refined and debated. But primarily the AMA decided it was acceptable for physicians to profit on their patients' treatments.

The final report noted that physicians, like all professionals, face a conflict of interest pitting the physician's financial self-interest against the interests of the patient. The way to resolve that, the AMA had decided, was not to return to its high-minded policy that said doctors should make money only from fees. Rather, the AMA in the mid-1980s echoed the past by decreeing: "Physician ownership in a commercial venture with the potential for abuse is not in itself unethical."[21] The way to deal with the conflict of interest that arises from owning a commercial venture is through disclosure, the council said. This position recalled the AMA's first response to fee-splitting at the turn of the century—the practice was okay as long as the doctor disclosed it.

The AMA added that doctors should not exploit patients by requiring unnecessary services such as tests or X rays, that doctors should not break the law, and that patients should be allowed to use facilities other than the ones owned by the doctors. And the guidelines added, "When a physician's commercial interest conflicts so greatly with the patient's interest as to be incompatible, the physician should make alternative arrangements for the care of the patient."[22]

At the *New England Journal of Medicine*, Relman saw encouraging signs in the new guidelines, but he again goaded the AMA to take a stronger stand. To declare once again that the patient comes first is good, he said, but it is not enough. In a *Journal* editorial, Relman wrote, "The AMA's present position has an even more troublesome aspect. In admitting that business deals create conflicts of interest for physicians, but arguing that we need be concerned only about arrangements that demonstrably lead to bad practice, the AMA's statement ignores the damage done to the public trust in the medical profession by even the *appearance* of conflicts of interest. That, after all, is a major problem with conflicts of interest." Relman held up as exemplary the statement adopted by the association of internal-medicine specialists, The American College of Physicians, which Relman called a firm and unequivocal statement. The ACP position stated: "The physician must avoid any personal commercial conflict of interest that might compromise his loyalty and treatment of the patient."[23]

The AMA responded through Dr. James Todd, who in 1985 had become second-in-command. He fired off an angry letter to Relman. "You are not the first to address this issue," Todd snapped. He said the AMA had repeatedly declared that it is unethical for doctors to put their own interests ahead of the interests of their patients.

"The AMA is working within time-honored ethical guidelines and does not believe that physicians . . . should be prohibited from making investments in, or participating in the ownership of facilities that function within the medical and health-care fields," Todd wrote. "Such a restrictive policy would impose unnecessary and unfair economic discrimination against members of a respected and respectable profession."

Relman tartly replied that a stronger stand against commercialism would "be a beacon to guide" doctors who were confused about the issue and would bolster the public's esteem for the medical profession. He added ominously: "If we [doctors] insist on exercising our right to invest in health-care facilities, the government and the public will inevitably treat us like commercial vendors rather than independent professionals."[24]

Hooked on Drugs[25]

The first big test for the AMA's new policy on conflicts of interest came in 1985 as delegates were putting the final touches on the guidelines. A survey of state pharmacy boards by *American Druggist* that year had discerned a new trend. Increasingly doctors, medical groups, and ambulatory-care centers were selling their patients prescription drugs. That meant a doctor would prescribe a drug for the patient's treatment and then turn around and sell that drug to the patient. Most doctors write a prescription and tell their patients to take it to a drugstore, where a pharmacist fills the prescription and sells it to the patient. Doctor drug-dispensing ends that arrangement.

Physician dispensing was not new. A quarter of doctors dispensed drugs in 1947; by 1967, with the proliferation of drugstores, only a tenth did.[26] Most doctors who dispense drugs said they do it for the convenience of their patients. They cite elderly patients and the parents of small children needing treatment—for them a trip to a drugstore could be an ordeal. Dispensing doctors also say patients benefit because they are more likely to fill the prescription if they buy the drugs at the same time the doctor gives them a prescription.

But opponents point to the other incentive for dispensing drugs: selling prescription drugs boosts doctors' earnings. That proved to be a powerful lure during the 1980s, when doctors worried about their incomes in the face of a greater push for controlling medical costs and increased competition among physicians. The danger inherent in physician dispensing is that a doctor might prescribe too many drugs to a patient, or prescribe drugs he or she had in stock even if another drug might be better.

The renewed interest during the 1980s in selling prescription drugs was inspired by several aggressive drug-repackaging firms. These companies bought drugs in bulk from pharmaceutical manufacturers and then resold them to doctors in convenient packages. For example, Doctors' Pharmacy, a St. Louis repackaging company, offered deals for a two-week supply of medicine for six different practices, such as ambulatory care and pediatrics. The Ambulatory Care package included twenty-two drugs at cost to a doctor of $1,537. Doctors who bought into the deal decided what to charge patients for dispensing the drugs, as well as the markup on the drugs themselves. The firm's brochure simply said, "Doctors' Pharmacy will increase the profitability of your practice."

But other sales pitches were more direct. One promised that "dispensing drugs offers a proven source of new revenue. Typically, about 15% additional net income." Another said, "A practice dispensing about 250 Rx [prescriptions] per week at $3.00 per Rx dispensing fee would earn $39,000 a year. At $4.00 per Rx dispensing fee, 250 Rx per week would yield $52,000 incremental profit." And the most direct said, "Each script [prescription] you write is like a check to the pharmacy; why not write that check to your practice instead?"[27]

Competing Interests

Pharmacists immediately saw the threat to their own well-being. If doctors sell prescription drugs, who needs pharmacists? The National Association of Retail Druggists (NARD), a trade group representing 30,000 independent pharmacists, sprang into action. John M. Rector, general counsel and chief lobbyist for NARD, recalled that his group met with the AMA during the summer of 1986 to discuss doctor dispensing. As a starting point, Rector said, he reminded Sammons of his opposition to physician ownership of drugstores and drug companies back in the 1960s.

"He was impressed we had done our research," Rector said. "It was obvious he was at a different place. I don't know that he had changed his view, but he had a different job. As a matter of fact, he did agree to a joint agreement that doctors should be doctors and pharmacists should be pharmacists."

In December 1986 the AMA's Council on Ethical and Judicial Affairs issued an update on the conflict-of-interest policy, and addressed doctor drug-dispensing. "Although there are circumstances in which physicians may ethically engage in the dispensing of drugs . . . physicians are urged to avoid regular dispensing and retail sale of drugs . . . when the needs of patients can be met adequately at local ethical pharmacies," the report said. In February 1987 the AMA again publicly backed the doctor-pharmacist system in a statement with NARD and the National Association of Chain Drug Stores.[28]

As the drug-dispensing issue heated up, several state legislatures began examining the issue. But the Reagan administration's Federal Trade Commission said doctor dispensing provided competition for drugstores and pharmacists, and deemed moves to limit the practice anticompetitive. In November 1986 the FTC sent a letter to the Georgia State Board of Pharmacy, opposing its proposed rules that would restrict physician dispensing. In the next month the FTC issued a similar letter to the Maryland State Board of Medical Examiners. The FTC's message was clear: state moves to limit doctor dispensing might invite FTC antitrust action.

Representative Ron Wyden (D-Ore.) tried to take on the FTC by attaching an amendment that would prohibit doctors from dispensing for profit to another bill. But a congressional committee rejected the amendment. The AMA took credit for its defeat, saying it had vigorously opposed the amendment.[29] The day after the amendment lost in committee, Wyden introduced a bill to ban doctor dispensing. His bill was brief and to the point. It said physicians could not dispense drugs for a profit except in certain cases. Those exceptions included the giving of shots and vaccines, emergencies when the nearest pharmacy was fifteen miles or more away, and rural or Indian clinics. The bill, of course, had the full backing of Rector and NARD, but not the AMA.

"Sammons always felt like we had picked his pocket," Rector recalled. Although the AMA had entered into an agreement with the druggists and the chain drugstores to in part head off any legislation on the federal level, Sammons felt he and the AMA had been taken advantage of," Rector said. "Here was Wyden coming up with a bill based on our agreement."

At a hearing on the bill, Dr. Nancy W. Dickey, chair of the AMA's Council on Ethical and Judicial Affairs, testified that the AMA discouraged doctor dispensing, but nevertheless opposed the bill. She said there was no proof that a federal law was needed because of widespread problems. An estimated 5 percent of the doctors dispensed. Besides, regulation of doctors properly belonged to the states, she said.[30] The Energy and Commerce Committee supported the bill but it never passed Congress.

Saying Yes to Drugs

The battle was not over. At the AMA's annual meeting in June 1987, some delegates took umbrage at the AMA position on drug dispensing, and introduced two resolutions asserting a physician's right to dispense drugs. About twenty-one physicians rose to speak on the question at the AMA's reference committee hearing, and they all supported drug dispensing. Dr. Whitney G. Sampson, an ophthalmologist, said, "I would say that the AMA needs an attitudinal adjustment, because up until now it has been reluctantly tolerant rather than supportive of dispensing."

The AMA delegates with little other debate had reversed the AMA's position on an ethical issue favored by the AMA's leaders and Judicial Council. Instead of the principled stand discouraging drug dispensing, the delegates took the opposite tack. To replace the offending language adopted just six months earlier, the delegates approved the following language: "The American Medical Association supports the physician's right to dispense drugs and devices when it is in the best interest of the patient and consistent with the AMA's established ethical guidelines."[31] Of course, the language left doctors in charge of deciding just exactly what is the patient's best interest.

Meanwhile, Relman's thinking on controlling conflicts of interest had undergone an evolution. At the beginning of the 1980s, Relman had put his faith in the ability of the ethical codes of the major doctor organizations, and especially of the AMA, to protect the professional status of physicians. Now he believed the AMA and others could not do it alone.[32]

The AMA, in particular, seemed to be having a difficult time sticking to a consistent position. And the medical association faced a confused approach by government, whose different branches often pushed in different directions. So now Relman still urged the AMA and other associations to hold up high ethical principles for all to see. But, Relman decided, physicians needed the protection of the law.

In a tone far different from that arguments heard on the floor at the AMA meeting, he concluded: "Trust in one's physician is an essential but fragile ingredient of good medical care. It may not withstand the conversion of physicians into vendors of drugs for profit."[33]

PROFITABLE SELF-DEALING

The rapid development of medical technology in the 1980s not only saved lives, but it also enriched those who owned it. An array of high-tech devices appeared, from easier-to-use equipment in doctors' clinical labs to more exotic apparatuses, such as magnetic-resonance imaging (MRI) scanners. And, like the pharmaceuticals and drugstores of the 1950s, they proved to be tempting investments for doctors with money to spare and a knowledge of the use of the high-tech machines.

In March 1989 Representative Fortney "Pete" Stark, a liberal Democrat from Oakland and chairman of the health subcommittee of the Ways and Means Committee, held a hearing on legislation aimed at banning Medicare payments to doctors from referring patients to facilities they owned. He quoted a *Wall Street Journal* article that had just appeared.

The article cited a Michigan Blue Cross and Blue Shield survey of forty diagnostic laboratories—twenty owned by doctors who referred patients to them and twenty owned by nonphysicians. At the doctor-owned labs, the average payment was $45 and the average number of tests per patient was 6.23. At the other labs, the average cost was $25 and average number of tests per patient 3.76. The conclusion was that physician ownership leads to more testing.

The article also described how in New Jersey the twenty-six doctors who invested in an MRI imaging center appeared to have struck it rich. Each partnership share cost $25,000 in 1986. By June 1988 a financial report showed a six-month return of nearly $10,000. The venture's prospectus projected that the annual return by 1995 would be about $35,000 per share and that ten years after initial investment total profits would be nearly $250,000.

And it mentioned how one consultant based in Southern California boasted that the seventy MRI centers he had helped set up with physician investors averaged 400 scans a month and more than $1 million in pretax profits. The national average for such centers, he said, was about 260 scans a month and pretax profits of $400,000. The key to success was involving the physicians who refer patients. As he put it, "Greed is a powerful motivator."[34]

In his opening remarks, Stark said, "All partnerships, no matter how well-intentioned, involve a serious conflict of interest that threatens the doctor-patient relationship and poses a risk of overutilization, substandard care, and unfair competition. Patients are anxious about their health and bewildered by the complexities of modern health care. They need to trust someone. . . . It's difficult for patients to second-guess their physicians. And, physicians, through self-dealing arrangements, should not put their patients in the position where they are forced to question their doctor's advice and loyalty."

Laws already existed to handle the most egregious kinds of kickbacks. Congress had first passed a Medicare antifraud law in 1972, which prohibited rebates and kickbacks for patients or business paid for by Medicare or Medicaid. In 1977 Congress strengthened the law by outlawing any "remuneration," direct or indirect, for referrals of patients or business under Medicare or Medicaid. The law also stiffened penalties, raising them from misdemeanors to felonies, upping the maximum jail terms from one to five years, and hiking top fines from $10,000 to $25,000. In 1980 Congress required prosecutors to prove the accused's intent, that is, he "knowingly and willingly" broke the law. And in 1987, Congress added a "professional death sentence" by allowing the Inspector General of the Department of Health and Human Services to bar guilty doctors and other providers from Medicare.

To help doctors, though, this law required the Inspector General to describe in federal regulations what financial arrangements—called "safe harbors"—would not be prosecuted. But these guidelines did not appear for comment until January 1989 and were not finally implemented until 1991. Meanwhile, some lawyers for doctors complained the safe-harbor regulations did little to clear up the murky waters. Stark complained many of the financial arrangements in self-referral schemes had found a loophole in the federal antikickback laws. "What is needed is what lawyers call a 'bright line' rule to give providers and physicians unequivocal guidance as to the types of arrangements that are prohibited," Stark said. "If the law is clear and the penalties are substantial, we can rely on self-enforcement. Few physicians will knowingly break the law."[35]

AMA's Contradictory Stand

The AMA had staked out its position. It was not necessarily unethical to own and refer patients to a facility, the AMA said. But to avoid crossing the line into unethical practice, the doctor had to follow five guidelines. Among them was a requirement not to break any state laws regarding self-referrals. The AMA's reliance on state law confused some representatives at Stark's hearing on the issue.

Relman testified first at the hearing. His appearance marked the final step in his ultimate disillusionment about the power of organized medicine to protect itself and its values against commercialism. Relman came out for Stark's law, and he explained why to a committee: "The basic purpose of the bill is sound. It meets the basic principles of medical ethics and it is clearly in the public interest."

Representative Jim Moody (D-Wis.) seemed puzzled about the AMA's position. On the one hand, he said, the AMA wanted no more federal laws defining ethical behavior—that should be left up to organized medicine. On the other hand, the AMA said if self-referrals were legal, they must be ethical. That, to Moody, seemed contradictory.

Moody asked Relman if he believed that the internal ethical procedures of organized medicine would eventually rule self-referrals out-of-bounds of ethical behavior. Relman replied, "I would like to think so, because I think the logic is inexorable." Moody pressed, "But you do not have the confidence that the profession itself will arrive there in a timely fashion?" Relman answered, "Correct."[36]

Dr. James S. Todd, the senior executive vice president of the AMA, downplayed the problem in his testimony. He said an AMA survey found that fewer than 10 percent of doctors had an ownership interest in health-care facilities beyond their own practices, and only about 7 percent of the doctors in this country referred patients to facilities in which they had an ownership interest. Todd also cited cases where physician investment in the facilities was good for patients, and he derided the evidence against doctor-owned facilities as anecdotal. "Legislation by anecdote is dangerous," he said.

Noting that both the Inspector General's office and the Government Accounting Office had studies due to be completed in two months, Todd argued that Congress should wait to see them before enacting a law. "It may well be that legislation in this area will be required, but at a time when the evidence is anecdotal," Todd said, "we believe any further legislation addressing a perceived problem is premature and probably overreaching."

He concluded that depending on the facts, "it could well be that a rifle shot" could hit the inappropriate practices, rather than the "shotgun approach" of Stark's proposed law.[37]

Representative Sander M. Levin (D-Mich.) asked Todd if the studies came back with results showing abuse in terms of substantial increase in referrals by physicians to facilities owned by them, would the AMA back a law containing a more generic approach than the "rifle shots" he suggested.

Todd replied, "If there are abuses and exploitation identified that cannot be handled by a rifleshot approach, of course we will support a more generic legislation because the profession does not want to allow these activities to continue if they truly are not in the best interests of patients."[38]

The Rifle Shot

On April 28, 1989, Inspector General Richard P. Kusserow released his study. Based on surveys of 4,000 Medicare providers and 1,100 labs, the study found a more widespread pattern than the AMA had of physician ownership of facilities, particularly independent labs, those not in doctors' offices. Kusserow's survey found that 12 percent of doctors who billed Medicare had ownership or investment interests in the facilities to which they referred their patients. And the study found that 8 percent of physicians billing Medicare had compensation arrangements with entities to which they referred. The report also found that referring physicians owned in whole or in part about a quarter of independent clinical and physiological laboratories. Finally, the study found that patients of referring physicians who had an interest or ownership of labs received 45 percent more lab services than Medicare patients in general. And the increased use of the labs cost Medicare $28 million in 1987.[39]

Responding to the study, Stark said, "Medicare patients, and the taxpayer, are paying tens of millions of dollars for needless tests caused by doctors referring patients to centers from which the doctor makes a profit because of the referral." Todd, however, presented a different interpretation, saying, "The Inspector General has shown nothing, other than by inference, to indicate inappropriate utilization." He cited the report finding that patients of self-referring doctors received 45 percent more lab services than the average Medicare patient. "That can be interpreted in two ways," he said. "The media interpret it as being bad. You could also interpret it as indicating there are a lot of Medicare beneficiaries out there who are not getting enough testing."[40]

Next, in June 1989, the GAO released preliminary results of its in-depth study of facilities in Maryland and Pennsylvania. In both states, physician ownership of labs and imaging centers was relatively recent: about four-fifths of the facilities in Maryland and two-thirds in Pennsylvania had begun in the past four years. As for the actual experience, the GAO found that in Maryland, physician-owners of laboratories tended to order about twice as many tests as doctors who did not own labs, as well as the most costly services. For imaging services, physician-owners ordered slightly fewer tests, but they tended to be much more costly, the GAO study found.[41]

But the AMA refused to believe that self-referral was a problem. At a hearing in June 1989 held by Representative Henry A. Waxman (D-Calif.) on Stark's self-referral bill, Todd repeated many of the statements he had made three months earlier to Stark's hearing. He listened as the studies of the Inspector General and the GAO were discussed. Then he said, "Studies as you have just heard have shown us the demography of the situation but without convincing conclusions. Anecdotes support multiple conclusions."[42]

The AMA was not alone in its stance. Joining it were the American Academy of Family Physicians, the American Academy of Neurology, and the American College of Rheumatology. But it found itself opposed by other medical groups, most notably the American College of Surgeons and the Institute of Medicine. The report of the latter on the effects of for-profit medicine on the quality of health care was widely quoted. "It should be regarded as unethical and unacceptable for physicians to have ownership interests in health-care facilities to which they make referrals or receive payments for making referrals," the institute said.

In the end, the AMA won a partial victory when a legislative compromise resulted in a watered-down version of Stark's bill. The House had passed a version of Stark's bill, but the Senate had held no hearings, nor did it pass any version of the legislation. To complicate matters, the bill was handled in the budget-reconciliation process, which meant that its fate was decided by the same conferees and at the same time as the massive revamp of physician payment under Medicare was hashed out in on-again, off-again style.

In December 1989 President George Bush signed the bill into law. As weak as the legislation was, it was the first federal law that deemed self-referrals a version of fee-splitting or kickbacks. Inspector General Kusserow described self-referrals as "business practices where the ultimate objective may be the same [as a kickback] but where the payments are masked as 'dividends,' 'rent,' or 'consulting fees.'" The law also laid the groundwork for a broader ban on self-referrals by inspiring a series of studies to figure out how many doctors had bought into the scheme.

CONFLICTING REPORTS ON SELF-REFERRALS

After passage of the Stark bill, the debate over how many doctors engaged in the practice of self-referral continued. In June 1991 the AMA released a study that found the practice was still not widespread, and was in fact declining. In a survey of about 4,000 doctors, the AMA's Center for Health Policy Research said it found only 8.2 percent of doctors had ownership interests in health-care facilities in 1990. That was down from the 8.3 percent in 1989 and 9.3 percent in 1988, it said. The AMA's top researcher tried to explain the drop by suggesting the investments were "perhaps not as profitable as [they] used to be." But longtime AMA lawyer B. J. Anderson suggested another reason to the *American Medical News:* "With all the congressional hearings and publicity, physicians aren't very trusting of any advice on whether it will be permissible or profitable to have an ownership interest."

But in August, a highly publicized study released by the Florida Health Care Cost Containment Board struck a blow against self-referrals. At the direction of the Florida legislature, the board hired Jean M. Mitchell and Elton Scott of Florida State University to survey some 3,000 freestanding medical facilities in the state. About 82 percent replied, a high rate resulting from the legislative mandate. From this survey Mitchell and Scott estimated that 7,600 doctors, or about 40 percent of the physicians involved in direct patient care, owned facilities to which they referred patients. Forty percent. That number dwarfed all previous studies, more than tripling the level found by the HHS Inspector General and quadrupling the AMA's findings.

Physician involvement in the freestanding facilities was significant. Doctors owned more than half of the existing facilities in the state in four of the ten types of facilities. Based on the survey, Mitchell and Scott concluded that abuses were most common in three types of doctor-owned arrangements: diagnostic imaging centers, clinical laboratories, and physical therapy–rehabilitation centers. They found that doctor-owned clinical labs performed almost twice as many tests as did independently owned labs. The average charge at the doctor-owned lab was $43, compared with $20 for other labs. Because doctors owned nearly all the MRI centers in Florida, the researchers compared the rates of use for the MRI centers in Miami with those in Baltimore, where two teaching hospitals are located. They found that MRI scanners were used 65 percent more often in Miami than in Baltimore.

The researchers rebutted the AMA's main argument for physician investment in medical facilities. The AMA said patients benefited from physician investments because they brought technology to areas that needed it. But they found physician-owned facilities "do not increase access to rural or underserved indigent patients." In fact, for the ventures with highest physician ownership—labs, imaging centers, and physical-therapy facilities—Mitchell and Scott concluded that they provided less access for elderly patients, used more services, billed at higher rates, and were more profitable than other independent facilities.[43]

The New Professionalism

AMA leaders took note of the fallout from the controversy over self-referrals. At its June 1991 annual meeting, the AMA's official line switched to emphasize "professionalism and the new AMA." In his inaugural speech the new president, Dr. John J. Ring, summed up the image the AMA sought to project: "It is time we prove to America, in deed as well as word, that we are a doctors' organization, working for the good of our patients, rather than a pressure group aiming for political power as a way to build organizational predominance, to create personal prestige or to line our own pockets!"[44]

The AMA even gave Dr. Relman a platform to express his views. In a *JAMA* profile, Relman said he understood the problems the AMA faces as a large umbrella organization. The AMA has the obligation to represent its members, he said, which means it must reflect the current attitudes of a variety of doctors. That means it will take the most conservative, most acceptable route. But that means the AMA must lag behind on some very important issues, such as conflicts of interest. Unfortunately, he said, that does not help the image of the AMA or doctors. "When the AMA is seen as serving the public interest, not just saying it serves the public interest," Relman said, "then I think that its image will improve."[45]

Meanwhile, the Council on Ethical and Judicial Affairs appointed a task force to reexamine the question of self-referrals. The AMA chose Dr. Russel H. Patterson, a Manhattan surgeon and the former chairman of the council when it developed the AMA's stance on self-referrals; Newton Minow, the AMA's lawyer in its battle against the FTC, who was better known for his attack on the "wasteland" of television during his chairmanship of the Federal Communications Commission in the early 1960s; and Robert Veatch, director of the Kennedy School of Ethics at Georgetown University.

In an interview later, Veatch said, "I invited them to use this as an opportunity to decide what their future image would be. You could choose either what I called the professional role, which holds forth the ideal that physicians do what's best for the patient and have no self-interest, or you could choose the entrepreneurial role, and be like businesspeople." It was the classic conflict between the two symbols of medicine: the single snake-on-the-staff of Asklepios the healer vs. the two snakes of Mercury, god of businessmen and profiteers.

Veatch said he was not committed to one role or the other. "I was prepared for them to go either route. I think once the choice was presented that starkly to them, they were in a spot where they couldn't say, 'We want to be entrepreneurial businessmen.' They clearly wanted to hold on to the idea of being a profession."

But the task force did not recommend a change in AMA policy to the council, according to Patterson. He had helped mold the AMA's previous stand, and the task force "took a much more permissive position as a group, at least as far as the ethics were concerned." He said he felt the level of abuse by self-referring physicians was "hard to pinpoint," and expressed concern that a shift in policy could result in fewer facilities. That would harm patients by restricting access.

The council, however, took a less permissive approach. "I think the position the council finally took was that even the appearance, or potential [of conflict of interest], was too much, and that therefore physician ownerships should be restricted," Patterson said. "The feeling on the council was that Caesar's wife had to be above suspicion." Patterson said that view was pushed by the "young physicians" in AMA membership and on the council. Both Patterson and Veatch raised questions about the council banning self-referrals to outside facilities while permitting them to continue inside the doctor's office. Patterson said, "I think the logic that has been used by Arnold Relman, the former editor of the *New England Journal,* is that the physician is directly involved in performing or supervising the performance" of the in-office test, diagnosis, or other service.

In December 1991 the council issued its report. "The Council believes that it is necessary to strengthen its opinion of self-referral," the report concluded. It cited two reasons. First, physician investments and self-referrals "have on balance been positive for patients and the nation's health-care system," the report said. "But anecdotes of excessive profit and utilization have been widespread, and the formal studies which have been done strongly suggest, although they do not prove, inherent problems with the practice." And second, the report cited a change in national priorities, placing cost control as the "dominant concern." Besides, the report noted, the United States already has "unparalleled" facilities and technology available.

"Physicians are not simply business people with high standards," the council concluded. "Physicians are engaged in the special calling of healing, and, in that calling, they are the fiduciaries of their patients. They have different and higher duties than even the most ethical business person." It added, "There are some activities involving their patients that physicians should avoid whether or not there is evidence of abuse."

The council noted for the first time that in self-referral arrangements "a potential conflict of interest exists." But it did not ban physician investment in health-care facilities; the council continued to support it. What the council sought to squelch was the practice of self-referrals: "In general, physicians should not refer patients to a health-care facility . . . when they have an investment interest in the facility."

In some cases, the council concluded, self-referrals were okay, but only if there is a need in the community and no other way to finance the facility. Even then, the doctor-investors had to meet ten standards before the self-referral would pass muster under the AMA's new ethical guidelines.[46]

The new guidelines left some physicians in the lurch. The council recognized the difficult spot entrepreneurial doctors were in, but could offer little comfort. Many physicians had invested in facilities under the AMA's looser guidelines adopted in 1986. The council suggested they reevaluate their investment and either divest or restructure the deal to meet the new guidelines. And if that wasn't possible, the council suggested physician-investors identify an alternative for their patients.

The delegates at the December meeting adopted the report, although some did so with great misgivings. The AMA stressed unity, but it was beset by undercurrents of discontent. Dr. Oscar W. Clarke, the council's chairman, said, "There is an ethical line we have to draw in the commercial world. We want to get that done before the public confidence is eroded, setting policy before someone else comes in and does it for us." Dr. John L. Clowe, the AMA's president-elect, added, "If Representative Stark and the Congress see that we have imposed these standards and the profession is complying with them, they will see that the necessity for additional legislation is not there."[47]

The Flip-Flop

In April 1992 the AMA tried to use its new image and new ethics to cut a deal with the Federal Trade Commission. Ever since the AMA lost its battle with the regulatory agency a decade earlier, its leaders had attempted to figure out a way to loosen the FTC's grip over physician activities. Part of the strategy was to show the government and the public that the AMA was a responsible organization that could regulate itself and be trusted not to put its own interest ahead of patients and the public.

The AMA sent an eleven-page letter to Janet Steiger, the FTC chairman, seeking the commission's support on a variety of "self-regulatory initiatives." Exhibit 1 in its appeal to the FTC was its difficult and unpopular new stand on self-referrals. "Professionalism, in all of its aspects, is a priority of the profession today," the appeal said. The AMA cited the December report by its Council on Ethical and Judicial Affairs, noting, "The treatment of the self-referral question has important symbolic significance for the public and policymakers with regard to which of two alternative conceptualizations of the physician's role—that of professional or that of entrepreneur—the medical profession will move toward the era of health-care reform."

But this new image was short-lived. A crack in the facade of physician unity appeared shortly before the AMA's annual June 1992 meeting. The Medical Society of New Jersey had adopted a resolution in May that was directly in conflict with the new AMA stand. Seeking to return the standard to the one AMA adopted in 1986, the New Jersey society's resolution said "a physician's referral to an off-site medical facility in which he has a financial interest is an ethical referral, as long as the patient is fully informed of the ownership interest and alternate facilities (if available) are named."

Dr. William E. Ryan, president of the New Jersey society and part owner of a clinical lab, said the stand was not a renunciation of AMA policy, but a reaction to the state of New Jersey's 1990 law barring self-referrals. The law, however, grandfathered in existing ventures. Ryan also said he did not see a conflict with the AMA ethical position, but an AMA physician-lawyer, Dr. David Orentlicher, disagreed. "If we are going to have an independent council deliberating and setting policy, we can't be putting ethics to a vote, and we can't be setting different guidelines for different states."[48]

But at the June meeting that is exactly what the AMA House of Delegates did: they put the new stricter policy on self-referrals to a vote. The New Jersey delegation introduced a proposal that allowed "medically necessary" self-referrals as long as the ownership interest was disclosed. The Florida delegation joined the New Jersey doctors in pushing for the policy reversal. The AMA's top leaders—Chief Executive Todd, President Ring, *JAMA* editor Dr. George Lundberg—lined up on the other side, seeking to preserve the ethical high ground. But over the objections of the Board of Trustees and the Council on Ethical and Judicial Affairs, the delegates overwhelmingly rejected the stricter stand and embraced the New Jersey proposal.

Dr. Ulrich F. Danckers, a member of the Illinois delegation, summed up the conflict: "We have embarked on a major effort to convince the Federal Trade Commission that the profession is able to control errant behavior of physicians. Our ethical statement is a major part of that effort, and we can't allow this resolution to blunt its well-balanced impact."[49]

But it had. Stark called the AMA delegates' action "an Oath of Hypocrisy," and said it would "disembowel their previous, admirable stand against the corrupting influence" of self-referral. One of the chief concerns voiced by many within the AMA hierarchy as well as among members was that the government would feel it must step in because organized medicine had failed to take a stand. The issue had gone beyond one of simple economics. Study after study showed that self-referral increased the cost of health care. Several states moved to ban self-referrals, the some state medical societies fought the laws. And soon the AMA would be tested by more attempts at federal legislation.

Reversing the Reversal

As the AMA Board and Judicial Council prepared to reverse the reversal at the December 1992 meeting, Relman urged them to retake the high ground. Although Relman supported the AMA's efforts to get concessions from the FTC and to boost its own self-regulatory structure, he warned against battling legislation that sought to ban self-referrals. As he put it, such efforts "merely strengthen the public's impression that physicians are more interested in pursuing their own economic interests than in preserving their good name or helping to keep costs down." Such efforts usually failed, he wrote, "leaving a residue of public cynicism and ill will toward organized medicine."[50]

The debate was heated and divisive. The New Jersey delegation was particularly adamant. But the AMA's leadership and trustees lobbied delegates aggressively. Ring, who had made the return to professionalism the hallmark of his tenure as AMA president, pleaded with delegates to take the high road. AMA president-elect Dr. Joseph T. Painter tried another tack. The profession cannot afford to be seen favoring profit over professionalism at a time when the AMA is seeking breaks from the FTC on self-regulation and the right for physicians to collectively negotiate with third-party payers, he said. And, as health-care reform became a national issue, the AMA had to avoid even the appearance of conflict of interest so that it would be taken seriously in the national debate.

The leadership prevailed. The delegates readopted the board's position on self-referrals. The final AMA position was not as pure as Relman had proposed, but it was closer than it had been at any time during the 1980s. Physicians could still own off-site medical facilities, but save for a few exceptions, they could not refer their patients to them, the AMA's ethical policy said. The policy also gave those who had invested under the AMA's old policy until 1995 to comply with the new guidelines. Relman complimented the efforts of Todd and AMA general counsel Kirk B. Johnson for taking the lead on the issue, but he still believed there were too many exceptions.

"There is still a rear-guard action that's being waged against this," he said, referring to doctors investing in such ventures as home-infusion treatments. "They write to me and they tell me that they're different, that they don't violate the principle of no self-referral because they really take responsibility for those patients. And by that reasoning of course a surgeon should be allowed to invest in ambulatory surgery centers because they take care of their patients in those centers. I don't buy that for a moment."

THE END OF SELF-REFERRALS

Representative Stark followed through on his promise and introduced a bill in January 1993 to ban all self-referrals, whether the tab was being picked up by the federal government or privately. The facilities targeted by the bill included clinical laboratories, physical-therapy services, occupational-therapy services, radiology services, durable medical equipment, outpatient prescription drugs, ambulances, home infusion therapy, and inpatient and outpatient hospital services. The new Clinton administration made clear that a ban on physician self-referrals was part of its overall plans for health-care reform. In its proposed budget for the Department of Health and Human Services, the Administration said by excluding self-referrals it would save $250 million over the next four years.[51]

The AMA's response was markedly different than in the past. After the bill was introduced, Dr. Nancy Dickey, an AMA trustee, did not outright reject the legislation. Instead, she said, "We look forward to talking with Representative Stark about the importance of exceptions which address unmet patient needs such as a community unserved or underserved were it not for the commitment of their physician citizens."[52]

At an April 1993 hearing held by Stark on his new bill, Dickey delivered the AMA's assessment: "The AMA believes that H.R. 345, as drafted, would establish an overly broad prohibition. The AMA would find the bill more acceptable if modified to meet certain conditions."[53] The AMA listed the conditions , and for all indications, Stark and his subcommittee seemed amenable to negotiating on the points raised by Dickey.

The "new" AMA attempts to avoid saying no. Instead, it says there is a better way. In an era of health-care reform, perhaps the AMA knew it would lose this one anyway. Yet it took the organization more than a dozen years to put the self-interest of its members aside and look the bigger picture. And then the AMA's action was not for purely ethical reasons, but for PR and as part of a strategy to play a more important role in the national health-care debate. But by the time the AMA leaders even recognized this need, damage had been done. Was it too late?

"I don't know that it is too late," said Relman. "I think that serious damage was done, which has not yet been undone. I think to the extent that the profession as a whole . . . is viewed with suspicion and with some hostility . . . I think [the AMA] position on self-referral was damaging. . . . I think it has hurt the medical profession as a whole. It has hurt the credibility of the AMA, and the respect with which the medical profession has been generally regarded."

As long as doctors have the potential to put themselves first and exploit their patients financially, from self-referrals or other conflicts of interests, patient-doctor relations will suffer. But Relman is optimistic: "I think that if the AMA continues to adopt publicly responsible and forward-looking policies, if it makes clear to the public and to government that it wants to help devise a health-care system that meets the public's needs, I think the damage can be undone."[54]

Medical Monopoly
Waging War on Alternative Medicine

Since its founding in the mid–nineteenth century, the American Medical Association, with its M.D.-knows-best doctrine, has attempted to root out quacks and snake-oil salesmen. Charlatans who prey upon the public ought to be eliminated. However, the AMA also had other, more selfish and cynical motivations in attacking all varieties of alternative healers, who after all competed to some extent with its members. These included protecting the financial interests of orthodox practitioners and supplying the divided factions within mainstream medicine with a common enemy against whom they could rally.

By helping medical doctors ascend the throne of medicine, politically and economically, the AMA has contributed to the elimination or suppression of competing healers. Because of these interventions, insurance covers unorthodox care only on a limited basis, if at all, and the research establishment has largely ignored what unconventional medicine might have to offer. Still, some alternative medical approaches have beaten the odds to survive in the shadow of a menacing AMA, and many Americans opt for alternative medicine because they find mainstream, AMA-style medicine unsatisfactory.[1]

The AMA has conducted a nearly 150-year war against alternative medicine. In its earliest years, the AMA, representing one of a number of competing medical approaches, led the so-called regular doctors to market dominance by the turn of this century. Despite the virtual monopoly of regular medicine, the AMA continued to battle the alternative practitioners. Having been badly bloodied in its defeat on Medicare in the 1960s, the AMA launched an all-out war on chiropractic, the most successful of contemporary alternatives.

DEFENDER OF THE TRUE FAITH

Most Americans see doctors who practice what technically is known as allopathic medicine. Allopathy, marked by the use of medicine and surgery and by an allegiance to the scientific method, holds itself up in near-religious terms as the one true faith, dismissing as cults groups that subscribe to other approaches. But allopathy actually is the majority party; there are now and have always been multiple schools of medical thought. Allopathy is simply the AMA brand of medicine, which experienced a serendipitous rise in an era in which scientific knowledge began to soar.

Before the AMA arrived on the scene in the late 1840s, allopathy was far from being assured dominance. There had been a teeming marketplace of medical theories: one school advocated a highly democratized system in which each person was his or her own physician; another promoted the use of plants as remedies; another used steam therapy and Native American medicines; and yet another, the "eclectics," borrowed from other sects whatever techniques they considered beneficial.

Dr. Samuel Hahnemann in the early nineteenth century founded the once very popular type of medicine known as homeopathy. Hahnemann's theory was based on the concept of like cures like. He and his colleagues developed an extensive catalog of remedies, which from self-testing they determined elicited symptoms similar to the diseases. Homeopaths (the term comes from the Greek meaning "like disease") gave their patients highly diluted doses of their remedies in hopes of effecting cures.

Hahnemann gave the competing school, allopathy, its name. In contrast with homeopaths, Hahnemann said allopaths (Greek for "other treatment," a put-down that stuck) gave their patients harsh purgatives and bled them to counter the effects of disease and injury. As a reform movement, homeopathy was in demand because its remedies did not have the dangerous side effects associated with allopathy, whose "heroic" treatments often were deadly.

Homeopaths underwent training equal to or even superior to that of allopaths. Not surprisingly, the popularity of homeopathy and other so-called irregular medical groups drew fire from allopaths, whose income and status were threatened. In forming the AMA, the allopaths nominally wanted to improve medical education and to fight quackery, but the counterculture of that era viewed these as wink terms for a campaign to wipe out irregular physicians, particularly homeopaths. At its founding in 1847, the AMA established ethical prohibitions against consulting with homeopaths and other irregular physicians. This policy led to a dispute *within* allopathy. The Medical Society of the State of New York was booted out of the AMA in 1882 because the group had dropped the ban against consulting with homeopaths. The next year, doctors attending the AMA meeting were forced to sign a pledge to adhere to the AMA's original ethical code barring such professional exchanges.

During its first half century, the AMA had failed in its anti-quackery efforts because it was unable to enforce its pronouncements against irregulars. Meanwhile, many allopaths, recognizing the success of the competition, dropped purgatives and bloodletting and adopted homeopathic remedies.

Ironically, the death knell for the strongest irregular groups sounded as allopaths joined forces with homeopaths and eclectics in the late 1800s to advocate licensing of doctors. In *The Social Transformation of American Medicine,* sociologist Paul Starr said regular physicians recognized that only by collaborating with homeopaths and eclectics could they "win licensing laws that would protect all of them against competition from untrained practitioners." His argument is that it is a myth that the dominant allopaths suppressed homeopaths and eclectics. Rather, he said, once homeopaths and eclectics gained licensing recognition and seemed more like allopaths, their public acceptance plummeted. By gaining mainstream recognition and becoming more like allopaths, the homeopaths and eclectics committed professional suicide.

Having divided and conquered the irregulars, the AMA was on its way to being recognized as organized medicine. By the turn of the century, the AMA and allopathic medicine had become king of the hill as the leading medical sects declined and were absorbed, and mainstream medicine was making and exploiting scientific discoveries.

New Enemies: Osteopaths and Chiropractors

By the time the AMA had succeeded with passage of state laws to license physicians, at the end of the nineteenth century, two other groups began to emerge to fill the void for those seeking alternatives. The two approaches, osteopathic medicine and chiropractic, both used spinal manipulation to treat disease. The AMA viewed both as quacks and did what it could to block them.[2]

Dr. Andrew Still, a frontier doctor, was dissatisfied with both allopathy and its irregular competitors. He set out to develop his own type of medicine. In 1874, based on a divine revelation and study of bones dug up from Indian burial grounds, Still left mainstream medicine behind and began advocating a nondrug, hands-on approach involving spinal manipulation, which he dubbed osteopathy. He contended that misplaced spinal bones interfered with nerves controlling the blood supply to the organs. Because Still wanted his followers to be general practitioners, osteopaths soon enlarged their skills by learning minor surgery and obstetrics. Eventually they became more like M.D.s, expanding their scope of practice to include major surgery and use of drugs. The osteopaths ultimately rejected some of their founder's theories and improved their educational requirements.

Despite its efforts to upgrade itself, osteopathy remained a pariah in allopathic eyes. In the 1920s the AMA began to describe osteopaths as cultists with whom AMA members should not associate professionally. The AMA, which viewed osteopathic education as second rate, barred doctors of osteopathy (D.O.s) from AMA membership and tried to block osteopaths from obtaining hospital privileges and participating in government-funded medical programs. The AMA was refining its bag of tricks to attack alternative healers. As much as the American Medical Association may have despised osteopathy, homeopathy, and other unconventional practices, it saved its strongest venom for chiropractic.

An Unscientific Cult[3]

The AMA considered all chiropractors quacks. In the AMA view, chiropractors were followers of an "unscientific cult" because they accepted heretical theories espoused by chiropractic founder D. D. Palmer. The one-time grocer—his enemies liked to dismiss him as a fishmonger—and "magnetic healer" held that disease had "one cause and one cure." The cause of disease, so chiropractic theory went, was subluxations, misalignments of the spinal vertebrae that interfered with the normal flow of nerve energy. Chiropractic's "cure" consisted of the forceful thrusts of spinal manipulation, known as "adjustments," to restore vertebrae to their normal position. In his 1925 book on quackery, *The Medical Follies*, Dr. Morris Fishbein, longtime editor of the *Journal of the AMA* and the person most identified with AMA views from the 1920s through the 1940s, described chiropractic as a "malignant tumor." Fishbein belittled chiropractic theory as a reversion to the original ideas of osteopathy, "so simple that even farm-hands can grasp it."[4]

Chiropractic also had a spiritual or metaphysical foundation, which made science-oriented physicians cringe. Once the spinal bones were in place, "an intelligent life-force," referred to as the "Innate" by Palmer, was unleashed and brought about healing. "Innate is part of the Creator. Innate spirit is part of Universal Intelligence," said Palmer. Chiropractors said they restored the normal harmony of misaligned bones to allow spiritual energy to heal the body.

However, in allopathic medicine's view, chiropractors, with their peculiar language and theories, might as well have been from another planet. Medical doctors, trained to consider themselves as scientists, spurned chiropractic theory as gibberish. The mainstream elite also looked down its nose at chiropractors because they underwent an inferior education, with many students in the early days entering chiropractic school with a high-school diploma. There also was a class difference because while many M.D.s came from the middle or upper classes, many doctors of chiropractic (D.C.s) came from blue-collar or rural backgrounds.

Medical doctors said chiropractic at best was a harmless placebo and at worst kept patients from potentially lifesaving therapy. They also were disgusted with chiropractors' penchant for advertising and promotion. While many M.D.s did not advertise at all and others restricted themselves to business-card ads listing name, address, and specialty, some chiropractors made flamboyant and even outrageous claims for cures for cancer and sponsored silly promotions, such as straight-spine contests.

With the outlook of the gentrified M.D. elite, Fishbein observed: "It has been said that osteopathy is essentially a method of entering the practice of medicine by the back door. Chiropractic, by contrast, is an attempt to arrive through the cellar. The man who applies at the back door at least makes himself presentable. The one who comes through the cellar is besmirched with dust and grime; he carries a crowbar and he may wear a mask."[5]

For most of its history, chiropractic represented only a minor annoyance to allopathy because there were relatively few D.C.s in the country, and they were largely confined to small towns in the Midwest and on the West Coast. But after World War II, veterans flooded chiropractic colleges, and chiropractic began to assume a higher profile.

CRACKING THE BACK OF CHIROPRACTIC

Chiropractors emerged in hordes in the 1950s and 1960s in Iowa, the group's birthplace. A worried Iowa Medical Society set out in 1962 to hobble chiropractic; it formed the Committee on Chiropractic to fight chiropractors' efforts to advance themselves in the state legislature. Robert B. Throckmorton, the medical society's general counsel, guided the anti-chiropractic campaign. The lawyer was especially concerned that the "mixers," a chiropractic faction, might be trespassing on medicine's territory by expanding its scope of practice. Mixers used spinal manipulation in combination with a variety of therapies, such as application of heat and nutritional treatments. In contrast, traditional "straight" chiropractors, who detested the mixers, used only spinal manipulation. The mixers were rapidly becoming the majority among D.C.s.[6]

Throckmorton was not troubled by the straights, whose practices were limited, but he feared the mixers would attempt to become *chiropractic physicians and surgeons*. Such a scenario had unfolded before with osteopathy, as one-time spinal manipulators metamorphosed into the equals of medical doctors.

Based on his efforts in Iowa, Throckmorton urged that the crusade against chiropractic go national. Speaking in Minneapolis in November 1962 to the North Central Medical Conference, a coalition of medical societies in the upper Midwest, Throckmorton issued organized medicine a call to arms against the "menace of chiropractic." He said medical societies had to address "the chiropractic problem" through a comprehensive program at the county, state, and national level. He said medical doctors had not taken chiropractic seriously: "To physicians, chiropractic is utterly ridiculous. Consequently, physicians have either ignored or ridiculed chiropractic and let it go at that. . . . The public is entitled to have facts, figures, and scientific information about this cult and its practices and limitations. The public does and should look to the medical profession for unbiased and authoritative information on this subject. Medicine has not fully met this responsibility."[7]

Throckmorton called for a "positive program of 'containment.'"[8] He ticked off a list of areas medicine should concentrate on to stop chiropractic: Oppose chiropractic efforts to be covered by health insurance and workmen's compensation. Oppose chiropractic efforts to get hospital privileges. Contain chiropractic schools. Encourage ethical complaints against chiropractors. Resist chiropractic efforts to enhance its position through legislation. Encourage disunity between the straights and mixers.

Throckmorton wanted to cut chiropractic off at each point at which it might better itself. He urged the AMA as well as local medical groups to form anti-chiropractic committees. He said: "Action taken by the medical profession should be firm, persistent and in good taste [and] behind the scenes whenever possible."9

Quackery? Or Rallying Point?

While chiropractic probably posed a real threat to medical doctors' pocketbooks in Iowa, the same could not be said in most of the United States. The ratio of medical doctors to chiropractors was 4 to 1 in Iowa, compared to 10 to 1 nationally. And there was no documentation that chiropractic presented a genuine public-health menace.

Still, Throckmorton's impassioned plea struck a chord in the AMA leadership, which viewed a campaign against chiropractic as a flag under which to rally the troops in troubled times when momentum was building for Medicare. Throckmorton's vision met AMA expediencies. Within a few months of his Minneapolis speech, he was hired as the AMA's general counsel. He was a man with a mission. The American Medical Association had always held itself up as a fierce foe of quackery and a proponent of high ethical standards. But by the 1960s, AMA leaders considered the departments that dealt with these issues to be comatose. Dr. F. J. L. Blasingame, the AMA's chief executive, described the two sections, the AMA's quackbusting Department of Investigation and the Department of Ethics, as "sleeping giants." Blasingame told Throckmorton his job was to "help these departments come alive."10

THE AMA CREATES A COMMITTEE ON QUACKERY

Like most institutions in the anti-establishment 1960s, the AMA found itself under attack. Its meetings were disrupted by angry medical students and were picketed by blacks, Latinos, the poor, and others with gripes against organized medicine. The AMA was losing its grip on medicine as well as being drained of its lifeblood—membership. Once an organization doctors joined as a matter of course, the American Medical Association was on its way to being unable to claim even half of America's doctors as members. The AMA's hard-won dominance of medicine was on the critical list.

AMA leaders recognized that they needed to rally the demoralized troops. They hypothesized that a divided house would pull together to fight a common enemy.11 When China is in trouble, it invades Tibet; when the AMA is in trouble, it often launches unifying campaigns to take on real or imagined enemies, such as competing health professions.

As early as September 1963, the AMA staff was gearing up to eliminate chiropractic, with the official rationale of protecting the public's health. Robert Youngerman, a Department of Investigation lawyer, said in a memo to Throckmorton that chiropractors "present a clear and present danger to the health and welfare of the public, and it would seem that as guardians of our nation's health, doctors of medicine should be dedicated to the *total elimination* of any such unscientific cult." (Emphasis added) To accomplish this goal, Youngerman suggested the formation of a "Committee on Chiropractic."[12]

The AMA Board agreed to the concept in November 1963, but chose a different name for the panel. "Committee on Chiropractic" sounded as though the AMA were establishing a diplomatic mission and extending an olive branch to chiropractors.[13] Instead, the AMA Board held out the iron fist. It ordered that the panel, made up of medical doctors, be called the Committee on Quackery. The goal of the new committee was no less than to "contain and eliminate" chiropractic.[14]

To energize the Department of Investigation and the new Committee on Quackery, in January 1965, Throckmorton hired as department director H. Doyl Taylor, an attorney by training and tough-talking city editor of the *Des Moines Register*. In his new post, Taylor enthusiastically went after all manner of quackery, from psychic surgeons in the Philippines to arthritis and cancer quackery in Mexico.

Despite his Iowa roots, Taylor professed to know nothing about chiropractors until he joined the AMA staff. "I didn't know a chiropractor from an antelope," he would say. But when his superiors told him chiropractic was a menace, he immediately recognized it as the "greatest hazard to the public health. . . . I opposed whatever the Committee instructed me to oppose."[15] One leading chiropractor later would portray Taylor as "the AMA's Adolf Eichmann," a bureaucrat who followed orders to destroy undesirables.[16]

The AMA Department of Investigation and the Committee on Quackery argued that existing AMA policy banning consultation with cultists was too vague to carry on the fight against chiropractic. They sought a *"necessary tool,"* an explicit anti-chiropractic position from the AMA's policy-setting House of Delegates.[17] Taylor helped fashion a position statement that for the first time specifically targeted chiropractors as a hazard. In the aftermath of the divisive Medicare battle, the AMA's House of Delegates in 1966 adopted the anti-chiropractic position, stating: "It is the position of the medical profession that chiropractic is an unscientific cult whose practitioners lack the necessary training and background to diagnose and treat human disease. Chiropractic constitutes a hazard to rational health care in the United States because of the substandard and unscientific education of its practitioners and their rigid adherence to an irrational, unscientific approach to disease causation."[18] With this single stroke, the AMA both declared itself the medical profession and tarred chiropractic as quackery.

Putting up Roadblocks

With AMA House endorsement, the Department of Investigation and the Committee on Quackery carried out their assignment with renewed zeal. Anywhere chiropractic made a showing, the AMA appeared—often covertly—using its influence to try to counter, block, and stop the enemy.

Taylor enlisted the support of hundreds of medical groups for the great war on chiropractic. He encouraged them to adopt ethical prohibitions against M.D.s either referring patients to or consulting with D.C.s The committee also worked to bar chiropractors from tax-supported hospitals, to which some D.C.s wanted to refer patients for state-of-the-art X-ray studies. When Congress began considering paying chiropractors for treating elderly patients under Medicare, the AMA collaborated with its traditional foes on the Medicare issue, including the National Council of Senior Citizens, the AFL-CIO, and the American Public Health Association, to put up anti-chiropractic roadblocks. The AMA urged these groups to take stands against chiropractic and then distributed their anti-chiropractic positions, creating an anti-chiropractic bandwagon.

When chiropractic organizations sought federal approval for programs to upgrade, standardize, and accredit chiropractic education, the AMA stood at the Department of Education's door to try to bar their way. Department of Investigation staffers even went undercover, taking assumed names with appended D.C.s to spy on chiropractic conventions.[19]

To "educate" the public and the medical profession, the Committee on Quackery organized "quackery conferences" around the country to focus on the menace of chiropractic. The AMA distributed anti-chiropractic literature by the gross. It purchased 10,000 copies of journalist Ralph Lee Smith's book *At Your Own Risk: The Case Against Chiropractic,* which exposed some tragic abuses at the hands of chiropractors, revealed the greed of some D.C.s, and ridiculed chiropractic training and treatment.[20] The AMA gave the book, which was partially based on Department of Investigation files and Smith's writings in an AMA magazine for consumers, to 1,000 of the nation's largest libraries.

In 1967 Congress asked the then Department of Health, Education and Welfare to appoint a panel through the Public Health Service to advise the government on whether chiropractors should be reimbursed under the new Medicare program. It was decided that to prevent the appearance of bias, no outside observers would be permitted, and that a proposed caucus with AMA representatives would not be allowed. However, as the study began in 1968, the AMA did everything it could to "coach" and persuade committee members that chiropractic should not be covered.

In a February 1968 letter, Taylor told Dr. Samuel Sherman, a member of HEW's Health Insurance Benefits Advisory Council with strong AMA links, "I'm sure you agree that the AMA hand must not 'show' in this matter at this stage of the proposed chiropractic study. . . . We must guard against the possibility that HEW may decide to do only what is politically expedient and include chiropractic 'as licensed at the state level'; or if a study is undertaken, admit chiropractic's totally unscientific testimonials."[21] Months before the study actually began, Sherman assured Taylor that the final decision would be based upon chiropractic's "lack of scientific merit."[22] And Dr. David Stevens, a member of the Committee on Quackery, said in a memo that a federal official reticently explained in a dinner meeting in October 1968 with Kentucky Medical Association officials that AMA testimony was "unnecessary as the final answer has already been determined."[23]

The AMA also used an insider to determine which panelists were "soft" on chiropractic so they could be "coached."[24] Panelist Dr. John McMillan Mennell, an expert on manipulative therapy from Jefferson Medical College in Philadelphia, complained of receiving phone calls "indirectly, but clearly inspired by the American Medical Association, implicitly suggesting what the tenor of my paper should be."[25] He was angered at the possibility that chiropractors might be penalized because of "the bitter bias of the American Medical Association, when there is substantial evidence that manipulative therapy brings relief to sufferers from mechanical pain."[26] In the initial vote on whether to recommend that Congress approve Medicare coverage of chiropractic, the federal panel split 4–4, but the final vote was changed to 5–3 against chiropractic coverage.

Chiropractic Cries Foul

The divided camps of chiropractic charged that the panel was "fixed." The International Chiropractors Association, representing the straights, and the American Chiropractic Association, representing the mixer camp, put aside their differences and released a May 1969 White Paper in which they outlined their charges against the panel. They complained that HEW's Ad Hoc Consultant Group and Expert Review Panel were dominated by medical doctors and included no chiropractic representatives.

The chiropractors said the federal report misrepresented chiropractic education, noting that nearly three-quarters of chiropractic colleges at the time required a minimum two years of prior college credit. The report also stated the four-year chiropractic-education program devoted more time to instruction in anatomy, physiology, radiology, rehabilitation, nutrition, and public health than did the four-year course in medical school. Further, the chiropractors rebutted the federal report by noting that organized chiropractic had formally rejected the "one-cause, one-cure" theory, which the AMA had long belittled.[27]

Congress demanded a response from HEW, which claimed every step possible was taken to prevent bias. In the meantime the AMA Department of Investigation added the panel's negative report on chiropractic to its so-called chiro kit, a package of anti-chiropractic materials it sent to consumers and others inquiring about chiropractic.

Throughout this period, members of the Committee on Quackery made disparaging speeches to build opposition to chiropractic. Dr. Joseph A. Sabatier, chairman of the committee, hailed from Louisiana, the only state in the early 1970s that did not license chiropractors. He told a gathering of medical society officials that "rabid dogs and chiropractors fit into about the same category. . . . Chiropractors were nice [but] they killed people."[28]

The Department of Investigation and the Committee on Quackery eventually backed off on the chiropractor-as-mad-dog-killer argument. Taylor advised a national insurance association that it would be playing "with dynamite" if it went after the chiropractors' record with malpractice suits.[29] After all, based on the larger number of medical doctors and the larger number of suits against them, the chiropractors were bound to come out on top. Like other health professionals, chiropractors put their patients at a certain amount of risk during treatment. A chiropractic adjustment of the neck in rare instances can cause a stroke. And some chiropractors resorting to ineffective or hazardous treatment could be putting patients' lives in jeopardy by keeping them from lifesaving medical therapies. But this problem was small in comparison to the dangers posed by mainstream medicine. Medical doctors more frequently than chiropractors engaged in potentially harmful, even deadly practices. Nevertheless, Taylor encouraged the AMA's consumer magazine to print articles—based on Department of Investigation files—showing the dangers of chiropractic quackery, such as chiropractors misdiagnosing cancers and other life-threatening ailments.

The chiropractors did what they could to counter the attack. They dispatched "truth squads" to tell their side to the press at hotels where the AMA held its annual National Congress on Medical Quackery.[30] Taylor, the former newsman, was shocked when the media started to give chiropractic equal time to answer AMA charges. The tide of battle was about to turn, though in completely unexpected ways.

THE AMA WAR BACKFIRES

In an unprecedented memo, on January 4, 1971, the Committee on Quackery reported to the Board of Trustees that it was well on its way toward achieving its first goal of containing chiropractic and was "moving toward the ultimate goal" of eliminating the competing healers. The committee also explained it had not submitted a progress report in the first seven years of its existence because "to make public some of [its] activities would have been and continues to be unwise."[31]

Around the same time, over in Davenport, Iowa, Dr. Jerome McAndrews, new on the job as executive vice president of the International Chiropractors Association, was pondering the fate of his profession. He had no way of knowing that an unusual parcel he received in the mail would have direct bearing on the future of chiropractic and its AMA antagonists. The package contained fifteen copies of a book entitled *In the Public Interest*.[32] The illustration on the book's cover immediately riveted his attention: a Nazi swastika was superimposed on the AMA's serpent-on-the-staff logo.

McAndrews, like most other chiropractors, believed his profession was the victim of clandestine maneuvering by the AMA. The AMA had long considered chiropractic quackery and an "unscientific cult"; however, this book appeared to document that the AMA was doing more than mouthing anti-chiropractic slogans. The book's thesis was that the AMA was plotting to eradicate chiropractic. It described the AMA's anti-chiropractic plan in detail and even reproduced internal memos supposedly obtained by an anonymous reform-minded physician on staff at the AMA. The paperwork from the AMA drones was enough to warm the heart of any conspiracy buff. The book purported to show that the AMA was intentionally wiping out a competing profession, not merely fighting quackery.[33]

The book began: "What you are about to read is not fiction. It is not the inside story of the rise of the Third Reich, nor is it a figment of a fanatic's fantasy of a communist conspiracy to take over America. What it is, is truth, fully documented, of how the powerful American Medical Association is going about doing away with one of the less powerful professions in the healing arts, chiropractic."[34] McAndrews could tell that whoever put together the book had an ax to grind, though he wasn't sure who the person was. He fretted that personal slurs aimed at AMA officials undermined the book's credibility.

Furthermore, McAndrews never heard of William Trevor, the book's author, nor Scriptures Unlimited, the book's Los Angeles–based publisher. The book acknowledged the assistance of an obscure organization known as Reform in Professional Organizations Freedom Foundation. Only years later would a lawyer point out that the group's acronym was an apparent joke—RIP-OFF. Though he couldn't be sure the material was authentic, McAndrews intuited a ring of truth. As he paged through the book, he realized it could help rally chiropractic's divided movement and could crack what he believed was an AMA-led boycott that deprived the public of the benefits of his group's unique type of health care.

When a representative of Scriptures Unlimited called to ask whether he had received the books and whether his association would like to reprint it, McAndrews arranged to buy the rights. He said a balding, middle-aged man, casually dressed, wearing a leather jacket, collected the $2,500 cashier's check from him. Fifteen thousand copies of the book were printed. McAndrews made only one change, he removed the swastika. *In the Public Interest* created a stir in chiropractic circles but received no attention elsewhere.

A Chiropractor Calls for a Suit Against the AMA

Dr. Chester A. Wilk, a Chicago chiropractor, was touched by the book. He had long held that medical doctors persecuted chiropractors and their patients. For instance, his patients had tremendous difficulty obtaining X rays at local hospitals in connection with chiropractic care, although the facilities had been built with public funds. He felt AMA prohibitions against professional cooperation between medical doctors and chiropractors was harming his patients. The activities of the AMA cabal outlined in *Public Interest* substantiated his personal experience.

A year before the Trevor book came out in 1972, Wilk had begun writing his own indictment of the AMA. The chiropractor, who has a copy of the Bill of Rights displayed prominently in the living room in his suburban Chicago home, in 1973 self-published *Chiropractic Speaks Out: A Reply to Medical Propaganda, Bigotry and Ignorance.*[35]

In his book, Wilk urged the AMA to stop engaging in monopolistic practices and join with chiropractic to help patients. As he went around the country promoting his book before local chiropractic groups, Wilk began beating the drums for a lawsuit to end discrimination promoted by the AMA and its fellow members of the medical establishment. Legal action against the powerful allopaths was an unpopular notion in organized chiropractic, which had lost an important lawsuit in 1965 before the Supreme Court, through which it had attempted to force licensure of chiropractors in Louisiana.[36] Nonetheless, at the grass roots, thanks to the feisty Wilk, a defense fund for a lawsuit was started in hopes of taking on the AMA.

"Sore Throat" Speaks

Wilk's efforts against the AMA got a boost in 1975 when an individual dubbed Sore Throat sent a torrent of purloined AMA papers to reporters at major media outlets, including the *New York Times,* the New York *Daily News,* the *Washington Star,* the *Washington Post,* and the *Chicago Sun-Times,* as well as to congressional committees and Dr. Sidney Wolfe, cofounder with consumerist Ralph Nader of Public Citizen Health Research Group. The internal documents revealed a pattern of seemingly underhanded activities, indicating possible postal and tax abuses involving the *Journal of the AMA,* apparent AMA manipulation of certain congressional leaders, and battle plans for the war to "contain and eliminate" chiropractic. Some of the documents relating to chiropractic were contained in *Public Interest,* but the theatrics of Sore Throat, whom reporters found to be highly credible because his tips usually checked out, thrust the issue into the media spotlight. Sore Throat, like the supposed source of documents described in the introduction to *In the Public Interest,* claimed he was a disgruntled AMA staff doctor who was trying to expose wrongdoing so that organized medicine could proceed with much-needed reform.

Bedeviled by leaks, which one AMA spokesman characterized as "death by one thousand cuts," the AMA was running scared. It hired a private eye to uncover who was behind the breaches. It purchased paper shredders to destroy documents. AMA spokesmen engaged in disinformation about Sore Throat, offering to reveal his true identity. One AMA spokesman told the press that Sore Throat was "a fruity chiropractor in Georgetown whose hobby is hairdressing."[37]

The AMA's detective, a former Secret Service agent, quickly traced the disclosures to a group the AMA had angered years before: the Church of Scientology. In addition, the AMA investigation found that Scriptures Unlimited was a small publishing house purchased by the Church of Scientology just to publish *In the Public Interest*.38

Scientology, a religion with a psychological bent founded by science-fiction writer L. Ron Hubbard in the 1950s, had a long-simmering grudge against the AMA. The sect believed the AMA had attempted to discredit the religion since its earliest days. And church members were angered by the publication in 1968 in an AMA consumer publication of an article entitled "Scientology—Menace to Mental Health," in which Ralph Lee Smith, a special target of derision in the Trever book, described the wealth gathered by Scientology's leadership and the problems the group had with the Internal Revenue Service. Smith dismissed Scientology's tenets as "simple—some say simplistic."39

In response, Scientology had issued a "doom program" to destroy the AMA.40 A Scientologist, who worked in the AMA's Drug Department, sometime between 1969 and 1971 had gone through AMA files and had discovered the mother lode of files on chiropractic, which formed the basis for *In the Public Interest*. During subsequent operations in the mid-1970s, papers relating to AMA lobbying efforts and business practices were uncovered and delivered by Sore Throat to the media, consumerists, and Congress.41

Ironically, only a few months before the leaked AMA documents began to show up in the press in the summer of 1975, the AMA dismantled the Department of Investigation and the Committee on Quackery. In the end, the department had described itself as a success, even though by the time of its demise Medicare covered chiropractic care to a limited extent and chiropractic was licensed in all fifty states. The main reason the AMA cited for closing the office was the AMA's financial woes, which had led to layoffs of several hundred employees in 1974 and 1975. But although the Department of Investigation and the Committee on Quackery technically were dead, they would continue to live on in another arena—the courts.

CHIROPRACTIC FIGHTS BACK

U.S. Representative John E. Moss, chairman of the oversight and investigations subcommittee of the House Interstate and Foreign Commerce Committee, was on Sore Throat's mailing list. And the California

Democrat was distressed at what he read. In October 1975 he sent the Federal Trade Commission copies of AMA documents pertaining to anti-chiropractic activities. He argued that the AMA efforts to eliminate chiropractic might constitute a group boycott, which was illegal under the Sherman Act. Moss pointed out that even though the AMA might find chiropractic undesirable economically or socially, Congress had included chiropractic treatments under Medicare coverage. He urged an investigation.[42]

But in the mid-1970s, the concept of prosecuting professionals, such as doctors, for antitrust was a new one, and the FTC failed to take on the case. However, Sore Throat contacted Wilk and other prominent chiropractors, giving the chiropractors' morale a boost. They decided to explore the possibility of an antitrust suit, acting under provisions in the federal law that allowed individuals to act as "private attorneys general." Wilk and the International Chiropractors Association's Jerome McAndrews consulted with attorney George P. McAndrews, Jerome's younger brother.

The younger McAndrews recommended eight Chicago law firms specializing in antitrust. These attorneys politely but firmly turned away the chiropractors. The firms felt uncomfortable with the unconventional chiropractors, and some feared that if they took up the chiropractors' cause, they might lose business from organized medicine, the many national medical associations based in Chicago. When the chiropractors informed him the suit would not be filed unless he represented them, McAndrews decided to pursue the case himself, obtaining assistance from Northwestern University antitrust expert Paul Slater. Chester Wilk, D.C., and three other chiropractors filed suit on October 13, 1976, against the American Medical Association and a Who's Who of major medical groups. All told, four AMA officials and eleven of the nation's most important medical groups were defendants, including the American Hospital Association, the American College of Surgeons, the American College of Physicians, the American Academy of Orthopaedic Surgeons, the American College of Radiology, and the Joint Commission on Accreditation of Hospitals. Ironically, the American Osteopathic Association had become so mainstream by that time that it was named as a defendant.[43]

As he went through his opponents' files during the pretrial discovery process, McAndrews, who had previously handled only antitrust issues connected with patents, thought he had a solid case since AMA documents repeatedly spoke of efforts to "contain and eliminate" chiropractic and outlined how this was to be accomplished, stating, "We can't let the public know what we're doing. The AMA's hand must not show." The

Trevor book and Sore Throat had provided the chiropractors with a smoking cannon.

A vast array of documents critical to the case was available, even though a top AMA official had advised state societies in 1978 to purge their files because of a pending federal investigation.[44] In preparing for the trial from 1977 through 1980, McAndrews visited thirty-four states and collected over one million documents and 164 depositions. The AMA couldn't have faced this legal challenge from Wilk, along with three other chiropractic restraint-of-trade suits, at a worse time because of the association's precarious financial situation. The AMA was trying to come back from near-bankruptcy, and its leadership and management knew the organization was looking at the expenditure of hundreds of thousands, if not millions, of dollars on its legal defense.

Hoping to make the suits go away, AMA leaders tried to blunt the organization's stand against chiropractic. The House of Delegates in 1979 adopted a board report, designated as UU, stating that *not* everything chiropractors did was without "therapeutic value." Rather than depict all chiropractors as cultists, the board said "it is better to call attention to the limitations of chiropractic in treatment of particular diseases." The report, however, reaffirmed that chiropractic theory was not supported by science, and the organization continued to stand by a section of its 1957 ethical code, which prohibited medical doctors from associating professionally with cultists.

Dr. James H. Sammons, the AMA's executive vice president, told delegates: "To deliberately place ourselves in violation of the antitrust statutes so that we can go home and self-righteously say that we have done so is sheer foolishness. It places every doctor in America in greater jeopardy than he is in already," said Sammons, a pragmatist who was willing to eat crow if it helped the organization survive. Dr. William S. Hotchkiss, an AMA Board member who had served on the Committee on Quackery during its final years, agreed, saying the board report should be supported as a defensive maneuver to save the AMA money. "If we could settle it all for a nominal sum, this would not be surrender, but would represent good common sense," he said.[45] The House of Delegates adopted report UU by a vast majority.

The AMA effort to rewrite history to head off lawsuits resumed the next year. In 1980, under the leadership of Dr. James S. Todd, a New Jersey surgeon and a rising star in AMA circles, the House of Delegates revised its ethical code, eliminating the section that banned consultation with unscientific practitioners. Legally, the AMA appeared to have sanitized the record of its anti-chiropractic stands, but its headaches were far from over.

The case of *Wilk et al. v. AMA et al.* finally went to trial before U.S. District Court Judge Nicholas J. Bua in Chicago in December 1980. A federal appeals court later described the trial as a "free-for-all between chiropractors and medical doctors, in which the scientific legitimacy of chiropractic was hotly debated and the comparative avarice of the adversaries was explored."[46] Bua told jurors they should not find the AMA guilty of wrongdoing if its actions were merely designed to inform the public about defects in chiropractic, adding that the AMA's advocacy was protected if it were aimed at lobbying for changes in law. After an arduous eight-week trial, the jury concluded the AMA's anti-chiropractic campaign was within legal bounds.

Afterward, two jurors, in tears, contacted McAndrews and told him they believed the AMA had done wrong, but based on the judge's instructions, they felt they had no choice but to let the physicians' group off the hook. McAndrews filed an appeal, arguing that Bua had erred in his handling of the case. In 1983 the Appellate Court of the Seventh Federal District agreed and ordered a new trial.

As the years ground on, AMA's codefendants in growing numbers settled with the chiropractors, creating ill will in the once-solid brotherhood. The AMA's battle became increasingly lonely.

U.S. District Court Judge Susan Getzendanner started a nonjury trial in May 1987. Much of the second trial was a rerun of the first. For their part, AMA attorneys argued that *if* there had ever been a boycott of chiropractic, it had ended in 1980 when the AMA adopted its new ethical standards. McAndrews countered that increased demand for chiropractic services and a significant spurt in chiropractors' incomes after liberalization of the ethical code were proof of the boycott's success earlier. He said the boycott still lingered because the AMA had never explicitly spelled out that physicians ethically could consult with chiropractors.

Chiropractic patients told the court how they were helped with headaches and back pain through spinal manipulation. Wilk described how his patients had been turned away from hospitals when he sent them there for X rays. He said he couldn't technically "refer" patients with medical problems to medical doctors but "transferred" them: "I turn them over and then I don't see them anymore."[47]

AMA lawyers put on the stand consultants who refuted the evidence by the chiropractors' experts that attempted to document that chiropractors were financially disadvantaged because of an AMA boycott. The AMA questioned the safety of practices used by chiropractors when they took X rays of patients without shields. Dr. William Jarvis, cofounder of the National Council Against Health Fraud and a faculty member at

Loma Linda University, criticized chiropractic's underpinnings: "As I see it, the major problem is a substitution of the chiropractic philosophy for science."[48] Chiropractors were also attacked for "practice building," procedures to boost their income by encouraging unnecessary patient visits. The chiropractors' attorneys were quick to point out that medical doctors, dentists, psychologists, and other professionals have been accused of similar methods.

In closing arguments, AMA trial lawyer Douglas R. Carlson said the AMA acknowledged that chiropractic was becoming more scientific and even took partial credit for improvements in chiropractic: "We suggest that one reason that it changed was because of the criticism of its bizarre methods."[49] The courtroom cracked up when McAndrews, in his closing, retorted that Carlson's position was akin to a German U-boat captain he met who took "credit for the American Olympic team being so good because . . . by sinking their ships, he taught them how to swim."[50]

The Conspiracy Unveiled

After a two-month trial, creating a record that included 3,624 pages of transcript, 1,265 exhibits, and excerpts from seventy-three depositions, Getzendanner, on August 24, 1987, ruled that the AMA and its officials "instituted a boycott of chiropractors in the mid-1960s by informing AMA members that chiropractors were unscientific practitioners and that it was unethical for a medical physician to associate with chiropractors. The purpose of the boycott was to contain and eliminate the chiropractic profession. This conduct constituted a conspiracy among the AMA and its members and an unreasonable restraint of trade in violation of Section 1 of the Sherman Act."[51]

Although the number of chiropractic schools, the number of chiropractors, and the number of visits to chiropractors grew during the boycott, Getzendanner accepted the Committee on Quackery's acknowledgment that it had succeeded in containing chiropractic. "These admissions were not mere puffery," she said. Although the AMA never disciplined any members for associating with chiropractors, the judge said the existence of the ethical stricture against such relations "is inherently a forceful mandator of conduct. . . . Enforcement was not necessary to obtain compliance with the boycott."[52]

Getzendanner shot down the AMA's claims that its anti-chiropractic policies were ancient history. She indicated that the AMA Board Report UU stating chiropractic was not entirely unscientific "was obviously written by lawyers in an effort to bring the AMA into compliance with the antitrust laws and not a bold change of position designed to reverse the attitudes of the AMA members formed, at least in part, by the then 11-year-old boycott."[53] The AMA's 1980 revised principles theoretically allowed AMA members to associate with chiropractors, but there was no explicit reference to chiropractors in the new code, the judge said. In her final case before retiring from the bench, Getzendanner said the AMA had failed to inform its members of the fact that it now recognized improvements in and benefits from chiropractic.

Getzendanner found the behavior by both the AMA and chiropractic to be a mixed bag. She said the AMA acted in the blind belief that it was protecting patient welfare by combating chiropractic. Meanwhile, she agreed that some therapies used by chiropractors were "alarming" and potentially harmful to patients. "I do not minimize the negative evidence. But most of the defense witnesses appeared to be testifying for the plaintiffs," she said.[54] She stressed that her ruling should not be construed as an endorsement of chiropractic, nor would she preside over a shotgun wedding between the professions. "Certainly no judge should perform that ceremony," she said.[55]

To combat the continuing effects of the conspiracy, she ordered the AMA to admit the "lawlessness of its past conduct" and to alter its official policy on chiropractic.[56] As a result, the injunction was published in the *AMA Journal* on January 1, 1988, with an editorial by AMA general counsel Kirk B. Johnson explaining why such an unusual document appeared in the scientific publication.

The judge also found the American College of Surgeons, the American College of Radiology, and the American Academy of Orthopaedic Surgeons guilty of joining the conspiracy; these groups reached out-of-court settlements with the chiropractors. The cases against the Joint Commission on Accreditation of Hospitals and the American College of Physicians were dismissed.

The AMA appealed the case. In February 1990 the Appellate Court upheld the lower court's ruling, and the U.S. Supreme Court let Getzendanner's ruling stand in November 1990.[57]

After negotiating for more than a year, the AMA in December 1991 agreed to make a $3.5 million payment for the chiropractors' legal costs and to publish a new position in its ethical opinions explicitly stating that medical doctors and chiropractors could associate professionally.[58]

Meanwhile, the old wounds between allopathy and chiropractic and other alternatives appeared to be healing. Mainstream physicians appeared to be more open to patients receiving care from nonphysicians. Several studies on the benefits of chiropractic were published in highly respected *medical* journals. In 1992 Congress, pressured by advocates for alternative medicine, directed the National Institutes of Health, a bastion of orthodox medicine, to launch a new venture that would not have been possible in the pre-Wilk era: the NIH Office for Alternative Medicine.[59] The AMA seemed to be moving on. It converted the voluminous files from the defunct Department of Investigation, which had hunted chiropractic, into a research archive in the organization's headquarters.[60]

PROTECTING THE MONOPOLY

The peaceful spring did not last long. The war against alternative healers was reignited in the fall of 1993. As in the years before Medicare was adopted, organized medicine was feeling the strains of change brought on by the health reforms proposed by the Clinton administration. Once again the AMA's own forces were divided and demoralized. They needed an enemy around which they could rally. The AMA took on a new threat to its control of the health field: nursing.

In *Witches, Midwives, and Nurses: A History of Women Healers,* Barbara Ehrenreich and Deirdre English note that the male-dominated medical profession afforded a subservient role to female-dominant nursing. Nurses were "ancillary," from the Latin for maidservant. Nursing work was "just low-paid, heavy-duty housework."[61]

They note that modern scientific doctors relied on nurses: "[He] was even less likely than his predecessors to stand around and watch the progress of his 'cures.' He diagnosed, he prescribed, he moved on. He could not waste his talents, or his expensive academic training in the tedious details of bedside care. For this he needed a patient, obedient helper, someone who was not above the most menial tasks, in short, a nurse."[62]

This role was institutionalized in state nursing-practice acts that in most cases restrict what nurses can do, preserving the doctors' monopoly. In effect, nurses in these jurisdictions are limited to providing care delegated by physicians.[63]

However, a cadre of highly trained specialists—known as advanced-practice nurses—has in recent years made some gains. In some cases these nurses are autonomous. They can diagnose and treat disease, prescribe medications, and receive reimbursement for their services.

The American Nurses Association sees as one of its key missions expanding the roles of these independent-practice nurses, including nurse-practitioners, nurse-midwives and nurse-anesthetists. With this in mind, the ANA increasingly has become politicized, having moved its headquarters to Washington from Kansas City in 1992. It was the first major health-care group to endorse the Clinton-Gore ticket.[64] (The AMA traditionally has not endorsed presidential candidates, concentrating its efforts on congressional races.)

In the health reform, nursing saw an opportunity to promote autonomy for nursing. Nursing was encouraged when the Administration said there was a shortage of primary-care providers—pediatricians, family physicians, and internists—to provide such care. The ANA charged that the majority of physicians had abandoned primary care for more lucrative specialty practices. It said if restrictions on nurses were lifted, advanced-practice nurses were up to the challenge of providing much of this basic care. The ANA's slogan became: "In the future your 'family doctor' may be a nurse." Nursing was among the first groups to endorse the early draft of Clinton's health proposal in September 1993.

Nursing argued that research showed nurses could provide up to 80 percent of care delivered by primary-care physicians, that care given by nurses was as good or better than physician-provided care, and that surveys showed the public was open to the idea of nurses furnishing more of this care. The ANA also contended that nursing care was less costly than that from physicians. Nurses earned less than doctors, $45,000 annually for nurse-practitioners vs. $111,800 for family physicians in 1992.

The Administration partially rewarded nursing in its final reform package, recommending that state restrictions on nurses be loosened and that Medicare reimbursement for nurse practitioners be expanded.[65]

A war of words ensued between medicine and its challengers, reminiscent of some of the battles between the AMA and chiropractic. Several state medical societies' political action committees warned in fund-raising letters sent to doctors that some "daffy ducks" were trying to "fowl up"—one state said "duck up"—medical care by lowering standards and allowing unqualified people to practice medicine. The nurses said these physicians were accusing them of being "quacks."

The AMA also went on the attack, questioning whether a shortage of primary care actually existed. And at the interim meeting in December 1993 in New Orleans, the AMA released a thirty-page report suggesting that giving nurses more autonomy "may increase the medical risk to patients and the ultimate cost of care." It opposed giving nurses more autonomy, including expanding their right to prescribe medicine and to be reimbursed directly for services. AMA leaders said they favored an expanded role for nurses so long as they work under the supervision of physicians. The report concluded: "Nurses in advanced practice are not educated to independently provide medical care to meet the broad spectrum of needs of patients in the community."[66] AMA leaders like to say that "nurses don't know what they don't know," and that nurses "ought to go to medical school if they want to be doctors."

The economic self-interest of physicians again blurred the AMA's claims that it was looking out for patients. As ANA president Virginia Trotter Betts put it, "The issue is control, especially control of dollars. The AMA wants physician supervision because then the physician gets the first dollar."

She noted that the AMA "has also opposed autonomy for any practitioner, whether that be nurse, podiatrist, psychologist, social worker or chiropractor."[67]

The AMA stands for the status quo, a physician-centered health-care system. It is unlikely that patients will suffer at the hands of highly trained nurses. But the AMA will not willingly relinquish the power, prerogatives, and pay physicians receive under the current medical monopoly.

CHAPTER 7

Smoking Gun
Playing Politics with Tobacco and the Public's Health

The AMERICAN MEDICAL Association holds itself up as an advocate for the public's health, but it has had an often shameful record on the biggest public-health catastrophe of our time, the tobacco epidemic. The death and disability from tobacco use is staggering. In this century, 14 million Americans have died from lung cancer, heart disease, and other tobacco-caused diseases. Each year in excess of 400,000 Americans die from tobacco-related disease, more than the combined death toll from AIDS, murder, accidents, alcohol and drug abuse, and suicide. The tobacco epidemic conservatively costs the economy $68 billion each year, in direct health-care costs, loss of productivity from illness, and foregone earnings of those who die prematurely from smoking-related causes.[1]

The AMA has had a long and intimate connection with tobacco, but unfortunately the nation's largest physician group, pursuing its own agenda, often has done more to promote tobacco interests than it has "the betterment of the public health"—one of its founding missions. The AMA's activities on tobacco can be divided into three periods. In the first, starting in the mid-1930s and lasting until the mid-1950s, at a time when the first scientific links between smoking and disease were being made, the AMA, through its journal, played a significant role in helping to promote cigarettes. Then, from the mid-1950s until the early 1980s, as evidence regarding the dangers of smoking became overwhelming, the

AMA not only maintained a virtual silence on tobacco, but collaborated with tobacco interests. In the third period, from the mid-1980s onward, pushed by idealistic medical students and young doctors, the AMA increasingly has spoken out against tobacco, but it generally has not used the full force of its political clout to persuade Congress to control the tobacco epidemic.

The AMA's savvy and resources have been sorely missed as smaller, less well-connected health groups have engaged in a monumental battle against an entrenched industry with a huge bankroll and a strong survival instinct. The American tobacco industry generates more than $50 billion a year in revenue and employs some 700,000 people. Legislation to restrict and discourage tobacco use usually does not get passed. Quite simply, because of politics and money, people are dying or becoming disabled by tobacco-caused disease.

CIGARETTE HUCKSTERISM AND THE AMA

Back in the 1930s, the AMA played a role in establishing cigarettes as a popular product. The AMA helped develop and then accepted in its journal advertisements that made cigarettes appear to be a physician-endorsed product. Coping with the hard times from the Great Depression, the physician group hit upon a previously untapped source of revenue: opening the *AMA Journal* to advertisements for nonmedical products. Soon, cigarette ads became a regular feature in the most widely read and highly respected physician publication.

By this time some researchers had begun to report in medical journals that lung cancer—then a rare disease—appeared to be linked to smoking. But this message had yet to penetrate the consciousness of doctors, let alone the general public.

In fact, cigarette makers laced their ads with health messages. "The American smoker during the '30s and '40s could have been forgiven for confusing his favorite brand of cigarettes with the latest wonder drug," said former senator Maurine B. Neuberger (D-Ore.), a reformed smoker turned smoking reformer in the 1960s. Examples of slogans were "Not a cough in a carload" for Old Gold, and "Not one single case of throat irritation due to smoking Camels."[2]

Philip Morris, a brand from an upstart cigarette manufacturer destined for market domination, ran perhaps the boldest, most successful campaign. In ads aimed at the public, diminutive bellhop Johnny Roventini, who belted out the signature phrase "Call for Philip Morris," hinted that his brand was "definitely less irritating." And in ads for the influential medical profession, Philip Morris used what it claimed was scientific documentation to hawk its smokes. Starting in November 1935, Philip Morris ads in medical publications, most prominently *JAMA,* touted an additive known as diethylene glycol, a chemical that moistened tobacco contained in cigarettes. Philip Morris said its research showed diethylene glycol made its cigarette milder than competing brands, which used another agent, glycerine.[3]

Unbeknownst to physicians and the public, America's most celebrated physician, a man intimately identified with the AMA, was working behind the scenes to help Philip Morris design its sales strategy. He was Dr. Morris Fishbein. Though the public came to think of him as being the AMA's president, he actually was the editor of the *Journal.* He was so well known in his time that the Marx Brothers casually used his name in a joke in their film *Room Service.*

When Philip Morris management first got fired up about diethylene glycol, company scientists approached Fishbein about the possibility of promoting the moistening agent in Philip Morris ads in the *Journal.* After examining the data, Fishbein told Philip Morris that the research failed to substantiate the company's claims. Fishbein told Philip Morris what steps to take to document the benefits of diethylene glycol.[4]

Philip Morris followed Fishbein's advice and paid pharmacologist Michael G. Mulinos, of the Columbia University College of Physicians and Surgeons, to conduct research on diethylene glycol. In his study, which appeared in the *New York State Journal of Medicine* in June 1935, Mulinos reported that of the unnamed brands, the one with diethylene glycol caused three times less swelling to rabbits' eyes than did those with glycerine.[5] Philip Morris made this research and some clinical studies in humans the basis for ad campaigns in *JAMA* and other medical journals from 1935 until the 1950s. The ads offered doctors free packs of Philip Morris along with reprints of the studies. Philip Morris' chief chemist and nine assistants attended all major medical meetings to explain Mulinos' research and to hype the supposed benefits of diethylene glycol. The company even dispatched representatives to doctors' offices to give them free cigarettes and a pep talk on diethylene glycol.[6]

The campaign was a major success, vaulting Philip Morris into the top ranks of cigarette sellers. Philip Morris was so grateful to Fishbein for guiding them that one of its managers offered him a retainer. (The executive later said the firm had $25,000 a year in mind, though the sum was not mentioned to Fishbein. At the time, Fishbein's annual AMA salary was $20,000 with $10,000 to $20,000 added from his books and other writings.[7] The *JAMA* editor declined, saying that helping the company was his pleasure.)

In the 1940s, other manufacturers copied the approach of using science and physicians to sell cigarettes. Ads for Camels, with Norman Rockwellesque scenes of wholesome children and kindly doctors, proclaimed: "More Doctors Smoke Camels Than Any Other Cigarette." The manufacturer in its ads invited doctors to visit Camels' scientific exhibit at the 1947 AMA convention.

Fishbein went out of his way to support Philip Morris in a few instances in which diethylene glycol was embroiled in controversy. In the most serious incident, a Southern drug manufacturer used the chemical, without testing, in production of a newly released liquid version of the first antibacterial medicine, sulfanilamide. Suddenly, in October 1937, people started dying; all told, more than 100 were killed, many of them children. The AMA help prove diethylene glycol was the culprit.

Philip Morris was quite disturbed by the episode because the moistening agent was the centerpiece of its physician campaign. Fishbein came to the rescue. In the midst of the tragedy, *JAMA* ran an editorial emphasizing that diethylene glycol was used safely in many places in industry, including as an ingredient in cigarettes.[8] With Fishbein's help, Philip Morris continued to advertise to doctors about diethylene glycol without the public being any the wiser.

Tobacco Dangers Nailed Down

In the 1950s the evidence started to become overwhelming that cigarettes caused not only lung cancer but heart disease and other ailments. But the AMA, and the federal government for that matter, had not taken the issue seriously. Meanwhile, the public was confused by the simultaneous appearance of scary studies in the press linking health hazards to smoking and upbeat ads for cigarettes.

In May 1950 *JAMA* published the first large study on tobacco. Medical student Ernst Wynder and surgeon Evarts Graham, of Washington University in St. Louis, found that 96.5 percent of patients with lung cancer in their hospitals had been smokers.[9] More research followed in the mid-1950s.

Finally, in 1957 the federal government took notice. Surgeon General Leroy Burney broke the government's silence, telling a televised news conference that longtime cigarette smoking caused lung cancer. This potential public-health bombshell was a dud because it failed to mobilize medicine's leader, the AMA, to tackle the tobacco issue. Diplomatically, Burney recalled that the AMA "had a rather detached, arms-length attitude."[10]

The risks were starting to penetrate the clouds of cigarette smoke, so commonplace in the 1950s. *Reader's Digest,* among the first publishers to refuse cigarette advertising, ran a string of frightening articles about smoking, such as one entitled "Cancer by the Carton." Tobacco sales leveled off and then declined slightly in the early 1950s. The tobacco companies were becoming as worried as the smokers.

The manufacturers recognized they needed to reassure consumers and tried a variety of tacks to create the impression that cigarettes were safe. One approach was to link cigarettes with health and doctors. Liggett & Myers' ads for its L&M brand claimed its filters were "Just what the doctor ordered." Philip Morris revived claims of benefits from diethylene glycol, this time plugged as "Di-GL" in ads aimed at consumers. In radio ads, Philip Morris bragged that Di-GL, found exclusively in its brand, "took the fear out of smoking."

The Micronite Filtered Truth: The AMA Connection

The AMA was considered such a patsy on the tobacco issue that one manufacturer ran a shameless campaign based on its commercial links with the AMA. However, to its credit, the AMA did for the first time resist the temptation of cigarette advertising, although more to placate its other advertisers than to protect the public from a health hazard.

In March 1952, P. Lorillard Co., manufacturer of Kent, sent letters to all American doctors to introduce them to Kent's Micronite filter, which Lorillard said offered "health protection," and suggested physicians prescribe these cigarettes to smokers with sore throats or other problems from smoking. Lorillard included free samples for the doctors to try.

Lorillard then made the AMA connection. It ran ads in *JAMA* in 1952 that mentioned the products' benefits had been authenticated in a booth at the 1952 AMA convention. Under headlines including HAVE YOU HEARD THE STORY OF NEW KENT CIGARETTES, DOCTOR? and DOCTOR . . . HAVE YOU TRIED THE NEW KENT CIGARETTE?, Lorillard told the readers of *JAMA* and other medical journals: "At the recent Convention of the American Medical Association, thousands of physicians heard the Kent story, and saw a convincing demonstration of the MICRONITE FILTER'S phenomenal effectiveness."

Some physicians complained about these tactics to the AMA. And some pharmaceutical companies were nervous that cigarette ads, which the AMA did not carefully scrutinize, might discredit drug ads appearing in *JAMA*. On October 31, 1953, the AMA acted. In a letter to tobacco companies, it said that beginning January 1, 1954, its publications would no longer accept their ads, and its scientific meetings would ban cigarette exhibits. The decision cost the AMA more than $100,000 a year in income.[11]

But the AMA had a hard time distancing itself from cigarette advertising because of an earlier decision to study some of the claims being made in the cigarette-filter wars. The AMA's Advertising Committee requested the AMA Chemical Laboratory, which primarily tested drugs for purity and potency, to study the effectiveness of filters. It was an area rich with advertising claims but with a scarcity of published data. Dr. Walter Wolman, former director of the AMA Chemical Laboratory, said the AMA Advertising Department wanted the filters studied as part of its efforts to sell advertising and to help keep ad claims "within the limits of AMA policy."[12]

The AMA Chemical Laboratory published its comparison of filtered and "regular" brands in July 1953. No filter was especially effective, but an unidentified filter on "Brand B-2" did better than the rest. From the description of the cigarettes, it was easy enough to determine which brand was which. The Kent Micronite filter, the only mineral filter in the study, was the most effective, though it still let through 59 percent of the nicotine and 56 percent of the tars.

Despite the unimpressive results, Lorillard latched on to the AMA study. Without AMA authorization, the firm in 1954 ran advertisements in *Life, Time,* and other popular magazines that cited the Micronite filter's supposed superiority in AMA lab tests. The ads, appearing to confer on Kent filters an AMA seal of approval, stressed that the AMA studies were "voluntary and independent," and claimed they "proved" the Micronite filter was "the most effective." It was cigarette puffery at its worst. The AMA was paying a price for its cozy relations with the tobacco companies.

In April 1954, in an editorial entitled "Cigarette Hucksterism and the AMA," the AMA and *JAMA* blasted Kent for unauthorized use of their names. They condemned the Kent ad campaign as "an outrageous example of commercial exploitation of the American medical profession." The editorial went on to belittle Lorillard's claims, saying that "a completely efficient filter would permit the smoker to inhale nothing but hot air!"[13]

Lorillard promptly rebutted the *JAMA* editorial with new ads that used the original ad as a backdrop to a text block that directed interested readers to the specific references supporting their claims in *JAMA:* "We have been told that the American Medical Association does not endorse any products in this field. But the type of filter that proved most effective in the tests is a type that is used only by KENT. . . ."[14]

(Ironically, Dr. Morris Fishbein, the former *JAMA* editor, who helped introduce the idea of using medical research to sell cigarettes, was a "research consultant" to Lorillard. Fishbein, who now received a $25,000-a-year retainer from the firm, tells in his autobiography of helping to design the clinical experiments with the Micronite filter that served as the basis for Kent's ads.)[15]

The AMA's decision to ban cigarette ads and to attack Lorillard represented the end of an era. No longer would the AMA be used blatantly to sell cigarettes. However, the AMA was far from making a clean break from the tobacco industry.

STRANGE BEDFELLOWS: THE AMA AND THE TOBACCO BARONS

By the early to mid-1960s, most health groups as well as the federal government recognized the time had come to take definitive action against tobacco. But the AMA did not join this effort; instead it collaborated with cigarette makers on projects the industry hoped would help keep the heat off them.

In 1963 the AMA announced and then backed down on a plan to study smoking. The AMA said it felt its study was superfluous because the Surgeon General, at the urging of President John F. Kennedy, was undertaking a large-scale study on cigarettes.

Then, on December 4, 1963, the AMA House of Delegates reversed itself and decided to launch an intensive basic-research program on smoking to "probe beyond statistical evidence" to determine whether smoking caused diseases. This sort of statement made the AMA sound a bit like the tobacco industry, which in the face of criticism always asserted that "statistical" or epidemiologic links between tobacco and disease did not prove tobacco causes those diseases. The AMA's goal, like the tobacco industry's, was to develop a benign cigarette, making smoking safe for America.

After putting $500,000 of its own into the kitty, the AMA set out to obtain additional research money from industry, health associations, and other sources. The Tobacco Institute was thrilled by the announcement—for years it had been looking for ways to work with the AMA, and now the opportunity was at hand.[16]

With release of the Surgeon General's report expected soon, the AMA was sending signals that it was willing to support the industry. AMA president Edward R. Annis in early January 1964 warned the state legislature in Kentucky that the government soon would present "insurmountable evidence that smoking causes cancer." He buoyed up the spirits of these tobacco-state legislators by saying that while his organization opposed disease, "The AMA is not opposed to smoking and tobacco."17

On January 11, 1964, Surgeon General Luther Terry released the study on tobacco and health. He considered the report so sensitive that he presented it on a Saturday when the stock market was closed.

Based on a fourteen-month review of thousands of previously conducted studies, including experiments on animals, autopsy-based investigations, and population studies, the panel concluded the evidence was strong enough to state that smoking *caused* lung cancer, an uncommon disease before the advent of cheap, mass-produced cigarettes. The panel also said the research linked smoking to emphysema, coronary artery disease, and a host of other diseases. The committee concluded that "remedial action," such as warning labels on cigarette packs and control of advertising, was in order.18

As expected, the tobacco industry questioned the validity of the report, saying that a statistical link between smoking and a disease was far from proving a causal relationship. But doctors were stunned when the AMA also downplayed the Surgeon General's report. AMA president Annis said *more research* was needed to discover "how tobacco smoke affects health, and, if possible, to eliminate whatever element may induce disease [because it is] unrealistic to assume the American people are suddenly going to quit smoking."19

On January 31, nearly three weeks after the Surgeon General issued his landmark report, the AMA Education and Research Foundation (AMA-ERF) appointed a committee to direct the research program, including three researchers who served on the Surgeon General's advisory committee and two who previously had done research sponsored by the tobacco industry. On February 7, 1964, the six major tobacco companies agreed to pay $10 million over five years for the AMA-ERF project.20

Because it accepted this tobacco money, the AMA was prevented from leading the charge against a public-health menace. Hence, the AMA presented a *neutral, balanced* message in a six-page brochure entitled "Smoking: Facts You Should Know," published in May 1964. The booklet stressed the dangers of burns and suffocation from falling asleep while smoking, and warned about the costly damage cigarettes could do to sofas, rugs, and clothing. But it characterized the major risks connected with long-term smoking about which the Surgeon General had warned as "suspected health hazards." The AMA brochure stated *some researchers* thought smoking "shortens life expectancy" and is "alleged to cause cancer of the lungs and bladder." On the other hand, the AMA said: "Some equally competent physicians and research personnel are less sure of the effect of cigarette smoking on health. Smoke if you feel you should, but be moderate."[21]

The House of Delegates was under pressure at its annual meeting in June 1964 to take a stand on the Surgeon General's report. Delegates had to reconcile Terry's warnings with the fact that AMA-ERF had accepted $10 million in tobacco industry funds. In the end, the House concluded smoking had a "significant relationship" to lung cancer, a weaker position than that taken by the Surgeon General.[22]

After three years, the AMA's research effort couldn't avoid finding health problems linked to smoking. In 1967 Dr. Maurice H. Seevers, who chaired the AMA-ERF committee and also had served on the Surgeon General's panel, said in the *AMA Journal* that "certainly there are no scientific data that would contradict the basic tenets of the Surgeon General's report." The University of Michigan pharmacologist said the AMA and the industry were committed, although for different reasons, to get to the bottom of issues of tobacco and health.[23]

So the money kept flowing to the AMA-ERF, which passed funds on to the researchers. In 1968 the tobacco companies committed $8 million more to the research. The advantages for the cigarette makers were clear. The project afforded them some cover for years. They could always point to the AMA-ERF project as evidence that not all the answers were in on tobacco's possible links to health problems.

By the early 1970s, the AMA was starting to experience some doubts about accepting the tobacco money, according to a confidential Tobacco Institute document. The memo revealed that on September 3, 1971, William Kloepfer, vice president of public relations of the Tobacco Institute, informed Horace R. Kornegay, the organization's president, that the research arrangement with the AMA was in danger. Kloepfer said Dr. Ernest B. Howard, the AMA's executive vice president, had told him the program was "a great liability . . . from AMA's view it has only caused further blackening of the AMA's image." The AMA wanted out, Kloepfer said, but the organization *"is most anxious to avoid any incident which will create displeasure with the AMA among tobacco area Congressmen— he said AMA needs their support urgently."* (Emphasis added)[24]

In Cahoots with Tobacco Congressmen

Years before this memo was written, the AMA had been accused publicly of being in cahoots with tobacco-state congressmen. This conservative bloc saw eye-to-eye with the AMA on such issues as restricting federal government controls in general and opposing the Medicare health program for the elderly. In a quid pro quo, the AMA helped its friends in Congress by taking positions on tobacco that from a public-health perspective at best were neutral, but at worst were at odds with those of other major health and medical groups. For instance, when the Federal Trade Commission suggested in 1964 that cigarette packages should carry warnings, the AMA shocked commissioners by opposing them. In a letter written three weeks after the tobacco interests funded the AMA-ERF project, Dr. F. J. L. Blasingame, the AMA's chief executive, told the FTC: "Since it is evident that cigarette smoking will continue despite any restrictive labeling that might be imposed, it is our opinion that the answer that will do [the] most to protect the public health lies not in labeling (which is likely to be ignored), but in research," he wrote, as if both approaches could not be undertaken simultaneously.

Blasingame parroted the tobacco industry stand when he stated: "More than 90 million persons in the United States use tobacco in some form; and, of these, 72 million use cigarettes. Long standing social customs and practices are established in the use of tobacco; the economic lives of tobacco growers, processors, and merchants are entwined in the industry; and local, state and federal governments are the recipients of and dependent upon many millions of dollars of tax revenue. For these reasons, it is most appropriate that a subject of this magnitude, regarding the labeling and advertising of tobacco, be controlled by the Congress of the United States in the form of enacted legislation, if any, rather than promulgated administrative regulations."[25]

The AMA position sent the medical world into a spin. The American Cancer Society, the Public Health Service, and many physician groups supported warning labels and tightening of regulation of cigarette advertising. Responding to the AMA's startling stand, FTC commissioner A. Everett MacIntyre said: "I'm really perplexed. Thousands of doctors and many individual medical societies favor the proposed warnings, but the AMA . . . [says] there is no further need for educational statements to the youth. This is precisely the position of the tobacco industry."

Dr. Alton Ochsner, an eminent chest surgeon from Tulane University School of Medicine, was angered. He was an expert on the cigarette–lung cancer connection, having noted as early as 1910 an unusual case of lung cancer in a smoker and reported on the link in the 1930s. He said the AMA was being "derelict" as a leader in health and its industry-supported research on tobacco was "just delaying tactics" because smoking was so obviously harmful. "Personally, I think the AMA is wrong in conducting more research. I think we have the answers right now," he said.

Blasingame shot back: "It seems to me that Dr. Ochsner and those who share his opinion are really advocating that an agency of the federal government be granted the power to destroy an $8 billion industry on the extreme theory that the American people need to be protected from themselves in the matter of smoking."[26]

U.S. Representative Frank Thompson Jr., (D-N.J.), an advocate for the Medicare plan to cover the hospitalization of the elderly, went for the jugular. He charged the AMA was siding with the tobacco industry in exchange for votes against Medicare. "It's an outrage and it's an obvious plot," he said. However, Representative Harold D. Cooley, a North Carolina Democrat, himself a tobacco grower, a leader in the tobacco bloc in Congress and chairman of the House Agriculture Committee, defended the AMA, contending Thompson's charges were "not only untrue—it is fantastic and an outrage to the House." Blasingame in turn told Thompson the charges were "slanderous . . . an unjustified assault on the integrity of the officials of the AMA and upon your colleagues in the Congress."[27]

As to the warning labels, the AMA strategy of having Congress decide won. In a classic deal, tobacco-state congressmen agreed to put warning labels on cigarette packs in exchange for a promise that warnings would be kept out of cigarette advertising for at least five years. Following this precedent, the tobacco industry has left its mark on virtually all legislation relating to tobacco and health, showing a willingness to concede on some points in exchange for not getting clobbered with something worse.

In exchange, tobacco-state congressmen helped impede passage of Medicare legislation. In the midst of their meeting in 1964, AMA delegates rose to their feet and cheered when it was announced that the House Ways and Means Committee had failed to pass Medicare.[28]

The AMA and the tobacco industry had become a mutual-aid society. Despite AMA denials of collusion with tobacco interests, the confidential memo from the Tobacco Institute reveals the AMA's extraordinary concern about offending tobacco-state congressmen. Muckrakers Drew Pearson and Jack Anderson described the AMA-tobacco industry relationship as "the weirdest lobbying alliance in legislative history." They said the doctors' lobby and the cigarette lobby worked in tandem: "The doctors were more concerned about Medicare, which they fancied to be a threat to their fees, than about the threat to the nation's lungs. So it happened that those who abet and those who cure illness lay down together in millennial bliss."[29]

The AMA Echos the Surgeon General Fourteen Years Later

Tobacco-industry-funded research under the auspices of AMA-ERF continued until 1972, having involved some 844 researchers who worked on 219 separate projects. In 1978, fourteen years after the original funding was obtained, the AMA released its concluding report, summarizing the AMA-ERF studies, most of which were six to twelve years old. The AMA group said its research "had not altered the conclusions of the 1964 report of the Surgeon General."[30]

But more interesting than the AMA-ERF report itself was the AMA's use of its release to harass the President. The AMA's report was publicized while Carter was visiting tobacco country. At the time, tobacco interests were up in arms over the campaign against smoking being waged by Joseph Califano, Jr., Carter's Secretary of Health, Education and Welfare. Califano, a reformed three-pack-a-day smoker, described smoking as "slow-motion suicide. . . . Public Health Enemy Number One." Politically, Carter must have agreed with bumper stickers cropping up in the tobacco belt: CALIFANO IS DANGEROUS TO MY HEALTH. On the defensive, the Georgia Democrat joked to a pro-tobacco audience that Califano had encouraged him to visit: "He said it was time for the White House staff to start smoking something regular"—a reference to media reports about marijuana use by members of his staff.[31]

Responding to the AMA-ERF study, Carter said: "Nobody need fear the facts about tobacco use. Certainly, no one need fear the emphasis on research that will make the use of tobacco in the future even more safe than it has been in the past." The Tobacco Institute said it could not have written it better.

But the institute contended that the AMA "contrived" release of the document to humiliate Carter. Dr. James H. Sammons, the AMA's executive vice president, denied these charges, claiming "a series of "unforeseen circumstances," including strikes resulting in delays in producing the clothbound cover and in obtaining packing material, an equipment malfunction in printing news releases, and an error in mailing. Whatever the reason, it served the AMA's purpose to embarrass Carter, who encountered AMA opposition to his plan to save billions in medical costs by capping hospital bills. Playing both sides of the fence, the AMA ultimately defeated the legislation with the help of Southern legislators.[32]

Meanwhile the AMA-ERF report gave the AMA some standing as a tobacco opponent, and the group in 1978 was invited to testify concerning its report on tobacco before the House Subcommittee on Oversight and Investigations. This was the first time the AMA had appeared before

Congress on this issue since Surgeon General Terry issued the first warning in 1964. Around this time, in a Senate Subcommittee on Health and Scientific Research hearing on a health-promotion act in 1978, the AMA revealed without fanfare that it favored legislation to create warning labels on cigarette packages with changing messages and other anti-tobacco measures. This was fourteen years after the AMA had first opposed warning labels. At last the AMA seemed to be acting like a group of doctors concerned about its patients' health. However, the AMA's powerful lobby did not pick up the ball and run on the tobacco issue. The AMA would not testify before Congress on tobacco issues again for another seven years, until 1985.

STUDENTS AND RESIDENTS REBEL
AGAINST AMA SILENCE

Meanwhile the AMA waffled on, failing to take the lead on the tobacco issue. In 1979 Congress had before it more than a dozen bills aimed at reducing smoking, an addiction the federal government then estimated was responsible for more than 300,000 deaths a year. The legislation attempted to strengthen warning labels on cigarette packages and advertisements, regulate smoking on airplanes, eliminate advertising expenses as a business deduction by manufacturers, prohibit cigarette makers from adding chemicals to prevent cigarettes from extinguishing themselves, and boost taxes on cigarettes in hopes of persuading smokers to quit.

By this time the AMA officially supported some of these approaches to control tobacco. But some medical-student and young-physician members of the AMA began wondering if the AMA was putting its legendary clout in Washington behind antitobacco legislation. Ronald M. Davis, the AMA student delegate, was outraged when he reviewed the AMA's list of statements to Congress and federal agencies. The University of Chicago student found the AMA had not testified on any of the legislation, and had not even written a single letter in support of the antitobacco bills consistent with AMA policy. The AMA had chosen to be silent and wasn't lobbying against tobacco.

The Student Business Section introduced at the AMA annual meeting in 1980 a resolution that Davis wrote, calling on the House of Delegates to "reaffirm its commitment to improving the health of the American people by commencing vigorous, persistent and ongoing lobbying for smoking-related bills." The get-tough resolution also called on the AMA to report annually on the status of smoking-related legislation and what AMA lobbyists had done regarding each of them.

There was a sinking suspicion among some students and physicians in training that the AMA was on the side of the tobacco industry. As a final "resolve," the students drew a line in the sand, demanding the AMA to show where it stood on tobacco. They pressed the AMA to acknowledge that it opposed the tobacco industry, and to affirm that "the health of the American public as a whole supersedes all other concerns."

The AMA had to think about the question, though. It had courted the students and young physicians, whom it desperately needed as members to sustain the organization, but older, established doctors generally did not share the young people's vision of what the AMA ought to be doing. After holding a hearing, a reference committee urged that the House of Delegates reject Davis's resolution. The committee argued that the AMA already had done its bit to fight tobacco. More seasoned delegates thought it would cause an undue burden on AMA lobbyists to fight for antitobacco legislation in the face of other pressing problems, such as Medicare funding and government regulation of medicine, with which it was contending at the time.

Sensing defeat, the students submitted a watered-down amendment that merely called on delegates to go on record as requesting the AMA's Washington lobbyists to *monitor* tobacco legislation and to inform delegates of any important developments. But even this amendment received a cool reaction. Dr. F. William Dowda, a delegate from Georgia, spoke out against adopting the resolution merely to "appease" the students. The Atlanta internist, a nonsmoker himself, said the AMA had only "so many Brownie points per year" it could use to gain access to Congress. "If the lobbyists became involved with smoking, then they are going to have to give up something in the health legislative line," Dowda said. "I realize that it is a windmill that the Student Section has, and of course I also have my own windmills. I respect theirs and I hope they respect mine, but I think at this time we should not do anything to impair the effectiveness of our Washington lobbyists. . . ."[33]

Some delegates were extremely callous about tobacco. One, a prominent university professor, said: "Smoking is not all that much of a problem because those who get cancer of the lungs don't last very long but other things [diseases] do." Comments denigrating the significance of the students' resolution and the tobacco issue embarrassed other delegates. The House of Delegates was humiliated into supporting the diluted resolution.

Dr. Daniel T. Cloud, a pediatric surgeon from Phoenix, who served as AMA president in 1981–82, discovered that the worst fears and suspicions of the students and residents about AMA lobbyists not pushing tobacco issues had a basis in truth. As he traveled around the country making speeches, Cloud pointed out that half of health-care costs were tied to preventable diseases, such as smoking-induced cancers and heart disease.

After one speech was reported in the press, Cloud recalled that the AMA received a letter from Senator Jesse Helms, the North Carolina Republican who was tobacco's No. 1 champion. Helms's letter expressed displeasure with the antitobacco positions being taken by some AMA officials. Cloud said the AMA's chief executive, Dr. Sammons, "was very distressed about the letter. He called me. He was upset that I might answer it, and he persuaded me not to write an answer. He said that Senator Helms had written it to satisfy his constituency and that no reply was needed. [Sammons] said, 'I've been in telephone contact with him. It's a done deal now. They've written their letter. They're going to show their people they wrote us and scolded us and now that's the end of it.'"

Cloud said it dawned on him that "this was sort of the game we were playing. I guess there had been a tacit understanding prior to that time between the tobacco-state lawmakers and the AMA that the AMA would lay off, if the tobacco people would support us in the fight against the government." He added, "We did have support [from the Southern bloc], and we got the support because of our laying off the tobacco issue," said the former AMA president. Smoking was striking down Americans by the hundreds of thousands a year, but, Cloud said, "We were not standing up. We were not doing what [Reagan-era Surgeon General C. Everett] 'Chick' Koop was doing and beating the drums against tobacco."[34]

INVESTING IN TOBACCO

The AMA not only got into bed politically with tobacco interests, but it even to a small extent bet its members' pensions on the economic success of the tobacco industry. In 1979 the resident physicians, under the leadership of Dr. Alan Blum, founder of Doctors Ought to Care (DOC), a health-promotion group, learned that the AMA's Members Retirement Fund owned $1.4 million in tobacco securities. The young doctors quietly tried to persuade AMA management to unload the stock. But AMA chief Sammons told the residents in a letter in October 1979 that it was not appropriate for the AMA to "inject itself into the investment field" and order its fund managers not to buy tobacco stocks. He was concerned that other special interests within the AMA would try to tell the organization how to invest. Sammons said that the point of the funds was to make money, and besides, the AMA-owned tobacco stocks represented less than 3 percent of the AMA portfolio.[35] In other words, the AMA was not about to sell the stock.

In summer 1980, disgruntled residents persuaded the AMA Resident Physicians Section to present a resolution to the House of Delegates declaring "that AMA fiduciary responsibility to the public is greater than its fiduciary responsibility to its investment portfolio." When the matter came up before the House in 1981, the residents were rebuffed by their elders. Dr. John J. Coury, Jr., chairman of the AMA Board's finance committee, argued that the purpose of the pension fund was "to make the biggest buck," not to make social statements. He contended that interfering with the investment managers would violate federal Security and Exchange Commission regulations. AMA officials also attempted to minimize the issue by noting that "tobacco" companies were highly diversified and were involved in many nontobacco industries.[36]

Advocates for selling the stock as a matter of principle lost the battle but they won the war. Newspaper editorialists and cartoonists had "a field day" with the AMA and its tobacco stocks, said an AMA spokeswoman. For instance, one editorial cartoon in the *Chicago Tribune* depicted a doctor speaking to a patient about his tobacco habit. In the background is a newspaper with the headline CIGARETTE STOCK IN AMA PENSION FUND. The doctor states: "I can't say this strongly enough, Mr. Morson. . . . If your cigarettes are made by anybody other than Philip Morris or Reynolds Industries, you've got to stop smoking!"[37]

The bad publicity was causing heartburn at AMA headquarters. Quietly, the portfolio managers sold off the tobacco stocks. In 1985, the AMA officially informed its investment brokers that tobacco securities could not be purchased without prior approval by the AMA Board or its finance committee. What the AMA leadership lacked in conscience, it substituted with sensitivity to public relations and image.[38]

THE TOBACCO-GROWING AMA PRESIDENT

The AMA leaders' resolve to fight tobacco was challenged in a very personal way at the June 1985 meeting. It was a turning point that resulted in the organization's going on the record with stronger antitobacco policy.

Dr. A. Stuart Hanson, an AMA alternate delegate from Minnesota, told a hearing at the meeting: "The AMA is an embarrassment to me. We need to have our own house in order." The Minneapolis lung specialist said AMA leaders ought to be at the vanguard in the war against tobacco. However, he said, two of the AMA's top leaders had difficulty refraining from puffing in public, and two AMA Board members, though non-smokers, owned a farm on which tobacco was grown. Hanson said the AMA leaders had to change their ways if they wanted the organization to retain any measure of trust from the public, the profession, and its own membership.

The AMA confirmed to the *Chicago Sun-Times,* the only general press covering the session, that two of its board members, Dr. Harrison L. Rogers, the AMA's president-elect, who was to be inaugurated two days later, and board member Dr. F. William Dowda, Rogers' longtime friend from Atlanta, owned a 200-acre farm near the Okefenokee Swamp in Georgia, on which a tenant farmer grew tobacco on seven acres. The AMA management defended the doctors' right to invest as they pleased. It also verified that its board chairman, Dr. Coury, and its outgoing president, Dr. Joseph F. Boyle, were "less than successful in their attempts to quit smoking."39

The AMA Board circled its wagons. But behind closed doors, Dr. Ronald Davis, who as a medical student had raised questions about the AMA's lack of action on tobacco and now was a resident-member of the board, offered an emotional and spirited defense of Hanson and expressed his own embarrassment about the situation. "I just defended him and the importance of symbolism," said Davis in an interview later. But his fellow board members essentially felt that their tobacco-farming and tobacco-smoking confreres had been victims of a "cheap shot." Outspoken opposition to tobacco had not yet become fashionable among the AMA's elite, who at the time still were provided their favorite cigarette brands while staying at the Needham House, the AMA's posh town house in Georgetown.

The symbolism of an AMA leader owning a farm on which tobacco was grown did not escape Rogers. He announced he was considering his options. He said in an interview years later: "I did not really want to remain in that position of having to go around the country and answer that question every time I hit some new town. You know, 'Why do you grow tobacco?'" After a few months, he sold his portion of the farm to Dowda.40

AMA Delegates Get on the Antismoking Bandwagon

At this same meeting, where AMA leaders were vilified for their tobacco ties, delegates began building a strong antitobacco platform. They churned out antitobacco resolutions at an unprecedented pace. Of the more than one hundred statements on tobacco listed by the AMA in its policy book in 1993, 80 percent were adopted from 1985 onward.

In June 1985 the House approved a package of resolutions aimed at fighting tobacco and polishing the tarnished image of the House of Medicine. Dr. Ed L. Calhoon, a delegate from Beaver, Oklahoma, and a member of the federal government's National Cancer Advisory Board, urged delegates to take a strong stance because the nation's largest medical group had been perceived by some of its members and the public as being "a bit negligent in trying to speak to this issue." Delegates passed a resolution introduced by Calhoon entitled "A Smoke-Free Society by the Year 2000," which put the AMA on record as undertaking "a major effort" to strengthen its antismoking activities.[41]

The AMA also decided to get its own house in order. Delegates urged all physicians to stop using tobacco products and ordered the association's top staff to discourage smoking inside the Chicago headquarters and offer assistance to employees to quit. The delegates adopted a resolution requesting the AMA to support programs to eliminate smoking indoors where it would be harmful to others. Following the June 1985 meeting, the AMA removed cigarette vending machines from its headquarters. Delegates also called for an end to federal price supports for tobacco. The AMA once again seemed to be on its way to combating the tobacco epidemic.

Opposing Lawsuits to Fight Tobacco

However, the AMA Board announced a plan at the December 1985 meeting that appeared to place the self-interest of physicians in preventing malpractice suits ahead of its opposition to tobacco. The new flap arose when the board issued a report calling for opposition to a campaign by some tobacco foes to urge that the victims of tobacco-induced disease or their survivors file liability suits against tobacco companies. The board report characterized the liability suits as "an ineffective and unwieldy tool for shaping public policy" that would cause "a prohibitively high cost to society." The board contended that education and legislation would have greater impact than costly suits, which it said had not proven effective in getting people to quit smoking.[42]

Advocates for the lawsuits came out swinging. They said they supported the suits because the litigation was designed to harm cigarette manufacturers and to try to price cigarettes out of the reach of smokers, especially children. Dr. Michael Charney, cochairman of the Tobacco Products Liability Project, said antismoking efforts would suffer a serious setback if the AMA opposed liability suits. Northeastern University law professor Richard Daynard, Charney's cochairman, speculated at the time that the AMA Board may have opposed the lawsuits because it needed tobacco interests as "lobbying buddies" on pet legislation, such as a federal bill to reform malpractice laws.[43]

At the AMA's December interim meeting, many delegates voiced concerns about the board report. Dr. Richard F. Corlin, a California delegate, said the conclusions were "a misstatement of fact" since the tobacco liability suits seemed to be changing public policy.

However, Dr. Robert E. McAfee, an AMA trustee and one of the organization's most outspoken critics of the tobacco industry, pushed "across-the-board" reform of torts—from liability suits against doctors to those against tobacco companies. He also complained that the same attorneys who sued tobacco companies were the ones who took on physicians. "Should [San Francisco attorney] Melvin Belli [the so-called King of Torts] be shaping the nation's health policy?" asked McAfee, a surgeon from South Portland, Maine, who would be AMA president-elect in 1993. Corlin replied, "When it comes to suing the tobacco industry, we should find something nice to say about Mr. Belli."

To make peace, the AMA House watered down the final version of the report so it essentially contained nothing controversial. Delegates deleted the offending lines questioning the value of the tobacco liability suits.[44]

BANNING TOBACCO ADVERTISING

While the AMA got heat on the liability issue, it generally won praise at the same meeting for proposing a ban on cigarette advertising. Ultimately, however, the campaign for an ad ban did not succeed as the AMA's Washington lobbyists, in a pattern that has repeated itself many times, provided little muscle. The AMA's failure to use its political leverage to fight tobacco interests is legendary among antitobacco lobbyists and congressional staffers.

The AMA Board asked the House of Delegates to support a ban on cigarette advertising in magazines and newspapers as well as other cigarette promotion. It was a potentially important approach to help prevent children and adolescents from taking up smoking. Antitobacco groups view cigarette promotion as the manufacturers' means to addict the next generation of smokers. AMA chief Sammons contended that ad-ban legislation and public education offered "a quicker resolution of the tobacco problem" than would a strategy of suits against tobacco companies.

It was apparent that bringing about a tobacco-ad ban would not be easy. The AMA might receive support from tobacco opponents, but other powerful special interests, including publishers, the advertising industry, and civil libertarians, would oppose a ban as a violation of constitutional guarantees of free speech. "We have a legal product. We work under the same Constitution as all those [medical] people," said the communications director for tobacco giant Philip Morris, which held itself up as a defender of free speech and in 1991 even purchased sponsorship of the Bill of Rights Bicentennial. Some legal scholars said if an advertisement was not deceptive, it should not be prohibited.

But the AMA dug in its heels. After having been criticized so often about being weak on tobacco issues, it hoped to persuade doctors and the public that it was a public-health advocate. AMA general counsel Kirk B. Johnson argued that an advertising ban would be upheld because cigarette ads use deceptive themes to create an image of "good health and youthful vigor" and because commercial speech does not have the same legal standing as personal speech. The AMA even hired two Columbia law professors to study the issue. Based on legal precedent, particularly a ban of advertising for gambling aimed at local residents in Puerto Rico that had been found constitutional, they concluded a cigarette-ad ban could be upheld in the courts.[45]

To sponsor the legislation, the AMA chose Representative Mike Synar, a Democrat from Muskogee, Oklahoma, with a reputation for antagonizing special interests and refusing funding from political action committees. The AMA pledged to work in the trenches on the issue and to have its grass-roots network of doctors pressure their federal legislators to vote for the bill. The AMA promise of help "was very explicit," said a lobbyist from another health group, who had discussed the arrangements with Synar.

The AMA helped draft the bill and testified before Congress. And to help publicize the legislation, the AMA, in an unconventional move for such a conservative organization, printed black-bordered "obituary postcards" which physicians could send to federal legislators to inform them of the death of a constituent from tobacco-caused disease and to ask them to support the ad ban.

But in the end, AMA lobbyists essentially were a no-show. Kim Koontz-Bayliss, Synar's former legislative aide on health, said the AMA did not provide the sort of "scorched-earth" campaign for which she had hoped. "I think they were very helpful, but it was not their first priority," she said.

Most involved agree that the AMA failed to use its clout in Congress to get votes required to pass an ad ban. Synar's legislation never even made it to a subcommittee vote.

The AMA Bails Out on an Aircraft Smoking Ban

The AMA would have made a logical ally to help push a ban on smoking aboard aircraft through Congress. After all, in 1986, as part of its plan for a "tobacco-free society by the year 2000" the House of Delegates endorsed such a ban. But in 1987, when Congressman Richard J. Durbin introduced a bill to prohibit smoking, the AMA again was absent.

When Durbin was a teen, his father died from tobacco-related disease. After Durbin was elected to Congress in 1982, the Illinois Democrat set out to do something to put a dent in the tobacco epidemic. A member of the House Appropriations Transportation and Agriculture subcommittees, Durbin decided exactly what to do after he was assigned, against his wishes, to a smoking section on a flight from Phoenix to Chicago. Backed by a National Academy of Sciences report about the dangers of cigarette smoke to nonsmoking airline passengers, Durbin dedicated himself to passing a prohibition of smoking aboard commercial aircraft.

The congressman introduced a broad bill to ban smoking aboard aircraft. But, facing major opposition from senior members of Congress from tobacco states, he couldn't move the bill out of committee. Durbin then wrote a more limited proposal to outlaw smoking only on flights lasting two hours or less, which represented about 80 percent of domestic flights. He wasn't optimistic, but he had a bold plan. He would do an end run around the subcommittee and committee and introduce the ban as part of the transportation spending bill.

Durbin's bill unexpectedly passed in July 1987 by a narrow margin. "It was amazing. No one had really taken the tobacco lobby on with a frontal attack like this before. They didn't take us seriously, which was their real misfortune because we won by five votes on the floor (198–193) . . . with a very strong coalition, Republicans and Democrats, liberal-conservative, east, west, north and south," said Durbin. The law was a popular one and was implemented without the chaos predicted by tobacco advocates. But it expired two years after it had passed. Legislation adopted in 1989 made the smoking ban permanent and extended it to about 99 percent of all commercial domestic flights.

The AMA claimed credit for the victory. The AMA in 1989 mailed recruitment letters that boasted about its role in getting the smoking ban on aircraft passed. This galled lobbyists from health groups active on the bill. Durbin said the Association of Flight Attendants and the Coalition on Smoking OR Health helped get the bill through. Durbin bluntly said that the AMA was "not there, and there was no evidence of any strong support for our effort from the American Medical Association."

Durbin saluted the AMA for cosponsoring legislative strategy sessions in recent years for antismoking forces. However, he added, "I think there's much more interest in the AMA in this debate on national health care and how it's going to affect the delivery of health services and the practice of medicine in America. When you start dealing with public-health issues, like tobacco, I don't believe that is the No. 1 item on their agenda. I think it frankly is down the list."[46]

THE PROMOTION BAN FAILS IN THE HOUSE

The next major tobacco issue to come along was the most comprehensive bill to fight tobacco promotion ever introduced. The AMA, which was committed on paper to such legislation, again failed to get involved.

After the ban on smoking aboard airplanes was made permanent, the spirits of antitobacco lobbyists were lifted. They began to feel a great deal more might be possible. Representative Henry A. Waxman, chairman of the House Subcommittee on Health and the Environment, introduced the most sweeping antitobacco legislation to date: H.R. 5041, the Tobacco Control and Health Protection Act. The legislation thumbed its nose at the $3.6 billion tobacco advertising and promotion industry. The bill would eliminate tobacco advertising and promotion as it had been known in this country, the $2 billion orgy of images of cowboys puffing on cigarettes in Marlboro Country, bone-thin Virginia Slims gals and Joe Camel, the James Bond–like cartoon character used to hype Camels, and the portraits of youthful swimmers, skiers, and other athletes enjoying a smoke—though their cigarettes rarely are lit. The legislation would have allowed print advertising to continue in the form of "tombstone" ads, showing a cigarette pack against a neutral background.

The bill would have prohibited tobacco companies from promoting athletic, musical, and artistic events, the nearly $1 billion effort to tie smoking to popular culture and the fine arts by placing signs for cigarettes in sports stadiums so that they are flashed on broadcasts of games, and associating cigarette brands with leading ballet companies and art exhibitions. In addition, the bill would have punched up warning labels by explicitly noting, other among things, that "Cigarettes Kill," stopped the insidious placement of cigarette products in movies and TV shows, and required states to enforce laws against the sale of tobacco to minors. The tobacco industry was expected to wage an all-out battle against the advertising provisions, again claiming Constitutional violations.

The Physician/Congressman from Tobacco Country

Waxman, who has worked closely with the AMA over the years, said he considered the AMA an "activist" on tobacco issues because it has strong antitobacco policies and because it has testified against tobacco before Congress.[47] But other congressional insiders insist that the AMA didn't deliver on Waxman's bill.[48] When it was clear that the vote on the Waxman bill was going to be close, the legislation's supporters asked the AMA to "get us" the vote of Congressman J. Roy Rowland, a close AMA ally and a member of the subcommittee. One of only two physicians in Congress at that time, Rowland had been effective in getting through a number of bills on medical matters, such as AIDS, infant deaths, and rural health. Rowland was a top recipient of donations from the AMPAC, and he had helped grease the skids in 1991 for AMA-designed "antihassle" legislation to reduce Medicare paperwork and regulation of doctors. Health lobbyists hoped that Rowland would promote antitobacco legislation. As a family physician, he had seen his patients suffer from cigarette-related disease. Concerned about the risks, he gave up smoking in 1967, three years after the first Surgeon General's report. But there was one obstacle to winning Rowland's support, and a major one at that—his voters: the thousands of tobacco growers and the employees of the cigarette factory in his district near Macon, Georgia.

Rowland's loyalty to his constituents rang out clearly during hearings on H.R. 5041, in the congressman's hostile questioning of supporters of the bill, during which he asked what they were going to do about the welfare of the tobacco workers who would be displaced by a smoke-free society. In an extraordinary exchange, famed cancer surgeon Dr. William G. Cahan, of Memorial Sloan-Kettering Hospital in New York, turned the tables on Rowland.

> Rowland: Are you doing anything to help these people who may lose their jobs? Are you addressing it from that standpoint at all?

Cahan: Mr. Rowland, I understand you are a physician. Is that true?

Rowland: That is true.

Cahan: Do you think smoking causes lung cancer?

Rowland: Absolutely.

Cahan: You do?

Rowland: Absolutely. I am supposed to be asking the questions. Not you. . . . I am concerned about the people having jobs in the district I represent.

Cahan: Are we talking in those terms? Are we concerned about the poor people in Colombia being laid off because of the lack of demand for cocaine? . . . You and I have seen too many lives destroyed by this to think about necessarily getting to the . . . point whether somebody's job is in jeopardy. . . . I think your higher interest, the Hippocratic oath so-called, is to "do no harm." As a physician to a physician, you and I are both trying to keep people well and alive. That is our prime consideration.[49]

The AMA did not bother to lobby Dr. Rowland on this bill. AMA chief Dr. James S. Todd, a registered lobbyist, contended the AMA works hard on tobacco issues, but views Rowland in particular as a lost cause on this subject. "We know Rowland is rigid on [tobacco]. We don't waste time on him. Why bang your head against a stone wall?" said Todd.[50]

When Waxman's subcommittee voted on the proposed advertising and promotion ban in September 1990, Rowland was involved in maneuvers to cripple and then euthanize the legislation. First, he voted for an amendment to remove the tombstone advertising provision. Then, when the revised bill came up, he voted against it. The legislation made it out of the subcommittee, but died of inaction before the full Committee on Energy and Commerce. Strategists contended the bill might have had a fighting chance if the AMA had leaned on Rowland and the congressman had came out in favor of the advertising and promotion restrictions.[51]

Despite his shortcomings on issues of tobacco and health, Rowland remained an AMA favorite. The AMA in recent years has bestowed upon those it considers to have worked for the public health the Nathan S.

Davis Awards, named for the AMA's founder and first editor of its *Journal*. The award has gone to the likes of Dr. C. Everett Koop, the former Surgeon General; Waxman; Senator Edward M. Kennedy; and Senator Orrin G. Hatch, all of whom have fought against tobacco. The 1992 Davis recipients included Representative J. Roy Rowland.[52]

Tobacco opponents were aghast. Clifford E. Douglas, then associate director of government relations at the American Lung Association, said, "Dr. Rowland has consistently championed the interests of the to-bacco industry. He has actively opposed measures designed to protect children from tobacco addiction and even voted against legislation to eliminate smoking on airplanes. It is hypocritical for the AMA to see fit to honor this Member of Congress with an award recognizing his contributions to betterment of the public health."

AMA chief executive Todd, who served on the "independent" panel that selected Rowland, stood by the award, saying Rowland has "a defect from the point-of-view of certain people, [but] on balance Roy Rowland has been a positive force for health in Congress. To deal with one issue only, that is a luxury the AMA doesn't have."[53]

Following the Rowland affair, the message to members of Congress was that it is possible to oppose responsible antitobacco measures the AMA tacitly supported and still be a hero to organized medicine. As a Davis-award recipient, Congressman Rowland has a Steuben crystal bowl engraved with his name to prove it.

AN ANEMIC RESPONSE IN THE SENATE

In the Senate, too, when the tobacco epidemic was being attacked, the AMA was cited for its weak performance. Senator Edward Kennedy, chairman of the Labor and Human Resources Committee, introduced the Tobacco Product Education and Health Protection Act of 1990 that would have created a center within the Department of Health and Human Services to regulate tobacco products, given grants to the states for antismoking activities, and strengthened health-warning labels on tobacco-product packages and ads. This bill was approved by Kennedy's committee but got no further.

The AMA endorsed the legislation, and so was asked to mobilize its grass-roots network of state medical societies to enlist cosponsors. But when Dr. Mona Sarfaty, then senior health-policy adviser to the Senate Committee, checked on the AMA's progress periodically, she got only "a lot of hemming and hawing." Finally the AMA asked its state affiliates to write letters to their senators in support of the bill. This was far less than Sarfaty expected, since letters, if written at all, would not have the impact of phone calls or visits. She said the AMA involvement on the bill "was anemic, there was no follow-up, there was no direct contact. There was no real effort to make a priority issue of it in any way, and I was very angry."

If the AMA was anemic in this instance, it could be characterized as comatose when Kennedy in 1991 reintroduced the Tobacco Product Education and Health Protection Act. The revised bill would have created a Center for Tobacco and Health in the federal Centers for Disease Control. The agency would have promoted public education about tobacco's dangers, conducted research on tobacco use and cessation programs, and shared information about tobacco hazards with foreign countries, particularly poor countries considered vulnerable to the lure of American cigarettes. The bill would have forced cigarette makers to disclose ingredients on cigarette packs and would have made warning labels more hard-hitting.

This bill also took on the advertising issue in a fashion thought to be more palatable to industry than a total ban or tombstone ads. It would have authorized $50 million for grants for public-service announcements and paid advertisements to discourage people from falling victim to tobacco addiction and to persuade them to quit, especially those from high-risk groups, such as youths, pregnant women, minorities, and blue-collar workers.

The AMA again was asked to pitch in and again disappointed. When it came time to plan strategy, call in chits, and wear out shoe leather, the AMA was nowhere to be found. Douglas, then of the Coalition on Smoking OR Health, said he helped organize three strategy sessions on Capitol Hill of antitobacco groups, none of which the AMA attended. "An especially diligent effort was made to get the AMA to send a representative to attend the second strategy briefing. Several telephone calls and an invitation sent via facsimile did not succeed, however, in getting an AMA representative to attend the meeting or even in getting the organization to respond to the invitation," he said.

A disillusioned Sarfaty said, "[The AMA's] policies, on paper, sounded good, and they were willing to lend their name when it came to endorsement, but when the question was whether there was really going to be some of the lobbying that needed to be done, or even participating in strategy sessions, anything that really would seriously advance the cause of the bill, they were just not present and not helpful. It was very difficult to recruit them into the effort in any meaningful way."[54]

THE DEVIL'S MONEY FOR THE LORD'S WORK

By the late 1980s and early 1990s, the AMA seemed to want to become a strong advocate against smoking. But the activists within its ranks still had nagging doubts about its commitment to the issue.

On the positive side, the AMA was cranking out policy after policy against tobacco. And the AMA's Chicago legislative staff in 1989 filed petitions with federal and state agencies against a "smokeless" cigarette being tested in two states by R. J. Reynolds. RJR ended up withdrawing the product. The AMA, which a few years earlier wavered about a policy of using liability suits to fight tobacco companies, surprised everyone in 1991 by submitting a brief in the Supreme Court appeal of the Cipollone case, the highest-profile liability suit and the first in which damages were awarded.

Despite such moves, critics still did not trust their own organization. They felt the AMA was a paper tiger, all talk and no action on tobacco. At the AMA meeting in December 1992, the antitobacco forces raised questions about whether it was appropriate for the AMA to accept advertising revenues and grants for its public-health programs from nontobacco subsidiaries, such as food companies, owned by the tobacco conglomerates. Tobacco opponents considered this trading with the enemy.

But AMA leaders disagreed. They believed the AMA in effect was taking the Devil's money to do the Lord's work, and told the House of Delegates that if the AMA stopped accepting funding from tobacco subsidiaries, the organization would lose significant revenues and would either have to increase dues or eliminate some public-health programs. Besides, AMA honchos said, the group had no definition of what a tobacco company was: it knew not to take money from Marlboro, but was it wrong to accept funds from the General Foods side of Philip Morris or RJR's Fleischmann's margarine? Activists contended that accepting funds from any segment of these firms ought to be prohibited. The AMA House of Delegates directed the AMA Board to come back in June 1993 with a definition of a tobacco company to help decide from whom the AMA could ethically accept money.[55]

At the same gathering, Surgeon General Antonia C. Novello, the AMA delegate from the Public Health Service, spoke to a small group of AMA members who had formed a coalition in 1991 in hopes of moving the AMA from merely passing and filing resolutions to becoming true activists on tobacco issues. After hearing coalition members' complaints about AMA inactivity on tobacco issues, Novello summoned AMA chief executive Todd, who was attending another session. When he appeared, coalition leaders confronted him. Novello joined in, saying the AMA needed to start using its clout and know-how in Washington to more aggressively attack the tobacco epidemic.

Dr. Joel S. Dunnington, a coalition member and also a member of the board of the activist group DOC, informed Todd: "We perceived that the AMA didn't do much on tobacco issues. We have 11 pages of resolutions of AMA policy on tobacco, and when you call the Washington office they have no idea what's going on. If you look at the AMA legislative guide, it didn't have the word tobacco in it. AMA staff in Washington have no idea what's currently going on relating to tobacco in Congress. Tobacco has not been a priority."[56]

Such confrontations concerning tobacco between health advocates and AMA leaders have occurred repeatedly over the past decade. But the AMA continues to try to project the image of the organization being in the forefront in the war on tobacco. In fact, days after President Clinton was inaugurated in January 1993, the AMA ran an ad in the *Washington Post* headlined, DISEASE PREVENTION MUST BE A MAJOR PART OF HEALTH SYSTEM REFORM: STOPPING TOBACCO DEATHS IS OUR FIRST PRIORITY. The AMA noted it supported the idea of imposing a steep increase on the tax on cigarettes to discourage teens from taking up smoking and to encourage current smokers to quit. The AMA's ad informed the new Administration that the tax increase could save millions of lives and generate billions of dollars, which could be applied to reduce the deficit, to reform the health-care system, and to educate the public, especially children, about the dangers of smoking.[57]

At the end of the piece, the AMA listed a toll-free number through which more information could be obtained about the AMA's reform proposals. When Dunnington tried the number, his call rolled over to an employee in the AMA's membership-recruitment operation. Dunnington said the staffer knew nothing about the AMA's plans to fight tobacco.

Married to the Tobacco Mob?

In June 1993 the AMA Board unveiled its definition of the tobacco industry. Under the definition the AMA could not deal directly with tobacco companies, but could continue to trade with the companies' subsidiaries so long as they were not involved in the promotion of tobacco products.[59]

During a hearing of the Public Health Reference Committee, the board's definition was attacked vehemently. Dunnington gave example after example of how subsidiaries fought on behalf of their sister cigarette companies. For instance, Oscar Mayer Foods Corp., a sandwich-meat maker under the Philip Morris umbrella, lobbied against an ordinance to make restaurants smoke-free in its headquarters city. And Nabisco, a subsidiary of RJR, pulled $84 million in cookie accounts from advertising giant Saatchi & Saatchi after the agency prepared a TV commercial promoting an airline's pioneering smoke-free policy in 1989.

Dunnington told the committee: "Think of the tobacco parent corporations as being similar to the Mafia. If the Mafia buys the local concrete company, does that make it an honorable and legitimate organization?" Was the AMA married to the mob? In an uncharacteristic move, the reference committee repudiated the Board of Trustees' recommendation and accepted the view of the critics. The committee urged delegates to expand the definition of a tobacco company to include all subsidiaries.

When the full House of Delegates gathered, some longtime critics of AMA tobacco policy took the floor again to oppose the board's narrow definition. Dr. Stuart Hanson, who had exposed AMA leaders' ownership of a tobacco farm in 1985, urged the AMA not to be involved in the "nicotine drug trade." Dr. Ronald Davis, who as a medical student led the charge against tobacco in 1980, said, "These so-called diversified tobacco companies use their non-tobacco products to support tobacco. . . . If RJR Nabisco is using Oreo cookies to support tobacco, then I do not want our AMA to take money from Oreo cookies."

The AMA House was divided. Antitobacco advocates were on one side. On the other were representatives of medical schools, more than half of whom accept grants from the industry-supported Council for Tobacco Research, and the AMA Board, which argued forcefully for continued acceptance of subsidiary funds.[60] Dr. William Stoneman III, delegate from the Medical School Section, contended that a company should not be penalized and put on an AMA "blacklist" simply because it was purchased by a tobacco firm. He said to critics: "I think you're trying to be purer than Caesar's wife on this. It doesn't make common sense." Dr. John Ring, immediate past president of the AMA, speaking for the board, said the association needed potential contributions from tobacco subsidiaries to conduct its public-health programs.

When the vote came, the board won. The narrow definition of a tobacco company was adopted, allowing the organization to continue to accept and pursue tobacco-subsidiary funding. At a press conference afterward, AMA officials said they currently received no sponsorship from tobacco subsidiaries and were unable to estimate how much advertising revenue from tobacco subsidiaries was brought in by the AMA's journals and cable television operation. AMA chief Todd promised that the organization would be careful to evaluate subsidiaries before accepting funds, rejecting any that promoted tobacco in any fashion. From the tobacco opponents' viewpoint, acceptance of Oreo cookie money was tobacco business as usual.

A LONG WAY, BABY, BUT A LONG WAY TO GO

The AMA has come a long way from the times when it helped promote cigarette sales and protected the tobacco industry by conducting research on its behalf. Indeed, in recent years, the AMA has been out front on policies to fight the tobacco epidemic.

The AMA got a boost in July 1993, when it received a one-year $460,000 grant to organize a national office for a $10 million tobacco-control program for the Robert Wood Johnson Foundation.[61] This was quite a contrast from 1964, when it accepted the tobacco industry's proposal for a $10 million research program on cigarettes.

And in late March 1994, the AMA launched what it called "its largest and most comprehensive antitobacco and stop-smoking program ever." In its "How to Quit" program, the AMA turned to modern marketing technology, complete with a half-hour "infomercial" and 800 numbers, to sell a $69.95 kit with video and audio instruction to get people to break their addiction to nicotine.

The AMA said it would use its share of royalties to fund public health campaigns, including antismoking efforts.

But critics weren't buying the AMA's high-profile campaign. They berated the AMA for hyping a product that had not been tested in a rigorous scientific manner. And they pointed out that the AMA was not using its own funds to propel the antismoking push.

Once again, the critics said, the true test of the AMA would be whether it used its money and clout to lobby for antitobacco legislation. And it didn't.

The AMA still has a long way to go. In some ways, nothing has changed since 1980, when the idealistic students and resident physicians started their antitobacco campaign within the House of Medicine. It could be argued that in the biggest arena for national policy, the Congress, where AMA considers itself a potent force, the doctors' group has been preoccupied with issues it considers to be a higher priority, such as reform of the health-care system and other physician pocketbook issues. To keep faith with the public as well as its own members and House of Delegates, the AMA brass needs to move tobacco to the front burner in Washington, to put political clout behind the AMA's rhetoric.

CHAPTER 8

A Doctor's Right to Choose
Putting Physician Choice First in the Abortion Crisis

THE American Medical Association presents a third side to the nation's bitter and divisive abortion debate. Pro-lifers of course strive to protect the rights of fetuses, considering each of the 1.6 million abortions performed annually in the United States to be a murder. Pro-choice advocates seek to protect a woman's right to choose abortion as a fundamental civil liberty necessary for women to control their bodies and lives.

The AMA completes the triangle. Like the Roman god Mercury, holding up his caduceus with the two snakes as a sign of being a noncombatant, the AMA today claims to be "neutral" on the abortion issue. The AMA says it uses science to guard the public's health. But the AMA's approach to abortion seems more based on political expediency and retaining members than applying scientific research, which indicates that access to legal abortion reduces death rates for women.

The AMA has had a checkered history on abortion, shifting with the political winds as it suited the organization's purposes. From the late 1850s until 1900, the AMA placed the abortion debate on the national agenda, successfully campaigning for criminalization of the procedure. Historians generally agree that the AMA used the issue as a political tool to promote legislation to license physicians and undermine mainstream physicians' economic competitors.

After being silent on abortion for close to a century, in the 1960s and

1970s, the AMA, like many other institutions, grappled with the difficult medical and moral dilemmas created by abortion. The AMA faced a tension between those who wanted to liberalize abortion and those who considered abortion morally and ethically unacceptable. But as availability of abortion was increased by state legislatures and the courts, the AMA was forced to remove ethical barriers to physicians who chose to perform abortions. However, from the early 1980s to the present, as times have become more conservative, the AMA has insisted repeatedly that it is "neutral" on abortion. Yet, its policies point to the organization being pro-choice, or at least for a doctor's right to choose.

THE AMA'S PRO-LIFE CRUSADE

The "regular" medical profession in the mid–nineteenth century, when the AMA was founded, was buffeted by powerful societal forces. Mainstream—allopathic—medicine had yet to establish itself as a dominant social and economic force.

Allopathic practitioners, predecessors of today's scientific doctors, were threatened by the popularity of "irregular medicine." Irregular physicians, "wise women," and folk healers offered complete care to their patients. This included abortions, which allopathic healers pledged under the ancient ethical oath of Hippocrates not to perform.

The regulars also took note of the nation's dramatically falling birthrates among "native" Americans, the term for white Anglo-Saxon Protestants born in this country. They blamed this change in the social order on abortion, a common and legally accepted practice early in pregnancy.

Also, the first feminist movement had an impact at the time. Women were becoming more vocal about obtaining rights, such as voting and owning property, and they were campaigning against prostitution and slavery. The male establishment, including the male-dominated medical profession, considered this movement a menace to the status quo. Times were ripe for a backlash from the regular medical profession.

The AMA Crusaders

Using a mix of scientific, moral, and other arguments, Dr. Horatio Robinson Storer, a young Boston obstetrician-gynecologist, in the late 1850s spearheaded what turned into an AMA crusade to oppose abortion. Storer considered the average American uninformed about scientific developments regarding the fetus as a living being and unthinking about destroying fetuses. He contended that the practice was causing a ruinous slide in societal values. Working through the AMA, Storer thought doctors could put a stop to it.

At this time the AMA was a new organization, only ten years old, dedicated to improving medical education and running those it deemed quacks out of business. The fledgling AMA had yet to test its wings. In 1857 Storer and other pioneering right-to-lifers persuaded the AMA House of Delegates to appoint a committee to investigate abortion "with a view to its general suppression."[1]

Storer served as committee chairman. His fellow committee members were other physicians well-known for their opposition to abortion. One was Dr. Thomas Blatchford, of New York, who had publicly attacked the notorious Madame Restell, operator of a large-scale abortion agency with several branch offices on the Eastern Seaboard. The agency coyly advertised in newspapers its services to remove "menstrual obstructions."

The antiabortion crusade was the first successful national lobbying effort run by the AMA. The new organization gave would-be medical campaigners a platform from which they could achieve goals on a national scale never before possible for the medical profession. In the years prior to the Civil War, regular physicians were taking their first steps toward professionalization, using the AMA as their vehicle to control medical practice.

Historians have asserted that the battle against abortion aided the AMA's efforts to destroy the regulars' competition. The regulars deemed the willingness to perform abortion as a mark of distinction between themselves and the irregulars and grounds for opposition.

One of the AMA's key points in addressing the abortion issue was attacking the public's and the law's view of "quickening"—the concept that a fetus was alive only when the mother could feel it move or kick, an event that did not occur until the sixteenth to eighteenth week of pregnancy. Before quickening, induced abortion was generally tolerated and considered legal in the United States. In light of scientific knowledge of the day, the AMA Committee on Criminal Abortion thought it scandalous that the public did not realize fetuses were alive before quickening. By emphasizing medicine's scientific expertise, doctors were attempting to elevate their standing as a profession.

The committee at the annual meeting in 1859 criticized common and statutory law for ignoring the medical evidence for fetal life. Storer and his colleagues called upon physicians to stop the "slaughter of countless children" as well as to protect women from dangers at the hands of abortionists.[2]

Following its committee's recommendations, the House of Delegates opposed abortion not only after quickening but *throughout* pregnancy, except to preserve the life of the mother. The AMA also committed itself in the name of its "grand and noble calling" to save lives by working through its state affiliates to lobby for tougher antiabortion laws.[3]

As part of the campaign, the AMA in 1864 announced an essay contest on abortion. Dr. D. Humphreys Storer, Horatio's father, headed the judging committee, which announced the results at the AMA's annual session in 1865. Perhaps not surprisingly, Horatio himself wrote the winning essay, entitled "The Criminality and Physical Evils of Forced Abortion," having entered the tract with his name hidden by a seal, only to be broken on the convention platform.[4]

The essay sheds light on nineteenth-century medical views of society. Storer noted that it appeared that family size was shrinking among the so-called natives. He said this group's family size was deteriorating drastically, not because of a loss of "procreative abilities" but rather because the "natives" resorted increasingly to abortion.

Storer fanned xenophobic sentiments, citing a contemporary study showing the foreign-born who did not practice abortion were giving birth to more children than were the natives. He contended that not only did abortion harm mother and child and undermine morals, but it "strikes a blow at the very foundation of society itself."[5] He said Protestant natives in an act of self-protection ought to follow the example of Roman Catholics, among whom abortion was rare.

Storer said "native" women owed it to society to increase their birthrate; otherwise alien races would populate the Far West and the South. "This is a question that our own women must answer; upon their loins depends the future destiny of the nation," he said.[6]

The AMA published an expanded version of Storer's essay as a book, *Why Not? A Book for Every Woman,* to persuade the general public, especially women, that abortion was an evil. The book helped harden professional and public opinion against abortion. Storer followed up with similar antiabortion books aimed at men in 1867 and for lawyers, legal scholars, and lawmakers in 1868. Because of his declining health, Storer left the country in 1872, but regular physicians and their medical societies kept promoting criminalization of abortion to the public and legislatures.

The AMA Campaign Succeeds

The AMA crusade against abortion gained momentum as doctors successfully lobbied state by state for criminalization of abortion throughout pregnancy, not just after quickening. "The pressure of their crusade pushed state legislators beyond expressions of cautious concern about abortion and its possible excesses to straightforward opposition to the practice," according to abortion historian James Mohr, of the University of Oregon.[7]

The AMA campaign successfully changed the nation's abortion policy as states and territories passed tough laws. The new laws, often passed with nativist zeal, made abortion a felony, eliminated the distinction of quickening to make abortion illegal throughout gestation, and for the first time set down penalties against the women who had abortions. Between 1857 and the turn of the century, all states, except one, passed laws to restrict abortion. The single holdout, Kentucky, joined the rest in 1910.

In 1871 the AMA made its final statement on abortion in the nineteenth century; it would be its last major statement on the issue for nearly 100 years. The Committee on Criminal Abortion condemned physicians who continued to perform abortions, holding that the doctor's role was to be the protector not the destroyer of life and the advocate for God and not Satanic forces. The committee called for professional self-regulation and purification to remove abortionists, whom it referred to as "executioners" and "paid assassins."[8] The crusaders said doctors should take matters into their own hands and organize "a special police to watch, and to detect and to bring to justice these characters [abortionists]."[9]

In the view of the AMA, which was male-controlled by definition because women were excluded for the most part from allopathic medical schools, women essentially were breeders, who by aborting fetuses ignored their destiny to reproduce. In 1871 the Committee on Criminal Abortion said a woman who aborts "yields to the pleasures but shirks from the pains and responsibilities of maternity. . . . Let not the husband flatter himself that he possesses her affection. Nor can she in turn even merit the respect of a virtuous husband. She sinks into old age like a withered tree, stripped of its foliage; with the stain of blood upon her soul, she dies without the hand of affection to smooth her pillow."[10]

Ironically, the feminist movement of the time supported the AMA's antiabortion campaign. Feminist reformers fought abortion for their own reasons. They wanted to halt such abuses as women being forced against their wills to undergo abortion, and they also sought ways to make men responsible for their sexual indulgences.

Based on the report, the House of Delegates again denounced abortionists. However, delegates said a physician could perform an abortion if at least one other medical consultant agreed it was medically necessary, "and then always with a view to the safety of the child—if that be possible."[11] The medical profession was looking out for the fetus, the pregnant woman, and society at large, but it also was defending its own interests.[12]

According to Mohr, as the AMA and regular physicians gained control of medicine in the United States by the end of the nineteenth century, they no longer needed to press for abortion laws as a means of attacking the irregulars. He said, "By 1900 abortion no longer seemed to be a threat to the native population, and regular physicians had already successfully accomplished most of their personal and professional goals."[13]

The AMA provided a base from which Storer and like-minded colleagues helped shape public opinion and policy to criminalize abortion. AMA-inspired legislation remained on the books well into this century. However, these laws were not totally effective, and abortion continued to be performed underground, with sometimes disastrous results.[14]

REFORMING ANTIABORTION LAWS

After its 1871 report on abortion, the AMA did not concern itself with the matter again until the 1960s. The medical profession and the public were by that time being increasingly sensitized to the abortion issue. Many physicians already were well acquainted with the pain and hardship women endured to obtain illegal abortions and the doctors' difficulties in caring for women who arrived in emergency rooms dying from septic shock.

Then, there was the highly publicized case of a woman who wanted to abort a fetus she feared had been damaged by a tranquilizer. America in 1962 was caught up in the travail of Sherri Finkbine, a children's television personality from Phoenix. Early in her pregnancy, Finkbine, twenty-nine, the mother of four, had taken thalidomide. She soon learned the medication had caused grotesque limb damage in some European children. Although the Food and Drug Administration had not approved the drug, some Americans, such as Finkbine's husband, had brought it back from Europe. Fearing the worst, and on the advice of her doctor, Finkbine scheduled a "therapeutic abortion" in a Phoenix hospital. Since the time of the AMA antiabortion crusade, abortion could be performed legally only for *therapeutic* reasons. In such cases a fetus was aborted to save the life of the mother. But many desperate pregnant women used any ruse they could to try to qualify for a therapeutic abortion.

Finkbine told her story anonymously to a local newspaper in hopes of warning other women about the drug's side effects. When the article came out, the hospital canceled the operation, and Finkbine's efforts to abort the fetus became national news. She finally obtained an abortion in Sweden, where a pathologist confirmed the fetus had been a "monster."

The Finkbine case was dramatic, though thalidomide was not a large-scale threat in this country. The case however was a lightning rod for a public debate on abortion.

In the early and mid-1960s, the discussion about abortion was further energized by widespread concerns about fetal damage from the epidemics of German measles—rubella. Women whose fetuses might have been deformed by rubella did not meet the requirements for therapeutic abortion because the virus did not cause serious health problems to the mother. Still, rubella could wreak havoc during early development. An infected fetus faced the potential for deformed limbs, brain damage, blindness, deafness, and other problems. Frightened about possible side effects, many women received a sympathetic hearing from doctors and hospital abortion committees. The hospital committees had been established in the 1950s to prevent hospitals from being used to perform abortions for nontherapeutic reasons.

By the late 1960s, abortion was permissible only in forty-five states to preserve or save the *life* of the mother; whereas the mother's *health* generally was not supposed to be a consideration. But that was not the reality of abortion in the mid-1960s. At that time, about 10,000 abortions a year were being performed in American hospitals, few of them to preserve or save the mother's life. They commonly were performed for "fetal indications," such as the fetus having possible damage from rubella.

Only five states and the District of Columbia permitted abortion to preserve *the health* of the mother. And doctors approved up to one half of abortions because the pregnancy posed a threat to the mother's *mental health*. [15] The claim was made in such cases that women were threatening to kill themselves unless they had an abortion.

The Finkbine case and the rubella outbreaks softened both the attitude of the public and doctors concerning therapeutic abortion. Couples seeking abortions were shocked when they experienced the humiliating ordeal of obtaining a legal therapeutic abortion. Physicians, lawyers, and other policy leaders began to think seriously about reforming, even repealing, the nearly century-old state laws passed in response to the AMA crusade.

The AMA Revisits Abortion

With the growing confusion about what to do about abortion, the conservative AMA Board of Trustees decided in 1965 to revisit the issue. It

appointed a Committee on Human Reproduction, chaired by a prominent Roman Catholic obstetrician/gynecologist, to investigate abortion.
The committee presented proposed guidelines on abortion to the AMA
annual assembly in 1965. The policy was primarily based on model legislation recommended in 1962 by the American Law Institute, a group of
judges, lawyers, and legal scholars that periodically proposes legal reforms. The AMA committee said legislation should be passed to allow
physicians to perform an abortion only under certain circumstances:
when it could be established that continuing the pregnancy would
"gravely impair" the mother's physical or mental health; when there was
a "substantial risk" that the child would be born with a "grave physical or
mental defect"; and when it was legally established that the pregnancy
resulted from statutory or forcible rape or incest. The committee also
urged that abortion be performed only in hospitals and that two physicians other than the doctor performing the abortion support in writing
the need for the operation.

The committee's recommendations went beyond existing legislation,
and would have placed the AMA in the position of recommending
changes in state laws. Many delegates did not want the organization to be
a leader on such a controversial and divisive issue. As a result, the AMA
reference committee, which heard discussion on the report, concluded
that the AMA ought to defer to the individual states and their local medical societies. The House of Delegates was left to sort out conflicting religious, ethical, and legal questions. In the end, delegates ducked the
controversy and referred the report back to the Board of Trustees to further explore the issues with the American Bar Association and other
groups.

As the AMA mulled over the issues the next few years, the states began reforming their laws. Colorado led the way with passage of the first
modern abortion law, basing it on the American Law Institute blueprint.
In April 1967 Republican governor John Love signed a bill allowing
abortions in hospitals for women who were at risk of permanent mental
or physical damage from their pregnancies or who had been impregnated through rape or incest. The next month, North Carolina passed an
ALI-type law.

Then, Republican California governor Ronald Reagan in June 1967
signed a liberalized law, supported by the AMA's California affiliate, permitting abortion when the mother's health was at risk and when the pregnancy was the result of rape or incest. The future pro-life President,
however, persuaded legislators to remove a provision that allowed an
abortion to be performed when the fetus was deformed.[16]

The AMA Board's Committee on Human Reproduction presented

delegates with a new approach in June 1967. The committee skirted problems it encountered on its first outing two years earlier. This time it did not recommend that state laws be changed. Rather, it urged that the AMA merely adopt a liberalized position on therapeutic abortion to serve as a guide to its affiliates in states contemplating reform. The House adopted the policy, the first change since 1871. It put the AMA on record as allowing *abortion* in cases when there was documented medical evidence that continuance of pregnancy threatened "the health or life of the mother," or when the infant may be born with "incapacitating physical deformity or mental deficiency," or when a pregnancy from a legally established rape or incest represented a threat to the woman's mental or physical health. The guideline also urged that two physicians endorse the appropriateness of the procedure and that the abortion be performed in a hospital.[17]

The committee acknowledged Roman Catholic opposition to all abortion, even to save the mother's life. "The Committee respects the right of this group to express and practice its belief. However, the Committee believes that physicians who hold other views should be legally able to exercise sound medical judgment which they and their colleagues feel to be in the best interest of the patient," the report said.[18]

During the floor debate, a single delegate spoke out "to prevent the record from showing unanimous approval." The AMA position would not prove acceptable to many Roman Catholic physicians or others with right-to-life views still attuned to the views of the nineteenth-century AMA antiabortion crusaders.[19]

THE ETHICAL DILEMMA

The AMA had been trying hard not to make radical changes in its policies, but events in 1970 were about to overtake it. A handful of states began repealing, not just reforming, their abortion laws. This meant physicians in these states were free to perform elective or nontherapeutic abortions, procedures the AMA considered unethical. A reluctant AMA was being pushed to make some new policy decisions.

Hawaii became the first state to eliminate criminal penalties for abortion as opposed to reformulating its statutes according to the American Law Institute model statutes. In Hawaii abortion could take place before the twenty-fourth week of pregnancy, after which the fetus was considered "viable" or able to live outside the womb with medical support. Hawaii also eliminated hospital abortion committees, though it still

required the procedure to be performed in a hospital. Hawaii's Democratic governor John A. Burns, who attended mass daily and once had
been named Roman Catholic layman of the year, let the bill become law
without signing it in March, because he considered illegal abortion dangerous and also because he believed legal silence on abortion was faithful
to separation of church and state. In April 1970 the New York legislature,
by a single vote switched at the last minute, repealed its abortion law, leaving abortion a matter between a woman and her physician through the
twenty-fourth week of pregnancy. Developments in populous New York
were too big for the AMA leadership to ignore.

Just before the annual meeting in June 1970, the board announced
in the AMA newspaper its proposals to liberalize policies beyond the
stands taken on therapeutic abortion in 1967. Sympathetic to the plight
of the physicians in New York and other states where the laws had been
repealed, the board said: "Many physicians find themselves unable to
perform a legalized medical procedure without violating the policy of
their professional association."[20]

On short notice, pro-life doctors in Boston scrambled to protest
the proposed stand. Dr. Joseph R. Stanton, an internist at St. Elizabeth
Hospital, on whose staff Horatio Storer had served a century earlier,
gathered 950 signatures on a petition opposing a policy change he considered to support abortion on demand. In his petition submitted at the
meeting, Stanton warned: "European and Japanese experience clearly
indicates that the people of this country will be ill-served and our profession irreparably damaged if medicine's time-honored position of pro-
found respect for and protection of human life from its inception to
natural death is altered in any way."

The reference committee held its hearing in June 1970 before a
packed room, where the testimony often was bitter. Dr. Gloria Heffer-
nan, of suburban Chicago, the only woman to testify against the board's
proposal, said, "The killing of the living inside the womb will open the
way to the execution of the living outside the womb."[21]

But Dr. Allan C. Barnes, obstetrics chairman at Johns Hopkins, observed that abortion helped treat "teenage illegitimacy . . . one of our
worst diseases." Dr. Josephine Renshaw, president of the American Medical Women's Association and a Washington obstetrician, said, "Over and
over again, I have seen boyfriends and husbands walking away from un-
wanted pregnancies, but women can't walk away."[22]

Behind the scenes, the AMA leadership was lining up the support it
needed to adopt a liberalized stand. Before the House of Delegates
voted, the AMA's Judicial Council, which sets the organization's ethical

standards, held abortion was ethical when performed legally and "in accordance with good medical practice." This statement rubbed salt into the wounds of the pro-life physicians, who argued that doctors themselves, not lawmakers, ought to determine professional ethics.

But by a 103–73 vote, the House of Delegates approved the new policy. The AMA was now on record as recognizing abortion as a "medical procedure" that should be performed by a physician "in conformance with standards of good medical practice" in a hospital after consulting with two other physicians. The policy also added a conscience clause saying no doctors, hospitals, or other medical personnel should be forced to participate in abortion if they were morally opposed to the practice. Dr. Wendell Scott, chairman of the reference committee, said the new guidelines moved abortion beyond being limited to cases where it was medically indicated. He argued that the phrase "good medical practice" permitted abortion to be performed for social and economic considerations, such as teen pregnancies or a family's ability to afford another child.[23]

The AMA held another hearing on abortion at its winter session in 1970. Stanton and others protested the policy change. "We had an incredible number of doctors speak at those hearings. But it was a stacked meeting. The AMA wrote us off," said Stanton, head of the Value for Life Committee, a pro-life group chartered in October 1970. "Medicine had lost its soul."[24]

The abortion policies took a toll on AMA membership, resulting in a significant number of doctors quitting the organization. For the previous ten years, the number of AMA members had been rising, but after the abortion policy was set, a precipitous slide in membership occurred. Though it is not possible to know how many left over this issue, some 20,000 physicians, about 9 percent of members, left the AMA between 1970 and 1972.[25]

THE SUPREME COURT UPS THE STAKES
WITH *ROE V. WADE*

The abortion debate intensified in the early 1970s. Reform and repeal efforts, boosted by a growing women's movement calling on women to control their own bodies, continued at the state level, with many states liberalizing their statutes along ALI lines or repealing them. New devices made abortion safer for women undergoing the procedure. At the same time, the pro-life movement had some success, having under the leadership of Dr. J. C. Willke, founder of the National Right to Life Committee, defeated referenda in Michigan and North Dakota to create abortion on demand through the twentieth week of pregnancy.

Then, on January 22, 1973, the U.S. Supreme Court changed everything. In a sweeping 7-to-2 decision, the Court declared unconstitutional all existing state abortion laws, ruling simultaneously on a Texas case, *Roe v. Wade*, and a Georgia case, *Doe v. Bolton*. In one wide-ranging decision, the Court made abortion on demand the law of the land for the first trimester and made it available with possible restrictions in the second and third trimesters, threw out requirements for supporting physician opinions, got rid of hospital abortion committees, and even abandoned the requirement that abortions be performed in hospitals. Physicians were given a certified right to perform abortions based on medical judgment that could take into account a broad definition of the woman's well-being, including shaky marital status and indigence. "This allows the attending physician the room he needs to make his best medical judgment," said Justice Harry A. Blackmun, the decision's author.[26]

"Jane Roe," an unmarried twenty-five-year-old pregnant woman from Dallas County, was denied an abortion under an 1857 Texas criminal abortion statute that permitted abortion only to save a woman's life. Roe's life was not endangered, but she contended she ought to be allowed to have an abortion. She claimed she had been impregnated in a gang rape, though years later she recanted the story.

The Supreme Court found Roe had the right to an abortion, under privacy protections provided by the due-process clause of the Fourteenth Amendment.[27] Blackmun wrote that "the right of personal privacy includes the abortion decision, but that this right is not unqualified and must be considered against important state interests in regulation."[28]

Blackmun, former general counsel at the Mayo Clinic in Rochester, Minnesota, presented a trimester scheme for pregnancy. During the first trimester, or about thirteen weeks' gestation, a woman—with a doctor's consent—could have an abortion without government interference. As pregnancy progressed, the state had increasing rights to intervene—to protect maternal health during the second trimester and even to proscribe abortion during the third trimester unless the life or health of the pregnant woman were at risk. Blackmun made the personal physician the prime authority in the abortion decision. He stated: "The decision vindicates the right of the physician to administer medical treatment according to his professional judgment up to the points where important state interests provide compelling justifications for intervention. Up to those points the abortion decision in all its aspects is inherently, and primarily, a medical decision, and basic responsibility for it must rest with the physician."29 The Court's majority felt Doctor knew best.

In dissent, Justice William H. Rehnquist said the majority decision to recognize trimesters and to define state restrictions during each period "partakes more of judicial legislation than it does of determination of the intent of the drafters of the Fourteenth Amendment."30

Blackmun presented a broad historic perspective, tracing thought on abortion from ancient times to colonial America to his own time. Pro-lifers later would criticize him for relying heavily on a history prepared by an attorney for the National Association for the Repeal of Abortion Laws.

In the majority decision, Blackmun said the Hippocratic oath's disapproval of abortion was unusual in the ancient world. Hippocrates, the ancient Greek physician whose oath long served as the basis of medical ethics, belonged to the minority pro-life Pythagorean school. In contrast, the heavyweight ancient Greek philosophers Plato and Aristotle were pro-choice. Blackmun contended abortion, particularly before quickening, was tolerated in America in colonial times under the common law brought from England. The laws criminalizing abortion, passed under the guidance of the AMA in the nineteenth century, were a historic quirk, according to the official Supreme Court version. "It is thus apparent that at common law, at the time of the adoption of our Constitution, and throughout the vast portion of the 19th century, abortion was viewed with less disfavor than under most American statutes currently in effect," Blackmun ruled.31 The decision also took note of the recent liberalization of AMA abortion policy.

In the companion case, *Doe v. Bolton,* the Court struck down provisions of an ALI-type law adopted by Georgia in 1968. The case involved "Mary Doe," a married woman, an indigent with a history of mental illness. Doe was denied an abortion at eight weeks' gestation because her desire to abort a child she and her husband could not support failed to meet the statute's criteria. The Court said the Georgia law's requirement that abortions be performed in hospitals violated constitutional due-process provisions. Blackmun said Georgia had failed to prove abortions were any safer in a hospital setting than anywhere else. This decision cleared the way for the creation of a new workplace for physicians: the abortion clinic.

The Court also made it possible for women to obtain abortions on the say-so of their personal physicians alone, removing the Georgia requirement that two other doctors pass on the recommendation. The Court said that a required approval of two physicians other than the woman's had "no rational connection with a patient's needs and unduly infringes on her physician's right to practice."[32] Further, the Court knocked down the Georgia mandate that a hospital committee, consisting of three staff physicians, rule on a woman's abortion request. It said the committees were "unduly restrictive of the patient's rights, which are already safeguarded by her personal physician."

The Court's abortion decision strongly upheld a physician's right to practice. This fed the AMA's traditional position of fiercely promoting and protecting the autonomy of physicians to treat their patients without state interference. In dissent, Justice Byron R. White, joined by Rehnquist, described the decision as "an exercise of raw judicial power."[33]

LINING UP WITH *ROE* AND *DOE*

At its June 1973 meeting in New York City, the AMA made its abortion policy consistent with *Roe* and *Doe*. The House of Delegates "reaffirmed" its 1970 policy but removed requirements that abortions be performed in "accredited hospitals" and that consultations be made with two other physicians. In an effort to placate pro-life physicians, the reference committee suggested that the House adopt a statement affirming "the traditional favorable attitude of the medical profession toward pregnancy and motherhood." Dr. Joseph Donnelly, an abortion opponent, felt this was hypocritical and angrily moved that the clause not be added: "There were more abortions in this city in the past year than live births," the New Jersey obstetrician said. "We can no longer say that the traditional attitude of the medical profession is in favor of pregnancy and motherhood. It doesn't tell it like it is."[34] Delegates noisily overruled Donnelly and adopted the resolution.

DOCTOR'S CHOICE, NOT PRO-CHOICE

Following the 1973 Supreme Court decision, however, the right-to-life movement grew more sophisticated and began chipping away at abortion rights. Pro-lifers succeeded in lobbying in state and municipal governments for laws that made access to abortion more difficult.[35]

At the federal level they were also able to pull off a coup with a ban on the use of federal funds to pay for abortion for the poor under the state-federal Medicaid program. The ban began in September 1976, when Representative Henry J. Hyde, a freshman Republican from suburban Chicago, cut off federal funding of abortion through Medicaid with an amendment tacked on to the Department of Labor Appropriations Bill. Jittery about the increasingly high visibility of the abortion issue and calculating the courts would throw out the amendment, the Senate adopted the Hyde amendment, but it added the proviso that funding would be available should the life of the mother be endangered. As expected, a federal judge in New York blocked implementation of the law until its legality could be determined.

While still awaiting a court decision on the original Hyde amendment, the House of Representatives and the Senate in 1977 engaged in one of the most bitter internecine battles in history as they fought over abortion restrictions for fiscal 1978 relating to the budgets for the Departments of Labor and Health, Education and Welfare.

Senator Edward W. Brooke, a Massachusetts Republican, organized a campaign in July 1977 to line up votes to support federal funding of abortion. He cast the issue as being one in which the doctor in consultation with his or her patient—not the government—should decide whether an abortion should be performed. As part of this effort, he approached the AMA, and the doctors' group, always a booster for physician autonomy, was more than happy to help. Dr. James H. Sammons, AMA executive vice president, told Brooke in a telegram that the AMA believed the government should stay out of the doctor-patient relationship: "An abortion is a medical procedure and as such can only properly be performed by a licensed physician. The performance of an abortion is a matter of determination by both the patient and the physician, and the procedure should be performed consistently with applicable law and good medical practice." He said Congress should not "substitute its judgment for that of the trained physician" by specifying medical conditions that made abortion a "medical necessity."[36] Brooke used Sammons' telegram as a sales tool to try to win Senate votes.

When pro-lifers obtained a copy of the Sammons wire, they rebuked the AMA leadership. But Sammons told one writer the AMA was standing its ground in opposition to Congress defining when a medical procedure was necessary: "I cannot help but believe that the Association's position on this point would, in fact, represent the views of a majority of all practicing physicians."[37] Dr. Joseph Stanton, president of the Value of Life Committee, responded that the AMA surely recognized that the government was already heavily involved in medicine, such as having third parties decide whether patients should be hospitalized under Medicare.

Fetal Life

In August 1978 a federal judge lifted his block of the first Hyde amendment, rejecting pro-choice lawyers' arguments that the law was "unconstitutionally vague." The running battle over federal funding for abortion resumed. By the early 1980s, the right-to-life movement shifted its attention to the Senate, where Republicans sensitive to their views had a majority. Conservative North Carolina senator Jesse Helms, a pro-life angel, had in the mid-1970s failed in his efforts to push a constitutional amendment that would recognize the unborn's right to life. But in 1981 he came up with a new angle. He planned to push an easier-to-pass statute to nullify *Roe v. Wade*. Helms introduced the Human Life Statute, which defined a fetus as a "person" from the moment of conception, an idea advocated by Dr. Horatio Storer in 1865.[38] In the modern twist, Helms theorized that if a fetus were extended status as a person, the 1973 Supreme Court *Roe* decision effectively would be negated.

Recognizing potential dangers to patient care, the AMA was in the forefront of the opposition to the bill. In June 1981, Dr. Joseph F. Boyle, chairman of the Board of Trustees, who had contemplated becoming a priest before choosing medicine, told the Senate Judiciary Committee's Subcommittee on Separation of Powers that the Helms bill incorrectly assumed there was a "scientific consensus" supporting the position that life begins at conception. If the Helms bill passed, Boyle warned, it would damage physician-patient relations by "creat[ing] endless medical, ethical, and legal difficulties for the people of this nation. A physician could face serious dilemmas in advising pregnant patients. Under the bill, the physician would be responsible for the welfare of every fetus whose legal and health interest would in the eyes of the law, be equal to, but in conflict with, those of the woman."[39]

With AMA assistance, the bill failed before the full Judiciary Committee. But soon, as conservative winds blew stronger, the AMA for the most part would avoid abortion issues except when vital to protect physician interests.

STAYING ON THE GOOD SIDE OF CONSERVATIVES

With the arrival in Washington in the 1980s of the Reagan/Bush administration, its conservative agenda, including pro-life positions, became more fashionable. Trying to remain on the good side of the White House and its congressional friends, the AMA became less visible on abortion and other issues that might offend conservative sensibilities. AMA chief executive Dr. James Sammons in 1982 went so far as to tell the editor of the *AMA Journal* to have his staff go easy on articles on particularly sensitive issues, including abortion, nuclear war, and tobacco.

However, the AMA still stood up for physician rights as it filed amicus—friend of the court—briefs, a position presented by a party not directly involved in a lawsuit, in several major abortion-related cases before the Court. But pro-choice advocates detected a weakening of the AMA's resolve, especially in lobbying on abortion issues. The AMA wanted to avoid the issue because of persisting memories of membership hemorrhage and because it considered other matters to have a higher priority in Congress.

A case in point involved the controversial "gag" rule, an order promulgated by Reagan's Department of Health and Human Services in 1988 that prohibited abortion from being mentioned as a birth-control option to patients in federally funded family-planning centers. Pro-choice advocates expected the AMA to immediately bring out its big guns in the courts and in Congress to oppose this affront to physician autonomy. But the AMA faltered.

Ann Allen, general counsel for the American College of Obstetricians and Gynecologists, said the AMA joined forces only hesitantly in an amicus brief in the *Rust v. Sullivan* case, an unsuccessful challenge of the legality and constitutionality of the gag rule. And within the brief, the AMA selectively opposed the gag rule on statutory grounds, standing apart from ACOG and other medical organizations' broader opposition to the gag rule on constitutional grounds, such as violation of free-speech guarantees.[40] The Supreme Court upheld the gag rule in 1990, leading abortion-rights and medical groups to begin lobbying for laws to nullify the regulations. After the AMA belatedly signed on, President Bush announced that physicians were not barred from counseling patients about abortion, though the gag still applied to other health workers who actually did most of the counseling. Many pro-choice advocates remain angry and distrustful of the AMA.

Kirk B. Johnson, AMA general counsel, insists the AMA has showed courage and leadership in filing briefs in abortion cases. He explained the AMA philosophy: "On the issue of whether or not a woman has a fundamental right to privacy and a right to obtain medical treatment, we are not neutral. We are as pro . . . I wouldn't say pro-choice . . . but as pro-right-to-privacy as you can get. And we've always felt strongly about that. It really goes to the very heart of the physician-patient relationship; the right of people to select their physicians and obtain medical judgments and legal medical procedures. And as long as abortion is a legal procedure you have to be entitled to exercise your right and you cannot be impeded."[41]

In the case of abortion, as in so many other issues, the AMA is playing politics rather than trying to do what is right or just. Rachael Pine, of the New York–based Center for Reproductive Law and Policy and formerly an attorney with the American Civil Liberties Union's Reproductive Freedom Project, questioned the AMA's commitment. "They have the right views, but politics really intervenes about when and where they'll express them," she said. "If they really want to be neutral, they would stay out of it."[42]

ABORTION-POLICY SHIFT?

AMA delegates attending the winter 1989 meeting in Honolulu, for the most part were caught up in a financial scandal involving some of the organization's top staffers. But they still found time to dabble in the abortion debate.

The California delegation introduced a resolution calling on the AMA to acknowledge a woman's right to an "early" abortion. The policy stated that "early termination of pregnancy is a medical matter between the patient and physician, subject to the physician's clinical judgment, the patient's informed consent, and the availability of appropriate facilities." During a hearing, Dr. James E. Davis, immediate past president of the AMA, urged delegates to back off. "This is apt to open up a lot of fruitless debate," he said. "The board does not think this issue needs to be re-aired."

Dr. Charles W. Plows, chairman of the California delegation, however, said the policy change recommended by his delegation would be a "warm and substantive" change from the AMA's "terribly cold and didactic" position on abortion, which did not directly recognize a woman's right to abortion. Plows was especially angered that disadvantaged women had difficulty obtaining abortion: "That rich women can get abortions and poor women can't is a lot of ca-ca."

Representing pro-life forces within the AMA, Dr. Edward G. Kilroy urged delegates not to "radically" change AMA policy. And another delegate insisted the "appropriate position is no position." Still, the California resolution was adopted. In the end, there was confusion about what transpired. Pro-lifers and pro-choicers said the policy had changed, but the AMA Board disagreed. AMA trustee Dr. Nancy W. Dickey said the new policy was merely a "reaffirmation" of existing policy.[43]

"Neutrality" in the War Zone

The AMA's policies in the 1990s on abortion send such mixed signals that the association angers people on both sides of the debate. Events occurring over a matter of days in the summer of 1992 highlight how the AMA's "neutrality" has resulted in its being attacked by both sides.

Abortion came up at the annual meeting in June 1992 in connection with a campaign to promote the health of teens. Delegates were discussing a policy that for the first time explicitly stated that physicians ought to be able to perform an abortion on an unmarried minor *without notifying her parents.* "This is new ground," explained AMA general counsel Kirk Johnson. "The old way was always to ask the parents."[44]

Still, the proposed position was actually an extension of an AMA policy in the 1960s that held doctors should be able to treat teens infected with venereal disease without parental notification. To protect the health of youths, the AMA felt it sometimes is necessary to sidestep the youngsters' parents because they otherwise might refuse needed medical care.

Despite this precedent, performing an abortion before notifying a minor's parent or obtaining parental permission remained a touchy matter. Surveys showed the vast majority of the public wanted parents involved when their minor daughters were scheduled to undergo abortions. Right-to-life groups saw the issue as a political wedge to put between the general public and the pro-choice movement. More than half the states had laws on the books requiring parental involvement or notification in abortion decisions by minors, though most of these laws were not enforced. Nevertheless, the issue was of more than symbolic significance because 11 percent of all abortions are performed on girls seventeen and under.

The AMA Council on Ethical and Judicial Affairs, which recommended the new policy regarding parental notification, said doctors ought to encourage minors to discuss their pregnancies with their parents or with a counselor or clergyman. The report said, however, if a pregnant teen did not want her parents involved, "Physicians should not feel or be compelled to require minors to obtain consent before deciding whether to undergo an abortion."

The contemporary AMA position on parental notification—as well as on abortion in general—relates to the AMA view of doctor-patient relations. The AMA above all else is an advocate of physician autonomy and works hard to keep anyone else out of the examining room. The AMA's objective in today's abortion controversy has been to protect a doctor's right to perform abortion, with a mind toward protecting his or her right to perform other procedures. Acknowledging state parental-notification requirements, the AMA said its policy applied only when it did not contradict local laws. The AMA was not going far out on a limb.

Attacked from Both Sides

As some delegates were cautioning the AMA hearing that the proposal could widen breaches among doctors, pickets marched outside the meeting headquarters. Members of the Pro-Life Action League carried mock tombstones with the names of 113 women who had died from legal abortions.[45] Protest leader Joseph M. Scheidler, director of the league and author of *Closed: 99 Ways to Stop Abortion*, said at the time that the AMA's policy intruded on the parent-child relationship by placing an exaggerated priority on the doctor-patient relationship. "My daughter cannot have her ears pierced without my permission," he said. "Now the AMA is saying that they want doctors to be able to take a girl in for major surgery without parental knowledge and consent."[46] The next day, June 23, the AMA House of Delegates adopted, without debate, the new policy in a victory, albeit a minor one, for pro-choice advocates.[47]

Then, only eight days after the AMA adopted this position, on July 1, 1992, a group convened by the National Abortion Rights Action League (NARAL), for other reasons, also condemned the AMA. Their beef was that the AMA was not aggressively supporting abortion rights at a time when the U.S. Supreme Court was expected to take away those rights by reversing its landmark 1973 decision, *Roe v. Wade*. The NARAL Commission on America Without *Roe* feared that women's lives would be endangered because they would be forced to seek illegal abortions. The group said organized medicine, especially the AMA, had abdicated its responsibility to ensure that women have access to the full spectrum of reproductive-health services.

The NARAL commission was incensed that the AMA had failed to file an amicus brief in *Planned Parenthood v. Casey*, the case expected to be the vehicle the Court would use to overturn *Roe*. In this suit, Planned Parenthood challenged a Pennsylvania law that required doctors to recite a script that pro-choice groups held was aimed at discouraging women from having abortions. The NARAL commission charged: "The AMA's failure to take a position in this critically important case reveals a serious lack of commitment to women's reproductive rights."[48]

The AMA's concept of neutrality is foreign to both pro-life and pro-choice advocates. AMA chief executive Dr. James S. Todd took it philosophically: "The pro-lifers pick on us, but so do the pro-choice people.

We're being attacked from both sides. That puts us in a neutral position, doesn't it? We can't win no matter what we do. And on this subject I think the less the AMA says [the better]."49

PUBLIC HEALTH VS. POLITICS

By turning abortion into a national issue for its own purposes almost 150 years ago, the AMA set off a series of events that helped create one of the thorniest controversies of our time. Perhaps now it could help lead us out of this maze.

In recent years the AMA has waved the flag of neutrality on the issue. But it ought to start acting like a group of doctors concerned about its patients instead of like medical politicians. The AMA likes to say that it sets its policy based on science. It also likes to say that it promotes the "betterment" of public health.

That being the case, if the AMA is willing to assume a leadership role, its own policies already contain the seeds to help make access to abortion a matter of good medical-patient care. The AMA of course has submitted, albeit somewhat reluctantly at times, amicus briefs on the pro-choice side in the courts. It also has advocated positions totally unacceptable to pro-life forces, such as research on and, if justified, use of the "abortion pill," RU-486, and also research on transplantation of fetal tissue.

But more fundamental than these is an AMA report, adopted in 1992, that received little notice except among pro-life critics. In its report, the Council on Scientific Affairs, the AMA's science arm, showed that since the Supreme Court ruled in the *Roe* case in 1973, abortion-related death rates had dropped more than fivefold. In fact, the report stated that the risk of dying from childbirth and pregnancy was twelve times greater than that of dying from an induced abortion. Quite a contrast from crusader Dr. Horatio Storer's claims in 1865 that more women died from abortion than from childbirth.50

The 1992 report went on to say that restrictive abortion regulations, such as mandatory waiting periods and the shortage of abortion doctors, were dangerous because they increased the gestational age at which abortion occurs. The council concluded that further restrictions on women's access to abortion could lead to "a small but measurable increase in mortality and morbidity among women in the United States."51

This means that loss of abortion rights poses a public-health threat. If the AMA is serious about safeguarding the public health, it ought to try to protect the health of American women. It could promote training of more doctors to provide what most Americans consider an essential medical service. It could advocate steps to prevent unintended pregnancies. Of course, it should continue to support "conscience clauses" that respect the right of pro-life doctors and other health professionals not to be involved in abortion. Pro-choice does not necessarily mean pro-abortion. The AMA, which started this fray so many years ago, could show the way to a new era by promoting not only a doctor's right to choose to perform abortions, but also a woman's right to have one.

Political Science vs. Medical Science

Bungling Health Policy on the AIDS Epidemic

LARRY KRAMER WATCHED power-lessly as friends died from a strange new infection afflicting young gay men. A physician who cared for many of these men prodded the New York playwright to sound the alarm in the gay community about the dangers of unprotected, promiscuous sex. In his 1985 play *The Normal Heart,* Kramer recounts the incident: Emma, the physician, chides Ned Weeks, a stand-in for the author, for his less-than-successful efforts to get the word out. Weeks angrily asks the physician what her medical brethren were doing to fight the growing epidemic: "What the fuck is your side doing? Where's the goddamned AMA in all of this?"[1]

It was a good question. Instead of being in the forefront of fighting the disease, the AMA sat on the sidelines, with much of the rest of organized medicine and the government, and failed to respond quickly to this modern plague. As gay men and then intravenous drug users were infected and died, the medical establishment, which should have shown compassion and attacked the problem the best it could, looked the other way. AIDS did not become a public concern until years later, when the "innocent victims" were recognized: heterosexuals infected by the tainted blood supply, hemophiliacs, and babies born to infected women.

It was not until 1987, six years into the epidemic, that the AMA adopted its first comprehensive package of policies designed to help the profession and the public deal with the outbreak. AIDS proved to be difficult for the American Medical Association to tackle in part because it involved sexual transmission of disease—and homosexual sex at that. Doctors and doctor organizations appear to be just as squeamish about sex as the rest of society, a situation that fosters ignorance and the spread of disease. In the aftermath of this public-health-policy fiasco, by October 1993, 339,250 Americans had been diagnosed with AIDS and 204,390 had died. Another one million had been infected with Human Immunodeficiency Virus, the so-called AIDS virus.[2]

A VICTORIAN MIND-SET ON SEX

The AMA has a history of mishandling sexual issues. In the Victorian Age, Dr. Denslow Lewis broke new ground when he studied sexual response in men and women. The Chicago sexologist presented his landmark findings at the annual scientific conference of the American Medical Association in 1899, scandalizing many attendees.

Scientific reports presented at the meeting ordinarily were included in the Proceedings of the AMA carried in the *Journal of the American Medical Association.* But after some outraged doctors declared the research obscene, the study was suppressed. However, in the 1970s, a Nashville psychiatrist discovered the injustice done to Lewis and championed his cause. Finally, eighty-four years after Lewis originally submitted his manuscript and seventy years after his death, the sexologist received his due. Dr. George D. Lundberg, *JAMA's* editor, published Lewis's findings in July 1983 under the heading "Delayed Communications." In an editorial in the *Journal,* Dr. William Masters, the famed sexologist, said that if Lewis's research had been published earlier, much suffering over sexual matters could have been avoided.[3]

In more recent times, the AMA blushed about sexually transmitted diseases. The organization launched a public-service campaign on television to attack the rising incidence of venereal disease in the sexually switched-on sixties. But when the networks leaned on the physician group, AMA officials eliminated from a sixty-second animated announcement specific mention of syphilis, gonorrhea, and the expression "intimate contact."[4] Victorian sensitivities prevailed once again.

OUT OF THE CLOSET,
ONTO THE EXAMINING TABLE

If the AMA had trouble dealing with heterosexual sex, homosexual sex was even more difficult. During the early years of the "gay liberation" movement in the late 1960s and early 1970s, homosexuals protested being stigmatized not only in society at large but in medical offices. Psychiatry, which labels what is "normal," had for a century officially defined homosexuality as a type of mental illness. If a physician took a sexual history, a rare occurrence in itself, he or she would consider a homosexual abnormal by definition. And, if the doctor did encounter a gay patient, he or she probably would not be aware of the special health problems connected with homosexuality, such as gastrointestinal diseases and sexually transmitted infections linked to anal sex.

The AMA began to consider addressing the issue of gays in the early 1970s. It was a reflection of a time when legislators in some states had removed from the books antisodomy statutes that had prohibited sexual relations between consenting adults of the same sex. AMA delegates considered a resolution in December 1974 calling for decriminalization of homosexual relations between consenting adults. But conservative elements shot down this policy because they feared AMA support "might be misinterpreted as an endorsement of prostitution."[5] The House of Delegates the following June found a way around this, declaring they supported "in principle repeal of laws which classify as criminal any form of noncommercial sexual conduct between consenting adults. . . ."[6]

Six years later, in December 1981, AMA delegates passed their first policy concerning homosexuals' health-care needs. The AMA said "nonjudgmental recognition of sexual orientation enhances the ability to render optimal patient care," especially in care of homosexuals. Gays praised the organization for saying that physicians should be educated to be "attuned" to the special medical and psychological needs of homosexuals. But activists were incensed when the AMA said it would encourage development of programs to make gays aware of "the possibility of sex preference reversal in selected cases" using aversion therapy, such as with electrical shocks.[7]

The 1981 AMA report on homosexuality made brief mention of some unusual diseases, referred to as "opportunistic infections," that seemed to be related to immune-system problems in gay men. AMA delegates did not know it, but they were witnessing a volcano about to erupt.

AIDS: THE EARLY YEARS

On June 5, 1981, in its publication *Morbidity and Mortality Weekly Report*, the federal Centers for Disease Control, the government's top disease watchers and fighters, reported on the appearance of opportunistic infections in five young Los Angeles men. They had been diagnosed with

Pneumocystis carinii pneumonia and other viral and fungal infections ordinarily found in people such as those with cancer or who had undergone organ transplants, people whose immune systems had been severely suppressed. Two of the gays had died, according to the report.

The collection of symptoms initially was referred to as GRIDS: gay-related immune deficiency syndrome. The name for the disease was changed to AIDS—acquired immune deficiency syndrome—when doctors found the condition also occurred in heterosexual intravenous drug users who shared needles. Blood and semen were the carriers of the virus that caused the disease.

The AMA staff considered the new disease a mere curiosity. It did not expect the outbreak to become a worldwide pandemic. Dr. Norbert Rapoza, a virologist who joined the AMA Department of Drugs in spring 1982, told *American Medical News* that the AMA had been "slow on the uptake—we thought [AIDS] would be confined to maybe 5,000 cases and would disappear."[8]

Dealing with an emerging epidemic, the AMA, which claims to be concerned about the public's health, was indecisive. Dr. Leonard Fenninger, AMA vice president for science policy at that time, said the organization was divided internally over what to do. Physicians from areas more heavily affected by AIDS, such as California, wanted the AMA to make AIDS policy a top priority, while other factions downplayed its significance. The best the AMA could muster in its first policy statement, adopted in December 1983, was to support publication of information about AIDS for the profession and public, call for physicians to become aware of AIDS symptoms, endorse "nonjudgmental" care for patients, and to request doctors uninformed about AIDS or who "do not choose to provide . . . care" to know to whom to refer patients.[9]

Monumental effort was required to get the House of Delegates to adopt this innocuous statement, which had been strongly opposed by many rank-and-file delegates. The Council on Scientific Affairs, the House's scientific branch, and the staff had to twist arms to get even that passed.[10]

Fenninger, who before joining the AMA was assistant head of the National Institutes of Health, said the very nature of AIDS made it a tricky subject even for doctors. The problem was the disease was intimately linked to anal sex in homosexuals and to drug abuse in underclass African-American and Latino communities. It was not a subject about which the typical AMA delegate cared to know. By the time the AMA adopted its AIDS policy in 1983, the tally kept by the CDC had reached 2,841 people diagnosed with AIDS, 1,158 of whom had died.[11]

THE AMA FINALLY TAKES A STAND

Some people argue that no significant public-health efforts could have been undertaken to attack AIDS until the test for HIV antibodies was approved in March 1985. The test made it possible to screen the blood supply through which some patients had been infected. Also, for the first time, the test made it feasible for sexual partners of AIDS patients to find out if they had been infected—though no treatment was available. Still, the AMA did not act until two years after the test was approved.

In June 1987, six years into the AIDS epidemic, the House of Delegates for the first time was considering a comprehensive package of AIDS policies. At this time the CDC's AIDS count had reached 53,812 diagnosed cases, with 31,862 deaths.[12]

Dr. David Ostrow, an AIDS researcher at the University of Michigan and a member of an AMA advisory panel on AIDS formed in 1985, said the intent of the AMA policies was good. But he complained that it had been slapped together quickly by AMA staff a week earlier without consulting with the advisory panel or other AIDS experts. "This is going to be the first time that the AMA has said what it thinks about AIDS, and the report was done without the input of the experts," he said.[13]

With an unusually large contingent of press in attendance, America seemed to be awaiting word of the AMA view on AIDS. The AMA unveiled a complex package of forty recommendations to attack the disease. It supported education programs to prevent the spread of AIDS, extension of anti-discrimination laws to cover people infected with HIV, review of research on how to prevent HIV among intravenous drug users, and development of methods for public-health officials to warn sexual partners of HIV-infected people.

The cornerstone of the policy package was testing for antibodies to HIV. AMA delegates endorsed routine antibody testing in clinics for people with sexually transmitted diseases, those seeking family planning services, and pregnant women in the first trimester. The AMA supported mandatory testing of prison inmates, immigrants, and military recruits. The AMA contended voluntary testing should be encouraged for homosexuals, bisexuals, and intravenous drug users, and their sexual partners.

Significantly, the delegates came out for routine, voluntary testing of patients requiring invasive procedures or surgery if they lived in areas with a high incidence of AIDS or who were homosexuals or drug abusers. If voluntary patient testing were refused, delegates urged that hospitals and doctors consider mandatory testing. In other words, patients were seen as a potential source of HIV for doctors. It had not been stressed yet what the experts already suspected: HIV spread could be a two-way street.

Surgeon General C. Everett Koop, a conservative praised for his approach to caring for AIDS patients, endorsed the AMA's policies: "Imperfect as they may seem to some, [they] would be a good start on a national policy."[14] But some experts warned that AMA policy could be used to justify abuses such as removal of doctors from their jobs, as had happened in a recent incident at Chicago's Cook County Hospital. "They [AMA delegates] recommend routine testing of all health-care workers and don't give reasons for that," researcher Ostrow said. "They don't say anything about the right of an infected doctor to work."[15] The AMA, in fact, was laying the groundwork for an AIDS policy disaster.

DEFENDING A DOCTOR'S RIGHT TO CHOOSE A PATIENT

A few months earlier, Dr. W. Dudley Johnson, a Milwaukee surgeon who pioneered heart-bypass techniques, shocked many when he revealed that he and his partners had refused to treat two patients infected with AIDS. Since the spring of 1986, Johnson and his partners had begun screening the blood of all prospective patients for HIV antibodies. He told the *Milwaukee Journal* that he did not know of any surgeons who had contracted HIV from infected patients: "I want to keep it that way." After that, several other health-care workers admitted they had refused to care for AIDS patients.[16]

Some doctors feared that their lives and their livelihoods—with potential lifetime earnings in the multimillions—could be jeopardized by an accidental stick with a needle smeared with HIV-infected blood or a bloody bone fragment slicing through their gloves during surgery. Furthermore, studies showed that many doctors preferred not to treat HIV-infected patients and homosexuals in general.

Mindful of the negative image of doctors refusing care to sick patients, the AMA Board of Trustees in November 1987 declared doctors had an ethical obligation to care for patients with HIV/AIDS. Dr. Russel H. Patterson, vice chairman of the AMA Council on Ethical and Judicial Affairs, said: "For centuries, the medical professional has taken care of patients with contagious diseases—smallpox, bubonic plague, whooping cough, to name a few. Society has accorded physicians a special place in life, and, in return, has come to expect that even at some risk to themselves, physicians will take care of patients. The Judicial Council believes nothing has changed. Doctors should be expected to take a degree of risk in caring for patients with AIDS."17

Buttressing its case, the AMA Board proudly pointed to the organization's original Code of Ethics from 1847, which stated: "When pestilence prevails, it is their [physicians'] duty to face the danger and to continue their labors for the alleviation of the suffering, even at the jeopardy of their own lives." The policy was unprecedented in medical annals. In fact, in earlier times, many physicians, including revered figures such as Galen, the second-century medical scholar and physician to Roman emperors, ran away from plagues. Because doctors fled from towns devastated by the Black Death, some European governments enacted laws in the fourteenth and fifteenth centuries to forbid such behavior.

The AMA Offers an Escape Route

The AMA's citation of the 1847 statement on physicians facing down pestilence sounded noble, but it was misleading. When the organization streamlined its Principles of Ethics in 1957, mention of the duty to care for patients during contagious outbreak was dropped.18 No one had foreseen a plague like AIDS.

Furthermore, despite its apparent high-minded stand, the AMA gave doctors a different message out of the other side of its mouth: physicians could excuse themselves from caring for patients whom they considered themselves "not competent" to treat. Dr. Alan R. Nelson, AMA Board chairman, put the most positive spin on this by saying a referral may be in the patient's best interest "when caring for that patient is not within the current realm of the physician's competence."19 This view was consistent with Principle VI of AMA's Principles of Ethics, which has held since 1912 that except in emergencies, physicians should be "free to choose whom to serve, with whom to associate and the environment in which to provide medical services."20

If a doctor felt that continuing caring for an AIDS patient was beyond his skills and knowledge, he only was bound ethically to try to find the patient a new physician or to give the patient reasonable notice that he was being dropped. Society holds soldiers, policemen, and firemen to a higher standard than the AMA held physicians in this medical crisis.

Dr. David Rogers, vice chairman of the National Commission on AIDS, said doctors refer patients routinely to consultants with special expertise. For example, neurosurgeons are not qualified to perform hysterectomies. But Rogers contended that the AMA position provided doctors with an "ethical" excuse to keep AIDS/HIV patients out of their offices. He said patients with HIV sometimes need specialized care, but "80 percent-plus of their treatment ought to be in the hands of ordinary working-stiff doctors." Jeffrey Levi, government relations director of the AIDS Action Council, agreed. "I don't know of any other disease for which there is that kind of bail-out option."[21]

The AMA's position on physicians' obligation to patients with HIV/ AIDS posed a deeper dilemma, one that goes to the very root of the AMA philosophy toward patient care. Ethicists said that the AMA policy flowed from the "contract model of medical care." With this approach, care for patients in effect is a commodity, and physicians are not required to practice medicine in a *moral* fashion. Under AMA ethics, with the exception of emergencies, doctors could pick and choose which patients they were willing to treat. In the AMA's own *Journal,* medical ethicists Dr. Abigail Zuger and Steven H. Miles urged the profession to change its approach. They called for a "virtue-based medical ethic," under which patients with AIDS or other dread diseases would be cared for because it was the right thing to do.[22]

But the AMA is not about to budge on its philosophy. It may condemn the sin of refusing compassionate care to patients with HIV infections or full-blown AIDS, but the sinner is, as the AMA puts it, "free to choose whom to serve."

DOCTORS WITH AIDS

One of the AMA's brightest moments during the AIDS crisis was when it successfully went to bat in court for Gene Arline, a Florida teacher who was fired because she had experienced three relapses of tuberculosis. Citing AMA arguments, the Supreme Court for the first time created a standard for defining whether people with infectious disease were handicapped and therefore qualified for protection against discrimination under the federal Rehabilitation Act of 1973. Only if an individual's disease posed a *"significant risk"* to others was an employer justified in removing him or her from the job. Lower courts extended the finding to the HIV-infected.[23]

But the AMA seemed to ignore its own landmark case in the winter of 1991 when the CDC nailed down the first spread of HIV from a health worker, a Florida dentist, to his patients. Anticipating a public backlash against all doctors, the AMA reversed its position and called for the infected doctors and health workers to stop performing "invasive" or surgical procedures on their patients.

It all started in late July 1990, when the CDC issued a report on a dentist with AIDS who may have infected a young woman, designated as Patient A. Based on another, far more infectious blood-borne virus, hepatitis B, experts had long recognized the possibility of health workers infecting their patients.

Nobody was prepared for the fallout from the first HIV infection spread from doctor to patient. The public was panicky. Doctors tried to be reassuring, but they were not persuasive. Medicine was in deep denial.

The CDC convened experts in August 1990 to review the dangers infected health workers posed to their patients and what could be done to prevent HIV transmission. During the discussions, underlying differences of opinion became clear as representatives of various groups staked out positions on whether infected health workers should be restricted and how to define which procedures posed possible dangers to patients. Foreshadowing events to come, virologist Norbert Rapoza, the AMA representative, asked: "What does the HIV-infected health-care worker who gets cut during an invasive procedure tell the patient into whose open wound he has bled: 'I'm sorry but I've just killed you'?"[24] The position was consistent with 1987 AMA policy, which said an infected physician should not place his or her patients at risk. Until the implications of the dental case started to sink in, no one had paid much attention to the AMA policy.

Other health experts attending this session thought they could head off the AMA's propensity to restrict infected health workers. They pointed out that patients faced far greater risks from hospital-spread infections or from the unsteady hand of a surgeon who had been abusing alcohol or drugs or who was upset from an argument with a spouse earlier in the day. With little media coverage, the debate initially remained confined to the small circle of medical-association officials and CDC consultants.

However, the incident assumed a new urgency when Patient A went public with her story. She was Kimberly Bergalis, of Fort Pierce, Florida, a clean-cut twenty-two-year-old who had no known risk factors for HIV. She said she had never had sexual intercourse. Her only apparent means of catching the disease was from having been treated by Dr. David Acer, though investigators did not know and may never know precisely how the virus passed from dentist to patient. By chance, a state health investigator figured out the dental spread of HIV because Bergalis mentioned that Acer had extracted her molars, and he happened to know that the dentist had AIDS.

Acer, forty, died September 3, 1990; four days later, several Florida newspapers published a letter Acer had written to inform his patients about his illness and his contention that he had followed CDC guidelines, including wearing a mask and gloves. Some experts think Acer may have been less than scrupulous about following those guidelines or that he deliberately infected—murdered—his patients. More than 500 former patients soon came forward to be tested. On September 21 it was revealed that two more patients had been diagnosed with HIV. (Ultimately, six HIV infections would be linked to Acer.)

Meanwhile, Bergalis and her parents mounted a campaign calling for mandatory testing for HIV of all doctors to prevent a recurrence of what happened to Kimberly. They also urged that patients be tested to protect health workers. Bergalis was the first HIV patient to go public and complain bitterly about how the medical profession had responded to the AIDS epidemic.

While there were some calls for widespread testing and restriction of infected physicians, Dr. M. Roy Schwarz, AMA vice president for medical education and science, said such actions were premature: "Until science proves it unequivocally, we think . . . that it would not be wise to change the guidelines [for testing]—unless the CDC has evidence we don't know about."[25] This seemed to contrast with the sort of get-tough approach advocated earlier by AMA virologist Rapoza.

Internal Tension About Policy

The AMA was experiencing internal tension over the issue, and would soon take a course different from that suggested in the Acer case. Schwarz said the Acer case brought AIDS into focus for the AMA by raising questions about what should be done, on the one hand, with a doctor who was HIV-positive, and, on the other, to protect the public health. He said in an interview that some within the AMA felt strongly that this was an ethical matter: "Since we above all else try to 'Do no harm,' that in this case we'd err on the side of caution. If you were HIV-positive you should not do any invasive procedure, and if you did it, you ought to disclose to the patient and let the patient make their choice."

He said he was among those who believed there was no scientific evidence for limiting HIV-infected physicians. He compared this restrictive approach to "saying go ahead and burn the people at the stake because you think they're witches even though you haven't got any evidence for it. I was convinced that the risk [of doctor-to-patient transmission] was extraordinarily small . . . probably so small you could never measure it. And therefore you shouldn't jump to a blanket public policy requiring a whole bunch of things on what is primarily a theoretical risk."[26] This view would prevail, but only after a year and a half on a policy roller coaster.

PUBLIC RELATIONS VS. PUBLIC HEALTH

Shortly, events turned up the pressure, and AMA leadership felt compelled to adopt a strong public position. The CDC had found through genetic testing of viruses that three patients had been infected by virtually the same virus found in Acer, the *Los Angeles Times* reported on January 11, 1991.[27]

There was no public-health threat, but the anticipated public fear was palpable. The AMA wanted to stifle potential panic. Responding to the article, the AMA Board, which had been slow on the draw in the past, sometimes taking years to hammer out policy, was stampeded in a two-hour discussion to adopt a policy on HIV-infected health workers. The board chose to take what it described as an ethical stand. But in trying to reassure the public, it jeopardized the welfare of HIV-infected physicians.

In a statement on January 17, 1991, the day before the CDC officially published the latest findings in its *Morbidity and Mortality Weekly Report*, the AMA Board of Trustees said that because of "uncertainty about risks to patient health, the medical profession, as a matter of medical ethics, should err on the side of protecting patients. . . . Until the uncertainty about transmission is resolved, the AMA believes that HIV-infected physicians should not perform invasive procedures that pose an identifiable risk to transmission or should disclose their seropositive status prior to performing the procedure and proceed only if there is informed consent." Physicians at risk who perform invasive procedures should be tested periodically for HIV on a voluntary basis, the AMA said.

A high-level CDC official said, "I can only assume that when they heard what the report was going to say, they sort of said, 'Oh, oh, maybe it's right and what side of this do we want to be on?'" He contended that the board adopted the policy "for PR purposes. They feared the press would come out and say, 'Here are all these rich doctors protecting themselves. All they care about is themselves and their incomes. They don't care about patients.' They weren't going to be viewed as protecting the self-interest of doctors. They really went way beyond even what CDC was thinking of at that point." In fact, the AMA had set the tone for a monumental policy debate.

The board was retreating from the legal principle the AMA had established of a *significant risk* of disease spread being grounds for removal from a job. It now advocated a new standard, saying that any HIV-infected health worker who posed an *identifiable risk* to his or her patients should be removed. If anyone could come up with a scenario under which there was the remotest chance of HIV transmission from a doctor to patient, then the health worker would be prohibited from performing the procedure. To steady the public's nerves, the AMA was proposing an unattainable zero-risk standard. Schwarz explained at the time: "The board thinks we have to help the public to manage their fears."28

The AMA Is Assailed

The AMA had dug itself into a hole from which it would be hard to extract itself. It and the American Dental Association, which had taken a similar stand, immediately came under attack. Critics saw the AMA position as an unscientific, public-relations gimmick that was unworkable because physicians who disclosed their status would be committing professional suicide. No patient would want to go under the knife of an HIV-infected surgeon, though there was no evidence the patient was at a real risk.

The Centers for Disease Control conducted a conference in February 1991 at which representatives from medical, public-health, and labor groups thrashed out what should be done. The AMA and ADA stood alone in support of voluntary testing.

"Even if the policy is not universally effective, it is better than any of the alternatives," Dr. Nancy W. Dickey, an AMA Board member, told the hostile audience. "And patients are certainly better off knowing that the profession has publicly reaffirmed that their interests will always come first."29

In contrast, public-health groups, strongly influenced by advocates for people infected with HIV, took a "civil rights" approach and opposed even voluntary testing for fear it would lead to mandatory testing. They were concerned that such restrictive policies could result in infected doctors and other health workers losing their jobs and facing discrimination for no good reason.

The AMA was singled out for criticism at the session. However, the AMA attempted to create an image of AMA solidarity with the rest of medicine. *American Medical News,* the official AMA newspaper, reported that the AMA joined with other groups in opposing mandatory testing. But the truth was the AMA and the ADA stood alone, as the *Journal of the*

American Medical Association pointed out.[30] While the AMA and ADA wanted the Acer affair to serve as the basis for policy, other medical groups portrayed the case as a rarity, and hence a poor model for national policy.

The AMA claimed to be putting patients first, but there was another interpretation. By abandoning HIV-infected doctors, most of whom were gay, the AMA could quiet public fears and keep the heat off the rest of the profession.

SLAY THE AMA

The House of Delegates reviewed the board's actions during a particularly tumultuous time. ACT UP (AIDS Coalition to Unleash Power), an activist group famous for street theater, attacked the AMA's policies on AIDS, national health insurance, and alternative healing at the AMA's annual meeting in Chicago in June 1991. ACT UP staged what it called a "Slay the AMA" protest. Protesters marched on the AMA's meeting headquarters, carrying signs calling on the AMA to oppose mandatory HIV testing of physicians, and posters with pictures of board members with the word GUILTY stamped across their foreheads. As the more than 200 protesters marched, some spray-painted "Fight the AMA" slogans onto the street and buildings and shouted "murderer" at AMA delegates. One ACT UP member infiltrated the House of Delegates during a speech by Vice President Dan Quayle, shouting that "People with AIDS need national health care." The Secret Service whisked her away. Quayle told a press conference that he supported mandatory testing of doctors and patients.

Outside the hotel, more than two dozen protesters were arrested for mob action. ACT UP made it clear that it viewed the AMA as an obstacle to ensuring that people with AIDS as well as other Americans obtain medical care.[31]

"Tell or Quit": Getting Tough with HIV-Infected Health Workers

During the annual session, the House reaffirmed the policies on testing of physicians who performed invasive procedures the board had advocated the previous January. Board member Dr. Raymond Scalettar summarized the policy: infected physicians should "tell or quit."[32]

Public hysteria about iatrogenic or doctor-caused AIDS was growing. Dentists were buying advertisements announcing they had been tested to be free of HIV, a move that critics felt would create a false sense of security among patients. In some cases, infected physicians went public or were exposed in the press, with the result that they were fired or had to shut down their practices.

The CDC in July 1991 issued guidelines to encourage health workers who performed exposure-prone procedures to undergo testing for HIV, and those found infected were urged to stop performing such procedures unless they were counseled by an expert review panel on how to continue. The agency did not define which procedures posed a special risk, leaving that decision to medical, surgical, and dental societies and local hospitals. Board member Dickey said that the CDC guidelines were "close to AMA policy. . . . Speaking for the medical profession, we accept the charge to further identify exposure-prone procedures."[33]

Science may not have backed AMA and CDC policies, but the policies resonated with public opinion. Polls conducted in the summer of 1991 showed that the vast majority of patients wanted to know if their doctors were infected, and most said they would seek care elsewhere if their caregivers were infected with HIV. Likewise, the public felt that patients should inform their doctors if they were HIV-infected. Soon, the politicians, currying public favor, weighed in.

Congressman William E. Dannemeyer, the rock-ribbed conservative Republican from Southern California, introduced a bill in Kimberly Bergalis's name designed to establish mandatory testing of physicians who performed invasive procedures and patients scheduled to undergo them. The proposal also required physicians to be tested for HIV in connection with obtaining malpractice insurance and hospital privileges. Senator Jesse Helms, the conservative Republican from North Carolina, introduced an amendment to the House-passed Treasury Appropriations Bill. Helms's punitive legislation would have hit health workers with ten years in prison and/or $10,000 in fines for not disclosing to patients that they were HIV-infected.

The AMA favored controls and testing, but not the heavy hammer of criminal law. In a letter delivered to Helms the day before the vote, Dr. James Todd, AMA's chief executive, said, "The American Medical Association believes that only through application of sound medical principles, rather than through the arm of the criminal justice system, will we be able to confront the issues of HIV-infected health workers with compassion, dignity and rationality and thus ensure the safety and health of all our patients."

Helms's bill passed in summer 1991 by an 81–18 margin. As a backstop, by a 99–0 margin, the Senate also passed another amendment to the Treasury Appropriations Bill, developed by the Senate leadership, mandating that states receiving funding for health programs adopt CDC guidelines or their "equivalent" on health-care workers being tested and disclosing their status to patients. Weeks later, on a voice vote, the Senate passed another Helms amendment attached to the Commerce Appropriations Bill that required passage of state laws that would allow doctors performing invasive procedures to test patients for HIV without first obtaining specific consent, except in emergencies.[34]

SEEKING A CONSENSUS

When the AMA was called on to lead the way on developing policy on infected doctors, it gladly took on the role. But because it promoted a policy based on public relations rather than science, it seriously bungled the job, alienating other medical and advocacy groups and unnecessarily keeping the public on edge.

The CDC announced in August 1991 that with the help of medical organizations it intended to "quickly" develop a list of exposure-prone procedures, those in which a health workers' blood might come into contact with a patient's body cavities, mucous membranes, or tissue beneath the skin. The CDC, like the AMA, discouraged infected physicians from performing exposure-prone procedures.

In this guideline the CDC said it wanted the private sector, the national medical societies, to reach a consensus on which procedures were risky for HIV-infected doctors to perform. CDC planned to incorporate that information into its guidelines. CDC has no regulatory power, but its recommendations often are adopted as state or federal laws. However, bills before both Houses showed that some in Congress favored forcing the states to accept CDC guidelines for HIV-infected doctors.

Responding to the CDC, the AMA, nominal leader of American medicine, sponsored a conference, hoping to involve dozens of medical specialty groups in the development of a list of exposure-prone procedures. Going into the meeting, only a handful of groups, including the American Academy of Orthopaedic Surgeons and the American College of Obstetricians and Gynecologists, had declared their support for keeping HIV-infected members of their specialties out of the operating room, especially when exposure-prone procedures were being performed. They, along with the American Dental Association, had promised to develop lists of invasive procedures that posed the greatest risk.

With the press kept out, AMA leaders gave attendees lessons in public relations and AMA-style realpolitik. Todd, AMA chief executive, said: "There is a definite need to address and decrease the current public fear and panic." He emphasized that *no* documentation existed of a medical doctor infecting a patient with AIDS, and that any physician who admitted he or she was HIV-positive would be destroyed professionally. "However, it still seems reasonable and ethically correct to identify those few procedures where transmission might be possible and ask for self-restrictions. . . . If we make any error, it must be in favor of the patient," he said.

Scott W. Wilber, director of the AMA's Department of Congressional Relations, observed that Congress was in a mood to take some action: "They [Congress] have to do something this year. They have to show leadership and respond to their constituents." He told medical groups that they needed to create the perception that "medicine cares about more than their own self-status."[35]

Perception and image, rather than science, were serving as the basis for public-health policy at this point in the AMA mind. But it immediately became obvious that in this policy battle, the AMA was going to have problems trying to persuade the other groups to develop a list. The would-be leader had virtually no followers. The only thing those in attendance supported was the concept of educating the public and health workers about HIV, hardly a policy breakthrough. They could not agree on a list of "green light" or safe procedures, let alone on those that might be amber- or red-light procedures.

The AMA prefers to present a united front, but in this case seemed to be sending out conflicting messages. Board member Dickey said the AMA still was committed to the CDC plan to develop a list of risky, exposure-prone procedures "to help reassure our patients that it is their interest and well-being that AMA puts first." At the same time, AMA's science vice president Schwarz said compiling such a list could make "the situation worse, not better" by suggesting that the risk of contracting HIV from an infected doctor was higher than it really was.[36]

THE BERGALISES HAVE THEIR SAY

As hearings were being organized in September 1991 on his bill to control AIDS through mandatory testing of health workers and patients, Congressman Dannemeyer charged that Health Subcommittee chairman Henry A. Waxman, a liberal California congressman with a large gay constituency, was attempting to prevent the dying Kimberly Bergalis from testifying. Finally, Bergalis was scheduled to testify at the second hearing on September 26. With massive media coverage, Bergalis rode a train to Washington from her Florida home. Emaciated and exhausted, she had to be brought into the hearing room in a wheelchair. Bergalis's testimony was poignant, though brief: "I would like to say that AIDS is a terrible disease which we must take seriously. I did nothing wrong, yet I am being made to suffer like this. My life has been taken away. Please enact legislation so no other patient or health-care provider will have to go through the hell that I have. Thank you." It took fifteen seconds.

Her father, George Bergalis, minced no words: "Kimberly is the result of ten years of protection, of covert action, of unwillingness to address the real issue." He said Congress should start treating HIV/AIDS as a health issue rather than a civil-rights issue.[37] Others testified that widespread testing of doctors and patients would be too costly, costing billions and offering a false sense of security since HIV-negative one day could be HIV-positive the next. Dannemeyer and his supporters counterattacked, saying that testing can be done at a low cost as evidenced by the U.S. military's testing of recruits.

Congress in October rejected the restrictive Helms and Dannemeyer legislation. Instead, a bill written by the Senate leadership, which gave the states leeway in developing policy, was passed by the House and soon signed by President Bush. It required the states to adopt CDC guidelines on dealing with infected health-care workers and exposure-prone procedures or else lose vital federal funding. But the states were given considerable leeway by allowing them to adopt guidelines that were the *equivalent* of CDC recommendations. This provision also took some pressure off the CDC to develop a list of risky procedures, though the agency officially continued to try to do so.

Medical Groups Oppose the AMA Stand

Meanwhile, support for the list eroded even more among the medical societies. The American Dental Association, which for the previous ten months had repeatedly said it would produce a list of exposure-prone procedures, saw the weakening resolve of other groups and on September 30 dropped the quest. It said there was no scientifically valid way to compile a list.[38]

A month later the American College of Surgeons, the largest organization of surgeons, assaulted the CDC-requested plan, noting that a dental extraction "is the only procedure that can be logically called 'risk prone.'" The College said it was "dismayed that insurers, licensing bodies, government agencies and legislative bodies may propose regulations based on the CDC guidelines, because such actions are not based on direct scientific data; they are not cost effective; they are intrusive to the extreme; and they are unable to achieve their desired intent."[39]

Despite the rejection by other groups, the AMA kept trying to reassure the public by promising to make a list of exposure-prone procedures. Reacting to the American College of Surgeons' opposition, Dickey said: "The general public, in response to both their concern for the disease and how it has accelerated in response to the Bergalis case and others in Florida, really don't care what the numeric risk is. They want some form of guarantee. Until science can provide numbers that are reassuring to the public and dictate clearly to the profession, the AMA will probably continue its current policy."[40]

By November 1991, when the CDC had hoped to publish final guidelines, the AMA was the only major group left that endorsed the CDC approach to compile a list of exposure-prone procedures. The guidelines were ridiculed at a CDC-sponsored conference in November. Dr. LaMar McGinnis, Jr., chairman of the AIDS committee of the American College of Surgeons, charged that the plan involved "biopolitics" rather than science. At the meeting, one-time supporters of the plan, including the American Academy of Orthopaedic Surgeons and the American College of Obstetricians and Gynecologists, renounced the concept of listing exposure-prone procedures. By December 1991 the CDC was sending out signals that it too was going to abandon support for lists of exposure-prone procedures, and the AMA too was considering backing off on the plan.

THE AMA FLIP-FLOPS AGAIN . . . AND AGAIN

Kimberly Bergalis died December 8, 1991. Her father warned physicians and other health workers: "Someone who has AIDS and continues to practice is nothing better than a murderer." He again urged that HIV testing be required for both doctors and patients.

The next day, December 9, at the AMA meeting in Las Vegas, a committee heard support for a report that would have rejected making a list of exposure-prone procedures and would have made AMA policy consistent with other major groups. But then word came out on December 10 that three patients might have been infected with HIV by a Philadelphia surgeon. Mercy Catholic Medical Center, one hospital where the surgeon had operated, conducted a "look-back" study of

330 patients to determine whether any of the doctor's patients were infected. The research turned up the three surgical patients infected with HIV.

Could this be the long-feared case of a medical doctor spreading HIV to his patients? Should the AMA stand by its much-pilloried policy? Or should it drop the policy and rejoin the rest of medicine?

On the verge of reversing a controversial policy it had promoted for a year, the AMA leadership was spooked, even though the infections in all three Philadelphia patients could be explained by their having engaged in behaviors that put them at risk for HIV. The AMA Board met late into the night and decided to recommend that the organization, at least for the moment, should not drastically change its policies. AMA delegates went along with the board and merely asked the medical community to "determine if there is any scientific basis for the development of a list" of exposure-prone procedures.[42]

In the background, CDC officials had been conferring with the AMA staff to try to find a way for the AMA to gracefully abandon its by now highly embarrassing policies. In a memo to his staff, Dr. Gary Noble, deputy director of the CDC, said, AMA science vice president "Roy Schwarz called to say that, much to his chagrin" the AMA House had failed to drop the proposal. "He hopes this can be repaired by passage of a new resolution at the next meeting in June."[43]

The AMA was left holding the bag. It didn't officially give up on the concept until its annual meeting in June 1992, when it returned to the position of saying that HIV-infected physicians should not be removed from practice unless they posed a significant risk to public health, the standard used under federal laws. According to Schwarz, the AMA had "become more comfortable with the scientific conclusion that the risk was very small. When that point occurred, then the policy was clarified and everybody started singing completely from the same hymnal."[44]

In the end, the AMA had little clout in gathering medicine's forces in an important policy skirmish involving AIDS. Its position had been derided as unscientific and as a ploy to alleviate perceived public fears raised by an aberrational incident in which a dentist in an unexplained fashion gave HIV infections to six patients. Look-back studies involving more than 19,000 patients treated by infected surgeons have failed to turn up patients whose doctors had infected them.[45] The CDC eliminated its call for a national list of exposure-prone procedures, and the states had wide latitude to develop policy regarding HIV-infected workers. The CDC recommended that HIV-infected health workers be handled on a case-by-case basis and be permitted to stay on the job unless they posed a danger to patients.[46]

THE WRONG QUESTION

The AMA had improperly framed debate on the issue, putting the public and the medical profession through an unnecessarily difficult and rancorous process. Dr. Mervyn Silverman, president of the American Foundation for AIDS Research and former San Francisco health commissioner, contended: "The AMA was asking the wrong question: 'What do you do with the infected health-care worker?' They should have been asking, 'How do you reduce the spread of blood-borne illnesses in a health-care setting?'"[47]

Plastic surgeon Dr. Jane Petro, a lesbian and president of the American Association of Physicians for Human Rights in 1991, during the policy debate in 1991 said that as a result of the furor created by the Acer case there had been "a witch-hunt where a large number of people were fired, either because they were perceived to possibly be gay or perceived to possibly be HIV positive." Based on reports to her organization representing gay and lesbian doctors, the Lambda Legal Foundation, and to the American Civil Liberties Union, Petro estimated that up to 500 HIV-infected physicians lost their positions.[48]

The AMA's position of "tell or quit" contributed to the sacrifice of these vulnerable physicians. The AMA had used a tenet of the Hippocratic Oath, "First, do no harm," as its rationale to protect the public from HIV-infected physicians. But this public-relations posture mainly served to protect straight, uninfected physicians from mandatory testing. By isolating the infected minority, the AMA gave the oath a new twist: do no harm . . . to the profession.

The AIDS crisis showed how the game of medical politics could get in the way of sound public-health policy and medical science. The AMA argues that its response may have been slow, but no more so than other institutions. Roy Schwarz said, "I think the AMA wasn't much different than any other organization in society. First, we didn't know much about it. We tried to scramble to catch up. We tried to educate physicians to the best of our resources. We have not ducked a single tough issue in AIDS from a policy standpoint. It hasn't always been easy to get to a consensus and clear policy."[49]

After breaking a virtual policy blackout in 1987, the AMA has had a mixed record on AIDS, winning both high praise and scathing criticism. Former surgeon general Koop said he was delighted by the AMA's "aggressive action against AIDS and the willingness of the AMA Board of Trustees to expend large amounts of money on their AIDS Action Plan, which would include plans for education and projections about the spread of the epidemic. The AMA may earn its share of criticism, but it should be lauded for this private-sector effort of the doctors of America against AIDS."[50]

Advocates for people with AIDS also praised the AMA's 1987 amicus brief which the Supreme Court adapted to provide guidelines by which people with contagious diseases, including HIV, were protected against discrimination under federal laws defending the rights of the handicapped. However, responding to the Acer case in Florida, the AMA in 1991 ignored these standards in opposing HIV-infected physicians performing invasive procedures.

The AMA looked after *healthy* physicians, as reflected by the fact that in 1991 it established a disability-insurance program to safeguard the incomes of doctors who *become* HIV-positive. It has done little to help those unfortunate enough already to be HIV-positive. Benjamin Schatz, executive director of the American Association of Physicians for Human Rights in San Francisco, which runs a program to help HIV-positive physicians stay on the job, said the AMA "has taken their HIV-positive colleagues and thrown them to the wolves. They haven't done a damn thing for them." He said the AMA gave $10,000 to AAPHR's Medical Expertise Retention Program and refers HIV-infected doctors to his relatively small organization rather than offering them services.[51]

The AMA has issued many policy recommendations urging that funds be made available for education and prevention of HIV as well as calling for testing and protection of the rights of people infected with HIV. But, in some important instances, the AMA came down on the side of public relations and image rather than putting patients and science first. During the AIDS crisis, the AMA too often was guilty of public-health malpractice.

In Congress, the AMA received some credit for lobbying successfully on bills to fund AIDS research. But some lobbyists for gay groups contend that the AMA for the most part has been MIA, missing in action, on AIDS issues.

Larry Kramer, the playwright whose efforts led to the formation of a leading social-service agency for the HIV-infected as well as ACT UP, in an interview complained that doctors failed to use their considerable moral power to bring about change. "The AMA's record on dealing with AIDS has been frightful and shameful. More than anyone else, the doctors in this country know how awful AIDS is and how pervasive it is, and how dangerous it is, and how it is now a plague. And they have done precious little to use that knowledge to pressure government to do anything about it."[52]

Epilogue

As the 1990s began, the American Medical Association moved into an elegant mirrored-glass building in Chicago. The new headquarters is Japanese-designed and forward-looking, featuring sharp angles and a postmodern notch at the top. Left behind in the move was the AMA's old home, kitty-corner from the new one. It was a decades-old gray masonry structure, shaped like a squat square block, looking more like a fortress than the home of the nation's largest doctors' group. After the move, the AMA summarily razed the old building and paved it over for a parking lot.

At the same time, the AMA began refashioning its image in an attempt to bolster its sagging reputation. The AMA replaced the ornery Texas general practitioner, who ran the association with an iron fist until a financial scandal undid him, with his deputy, a smoother, Eastern establishment–type. It spent $800,000 on a campaign to enhance the organization's image, including doctoring the logo to make the snake-on-the-staff look friendlier and more trustworthy. And it spent more than $1 million more to buy ads in newspapers and magazines to boost the image of doctors and to stress that a "new" AMA had emerged in time to take part in the great national debate on health-care reform.

But try as it might, the AMA simply has not been able to bury its past, or many of its problems, in the rubble of its old headquarters. In its move to a new location, it has had little choice but to take with it a lot of old baggage. And that baggage is the foundation on which stands the AMA, its leaders, its policies, its politics, and its tactics.

Still, there *is* a new AMA. Throughout its history, the AMA has

217

reluctantly adapted to the change around it. When confronted by new technology, potent social reforms, or inescapable economic shifts, the AMA has taken the necessary steps to survive as an organization, to position itself, to maintain influence, and to protect the interests of its members. In doing so, the AMA also has abandoned positions or policies it no longer needs.

Take the AMA's current stand on the use of tobacco. After the Surgeon General issued his landmark condemnation of smoking in 1964 and on through the 1970s and into the mid-1980s, the AMA waffled. However, the AMA's line now is clearly antitobacco, although the organization itself is far from taking on the role as the ultimate antitobacco warrior. From a political standpoint, the AMA no longer needs to make the same trade-offs it once did with tobacco-state lawmakers who controlled Congress when the AMA fought to defeat, and then shape, Medicare. Now, on health-care legislation, the AMA must deal in the House with two liberal Democrats from California and two moderate Democrats from the Midwest, and in the Senate with two other moderate Democrats, one from West Virginia and another from New York. From the perspective of public relations, the AMA can gain points only by appearing to be health-conscious, rather than politically expedient. And, in the debate over sky-high health-care costs, the AMA can point to the expensive care required by smokers and claim it is fighting that public-health scourge. In contrast with the past, neutrality on tobacco issues no longer pays political dividends for the AMA. It adapted.

And the AMA even came around on the issue of whether physicians should be able to profit on the treatments they prescribe for their patients. After defending the rights of doctors to "self-refer" patients to clinical labs, MRI centers, and other physician-owned facilities, the AMA decided the negative publicity was not worth the trouble. In an effort to paint itself as an ethically responsible organization, the AMA imposed stricter ethical guidelines, although it did not ban self-referrals altogether. Besides, the AMA concluded that the main building boom of the most popular high-tech facilities, such as MRIs, was over.

But while the AMA shucks such stands, it stays close to its core positions. And that is where the "New" AMA vanishes and the "Old" AMA reappears. All that the AMA does, it does to protect those core positions. They are not all necessarily or inherently bad stands, but they are doctor-centered, not patient-centered. Those core positions include 1) protecting and extending the power of the AMA as an organization in and of itself; 2) defending the autonomy or independent authority of doctors over medical practice, 3) maintaining the AMA's and doctors' influence over the entire health-care system, 4) ensuring doctors still can operate under the fee-for-service system, and 5) enabling physicians to make as much money as possible. All of these positions are threatened by the prospect of serious, structural reform of the U.S. health-care system. That is why the AMA is a cheerleader for just enough reform to avoid a major overhaul.

The AMA is fighting a three-front war on health-care reform. First, it must battle with the Clinton administration and Congress to remove or soften changes that adversely affect doctors. Second, it must joust with other medical groups, including those nominally under its umbrella, that have embraced positions the AMA opposes. And finally, to maintain its membership and its status as a political powerhouse, the AMA must counter the impression that it is a fading organization.

Board members and staff have confided that some of the saber-rattling on health-care reform is calculated more at rallying a membership they perceive as highly conservative and frightened of even minor changes than in reflecting the beliefs of those who govern the AMA. Its leaders' public-relations efforts are designed to demonstrate to their special audiences that the AMA is doing something. The political pragmatists in the leadership are ready to make deals with the Administration and Congress, knowing that the terms will be unpopular among many members and that they will have to cajole these constituents.

AMA leaders are well aware that disgruntled members can vote with their feet. The AMA reported in November 1993 that its membership drive had for the year thus far fallen 3 percent short of the goal. The AMA plays to a hard-to-please membership: physicians are accustomed to having their way. Likewise, many members expect their leaders and lobbyists to have the ability to march into Washington and get whatever they want.

The "New" AMA's New Leader

The "new" AMA's leader is a Harvard-trained surgeon turned medical politician: Dr. James S. Todd. He already has brought a new attitude to the AMA, dropping the confrontational blustering of the past for a more conciliatory approach. Starting in the mid-1980s as the AMA's second-in-command, he helped shape the organization's response to many outside challenges. Now, in the 1990s, as the executive vice president, Todd has already begun reconsidering some of those earlier responses.

Todd faces a formidable task. He must restore the AMA's reputation, which the organization's own polls show to have reached a new low. He must rebuild the membership, which has drained away so badly that the percentage of doctors who are members has sunk to a level comparable to what it was at the turn of the century. At the same time he must hold together a profession split among factions of specialty and subspecialty groups. And he must steer the AMA through potentially the biggest change in the U.S. health-care system in more than a generation.

The sixty-two-year-old, white-haired Todd says he relishes his job, and would not give it up for positions for which he has been approached by executive headhunters, even one paying in the seven figures. He gained his first recognition within the AMA's hierarchy during the 1970s for his work on the malpractice-insurance crisis in New Jersey. But it was in 1980 that he rose to prominence within the AMA as the chairman of the committee that rewrote the Principles of Ethics. He served as board member from 1980 until 1985, when the AMA hired him as deputy executive vice president, the No. 2 staff position.

Todd made an unexpected early ascension to the top job at the AMA when a scandal forced the AMA's longtime executive vice president, Dr. James H. Sammons, to quit a year earlier than he had planned. Sammons backed Todd as his successor, and it didn't take long for the AMA to offer Todd a three-year contract, which in 1993 was renewed for another three years. Todd makes $442,000 a year in his position as the head of the $188-million not-for-profit membership association.

We had tried over several months to speak with Todd about issues discussed in this book. But he expressed a reluctance to be interviewed. Todd told us in a letter in fall 1993: "Under normal circumstances, I'd be pleased to cooperate unconditionally but, from all indications, your book about the AMA will hardly fit the definition of 'normal.'" He reiterated AMA concerns expressed a year earlier that our refusal to provide the organization with a copy of our book outline indicated we "had made up our minds about the AMA before completing the research and that, as a result, your research would focus on 'proving' your convictions." He stipulated he would consent to an interview only if he were permitted to review for factual accuracy the section of the book pertaining to this interview. We reluctantly agreed. More than a month passed before the interview took place.

We finally sat down with Todd for a one-hour interview on November 3, 1993, in the conference room adjacent to his sixteenth-floor office in the Chicago headquarters.

Todd assumed the job as the AMA's top doc at a time when the organization and the health-care system were being buffeted by talk about and perhaps the reality of reform. He has become a master of the rhetoric of change. The AMA chief executive often has talked about the AMA's House of Medicine being a House Divided and organized medicine being on the verge of civil war between feuding specialties. He has a plaque on a shelf in his office with a quote from Abraham Lincoln, who dealt with a nation divided and at war with itself. Said Lincoln: "Let neither a worship of the past, nor a confusion of the present, prevent us from preparing wisely for the future."

Behind Todd's desk is another framed saying. This one is from *The Prince* by the political theorist Machiavelli, known best for his philosophy that all necessary means should be used to maintain authority. Here there is a warning: "It must be considered that there is nothing more difficult to carry out, nor more doubtful of success, nor more dangerous to handle, than to initiate a new order of things."

Along these lines, one of the first things Todd did when he became executive vice president was to proclaim the creation of a "new" AMA. When asked what was wrong with the old one, Todd responded, "Nothing, but times change, and an organization that fails to stay in step with the times is doomed to failure." Todd looked back at his first year in his job: "1990, ten years to a millennium, tremendous change in the governance of this structure, tremendous change in needs of people for medical care. It just was time to make a statement that said we were concerned about all these things."

We wondered what about the AMA was new. After all, the same doctors essentially were running the AMA before and after it declared itself reborn. After a pause Todd replied, "I think it's more responsive. I think the doctors of this country realize that change is inevitable, that they want somebody or something that is going to help them accommodate to this change, that can be a visible symbol of what physicians are trying to do. You know that perception in this world is reality. You need to use the terms and fit your action to what is going on at that particular time."

We asked about the future of the AMA after the system was reformed. Some AMA staffers had suggested to us that the AMA might become irrelevant under certain scenarios. As to the future, Todd said, "The whole goal of the AMA at the moment, both at the board level and at the staff level, is to make this organization flexible, agile, responsive when necessary, out in front when appropriate." The AMA also is seeking government permission to reestablish itself as the enforcer of discipline of physicians, and at the same time to act as the doctors' bargaining agent.

We pointed out how the AMA's own polls show that the image of doctors and the AMA has slipped among most people. Todd acknowledged this and noted that this "distrust" on the part of the public is affecting other professions, including lawyers, clergymen, and businessmen. And he said other AMA polls show the public trusts the AMA more than the government. When asked about the size of the AMA's membership, he said it is proportionally higher than most other voluntary associations.

The name American *Medical* Association suggests a group that looks after the interests of both doctors and patients. And the AMA likes to say that that is what it does, though our conclusion is that the AMA is a doctor-first organization. We asked why the group shouldn't be called the American *Doctors'* Association. Todd answered: "Because it's more than that. The doctors belong to it. Doctors supply a considerable amount of their resources to help us do what it is we do. But we do a lot of things that are not directly for the benefit of doctors. I mean, the campaign against cholesterol. The campaign against violence. Adolescent health. And you could name, I suspect, women's health, our consumer publishing activity. We're more than a doctor organization."

When it comes down to the interests of doctors vs. the interests of patients, we asked which way the AMA would go. Todd finessed an answer. "Hopefully the right way," he said. We asked for an example. "A good example is the resource-based relative value schedule [sic]. The resource-relative value schedule was not fundamentally to the doctors' economic interest," he said. We asked why this was contrary to physician interests. After all, the chairman of the AMA Board had referred to this system as a means of preserving fee-for-service. Todd said: "Because fees were going to be limited, there was going to be a foundation upon which to judge the appropriateness of physicians' fees. But the basic issue was that neither the physician nor the public had any method by which to determine the appropriateness of fees or physicians to justify them."

We asked how this scale benefits patients. "Cost containment. Plain and simple," said Todd. But at the time the AMA made the decision to work for a fee schedule, the other options were fixed fees, known as capitation, or diagnostic-related groups (DRGs), both of which would have reduced payments to physicians even more. All the fee schedule does is preserve fee-for-service. Then we asked how does fee-for-service, a frequently chanted AMA mantra, benefit patients. "Sixty percent of the people in this country get their care under fee-for-service. It is the preferred mode of care delivery amongst all of the polls we do."

When asked why fee-for-service medicine is so important to the AMA, Todd said, "Before the government and the insurance companies got involved, it used to be a one-on-one relationship of mutual trust and responsibility. And that's fundamental in the healing process. Are you going to enjoy seeing a different doctor every time you go to your facility? Don't you want to develop a sense of trust, a relationship, a personal relationship?"

In other systems, such as health-maintenance organizations, we pointed out that patients don't necessarily lose that continuity. "You might, but you don't have to," Todd agreed. "But, you know, one size doesn't fit all. And yes, you can level some criticisms at the fee-for-service system; you can level some criticisms at the managed care-HMO systems. And I think that what we're trying to say is patients ought to have the information upon which they can make their personal judgment as to where they want to be."

We asked whether the AMA will outlive health-system reform. Todd said that the AMA's missions relating to science and medical education will help the organization survive no matter what. He expressed irritation about media views of the AMA that emphasize its political and socioeconomic activities over its other missions. He said that for every dollar the AMA spends on "socioeconomics," it spends two dollars on other things, including science and education. And he downplays the pacesetting millions the AMA's PAC spends on politics, calling the money it contributes to each politician's campaign fund as a "drop in the bucket."

Some observers say the AMA may be less relevant after reform. But Todd said, "I can make an argument it will be more relevant because the AMA is the only organization that is able to accommodate all of the diverse interests within the profession. We may not agree with them. They may be divisive, but we understand them and can explain them. And if you have increasing centralization of health care at the government level, the government is not going to want to deal with eighty-nine specialty societies. They are physically incapable of doing it. And therefore they are going to look to some sort of structure or organization than can embrace all of the diversity of medicine." He described the AMA as the "final common pathway" of all the conflicting agendas within medicine.

The interview occurred just days after President Clinton finally unveiled his 1,342-page Health Security Act. The Clinton bill not only would require at least one fee-for-service plan in each region, but would allow a physician organization like the AMA to negotiate on behalf of doctors. Todd said the Administration had made some changes the AMA had sought. Still, much remained unclear about what would transpire in the months ahead. Todd said this much: "I think this is going to be one of the greatest domestic debates this country has ever seen. It will far surpass Social Security, and I don't think we've seen anything close to what will eventually pass. I get the impression that something will happen next summer, next fall. The Congress can't go home without having done something on health-system reform."

THE AMA'S FUTURE

There is a saying within organized medicine that if there were no AMA, one would have to be invented. And for nearly 150 years, the AMA has struggled to hold together the often-warring factions within medicine. The outcome of the reform efforts will be important for us all, but for the AMA as a *political* organization it could be a matter of life or death. Even though the AMA has helped maximize doctors' earnings from Medicare, its membership dropped after its loss on this issue in the mid-1960s. If it cannot deliver for its constituents on the current health reform, its membership could further erode or even evaporate.

Hillary Rodham Clinton, the President's chief navigator for health reform, has predicted that under reform a "Darwinian struggle" will take place among health insurers. Reform also will bring to bear evolutionary forces on the AMA. And as it did after it lost its monumental battle over Medicare, the AMA is likely to sharpen its focus.

After Medicare, the AMA leadership faced two paths. One was to devote the organization to science and educational issues, doctoring in the purer Asklepian form, symbolized by the single serpent on the staff. The other was the political path, seeking the power to look after doctors' financial interests. Mercury, the patron god of businessmen, symbolized by the twin serpents of the caduceus, would favor this approach.

The AMA chose the second path, that of politics, transforming the organization into a big-time wheeler and dealer. The AMA says only one-third of its budget goes to politics. But as one of the country's largest PACs and a self-proclaimed 800-pound gorilla on Capitol Hill, it has no problem opening doors in Washington. AMA leaders even classify their meetings about physician pocketbook issues with politicians as being "educational." And over the years, the AMA has increasingly concentrated on defending and cushioning doctors against change.

Whatever happens with health reform, the AMA will survive in some form. It is well financed, has a strong survival instinct, and often has had its way. Hence, we advise the public: listen to what the AMA has to say, but consider that its message may not be as altruistic as it would have you believe. Remember it is a doctor-first organization, a special interest that may not put patient interests first. Recognize that though it uses the symbol of Asklepios, a minor god in the Greek Pantheon, that the AMA is as fallible as other human institutions, that it may blunder policies on health issues because of its own ignorance, bias, poor judgment, and political agenda. Beware the Serpent on the Staff.

Appendix

Dᴜʀɪɴɢ ᴛʜᴇ ᴘᴏʟɪᴛɪᴄᴀʟʟʏ tumultuous 1994 election cycle, the AMA as usual led the health field in political contributions, giving candidates for federal office nearly $2.7 million. At first the AMA's generosity was goaded by the Clinton's health-care reform plans, but later it was spurred on by the prospect of a Republican majority in the House and Senate. The resulting overhaul created a slight slip in the AMA's investment in the 104th Congress from $11.4 to $11.3 million.

Fifteen of the top twenty current recipients of the AMA's largesse are Republicans. And it is also notable that the new Republican Speaker of the House Newt Gingrich (R-Ga.) ranks 12th overall but first in direct contributions from the AMA's political action committee. And Senator Phil Gramm (R-Tex.), who is seeking the White House, now ranks fourth overall. His chief rival, Senator Bob Dole (R-Kan.), is way back in the field in 97th place.

Special interest groups give money to help politicians run their campaigns for election. Over the years the amount builds up becoming an investment by the interest group to ensure it has access to, and perhaps influence with a politician.

The following table updates the list published for the 103rd Congress. The figures are based on reports filed with the Federal Election Commission from 1975 through 1994, the Nexis database service, and the National Library on Money and Politics. The table lists the name of the politician the party affiliation and state, and four columns of dollar amounts.

The *Honoraria* column specifies the amounts, listed by Nexis, that the AMA or AMPAC paid politicians for speaking engagements or appearances between 1985 and 1990.

Independent Expenditures details how much AMPAC spent to independently boost a candidate's campaign. There is no limit on independent expenditures, which must be made without the knowledge or consent of the candidate. AMPAC made no independent expenditures in the 1994 cycle.

Direct Contribution is the amount AMPAC contributed directly to a candidate's campaign. Federal law limits PACs to one $5,000 contribution per election.

Total 1975–94 is the sum of Honoraria, Independent Expenditures, and Direct Contributions. This total represents the AMA's investment in each member of Congress.

AMA's Investment in the 104th Congress

NAME	HONORARIA	INDEPENDENT EXPEND.	DIRECT CONTRIB.	TOTAL
1. Rep. Vic Fazio, D CA	8,000	259,085	61,000	328,085
2. Sen. Bob Packwood, R OR		227,808	20,300	248,108
3. Rep. Scott McInnis, R CO		184,910	19,999	204,909
4. Sen. Phil Gramm, R TX		107,767	59,696	167,463
5. Rep. David E. Skaggs, D CO		109,480	41,050	150,530
6. James V. Hansen, R UT	1,000	65,359	69,000	135,359
7. Rep. Mike Parker, D MS	1,000	94,101	32,750	127,851
8. Rep. Gary A. Franks, R CT		81,254	30,200	111,454
9. Rep. Tim Johnson, D SD	1,000	64,410	43,249	108,659
10. Rep. Scott L. Klug, R WI		80,968	17,500	98,468
11. Sen. Daniel R. Coats, R IN	1,000	19,391	64,523	84,914
12. Rep. Newt Gingrich, R GA		1,000	80,636	81,636
13. Rep. Herbert H. Bateman, R VA		29,204	51,488	80,692
14. Rep. E. Clay Shaw, R FL		17,433	62,845	80,278
15. Rep. Bob Stump, R AZ		15,713	61,646	77,359
16. Rep. Jack Fields, R TX		8,829	68,152	76,981
17. Sen. Richard C. Shelby, D AL		26,858	48,600	75,458
18. Rep. Frank R. Wolf, R VA			74,850	74,850
19. Rep. Bill Emerson, R MO	500		71,305	71,805
20. Rep. Jerry Lewis, R CA	1,000		70,000	71,000
21. Rep. John Edward Porter, R IL	3,000		66,036	69,036
22. Rep. Carlos J. Moorhead, R CA		2,030	65,850	67,880
23. Rep. Harold L. Volkmer, D MO			64,950	64,950
24. Rep. Don Young, R AK			64,875	64,875
25. Rep. Henry J. Hyde, R IL			64,500	64,500

NAME	HONORARIA	INDEPENDENT EXPEND.	DIRECT CONTRIB.	TOTAL
26. Rep. Gerald B.H. Solomon, R NY	1,000		61,819	62,819
27. Rep. Pat Roberts, R KS			61,400	61,400
28. Rep. Robert T. Matsui, D CA			60,750	60,750
29. Rep. Bill Thomas, R CA			60,100	60,100
30. Rep. William F. Clinger, R PA		14,714	44,808	59,522
31. Rep. Ralph M. Hall, D TX			58,780	58,780
32. Rep. Ike Skelton, D MO			58,300	58,300
33. Sen. Olympia J. Snowe, R ME		14,581	43,325	57,906
34. Rep. Thomas J. Manton, D NY			57,500	57,500
35. Rep. Floyd D. Spence, R SC		500	56,450	56,950
36. Rep. Charles Wilson, D TX			56,272	56,272
37. Rep. Thom DeLay, R TX	1,000		54,650	55,650
38. Rep. Martin Frost, D TX			54,650	54,650
39. Rep. Jim Chapman, D TX	3,000		50,784	53,784
40. Rep. John Bryant, D TX			53,717	53,717
41. Rep. Jim Ross Lightfoot, R IA	1,000		52,434	53,434
42. Rep. Michael Bilirakis, R FL			53,250	53,250
43. Rep. Thomas J. Bliley, R VA	1,000		52,250	53,250
44. Rep. Charlie Rose, D NC	2,000		50,400	52,400
45. Barbara F. Vucanovich, R NV		15,187	37,100	52,287
46. Rep. Dennis Hastert, R IL			50,000	50,000
47. Rep. Harold Rogers, R KY			49,835	49,835
48. Rep. Jan Meyers, R KS			49,500	49,500
49. Rep. C.W. Bill Young, R FL			48,850	48,850
50. Rep. Constance A. Morella, R MD			47,634	47,634
51. Rep. Henry A. Waxman, D CA	3,000	2,000	42,250	47,250
52. Rep. Jim Bunning, R KY			46,750	46,750
53. Rep. Sonny Callahan, R AL			46,750	46,750
54. Rep. Doug Bereuter, R NE			46,500	46,500
55. Rep. Steny H. Hoyer, D MD			45,550	45,550
56. Rep. W.G. Hefner, D NC			45,225	45,225
57. Sen. James M. Inhofe, R OK			44,975	44,975
58. Rep. Curt Weldon, R PA			44,811	44,811
59. Rep. Joe L. Barton, R TX			44,067	44,067
60. Rep. Robert K. Dornan, R CA			43,500	43,500
61. Sen. Max Baucus, D MT		18,169	24,950	43,119
62. Rep. Jim Kolbe, R AZ			43,000	43,000
63. Rep. Dan Schaefer, R CO	1,000		41,500	42,500
64. Rep. Edolphus Towns, D NY	1,500		40,550	42,050
65. Rep. Louise M. Slaughter, D NY			41,449	41,449
66. Sen. Jon Kyl, R AZ			41,300	41,300
67. Rep. James H. Quillen, R TN			41,283	41,283

NAME	HONORARIA	INDEPENDENT EXPEND.	DIRECT CONTRIB.	TOTAL
68. Rep. Steve Gunderson, R WI	1,000		39,978	40,978
69. Rep. Dick Armey, R TX	2,000		37,950	39,950
70. Rep. John P. Murtha, D PA		618	39,250	39,868
71. Rep. Dan Burton, R IN	1,000		38,650	39,650
72. Rep. John R. Kasich, R OH			39,650	39,650
73. Sen. Charles E. Grassley, R IA			38,973	38,973
74. Rep. Bill McCollum, R FL	1,000		37,750	38,750
75. Rep. Nancy L. Johnson, R CT	2,000		36,067	38,067
76. Rep. Barbara B. Kennelly, D CT		9,968	28,050	38,018
77. Sen. Orrin G. Hatch, R UT			38,000	38,000
78. Sen. Larry E. Craig, R ID	1,000		36,964	37,964
79. Rep. Ronald D. Coleman, D TX	2,000		35,900	37,900
80. Rep. Norman Y. Mineta, D CA			37,800	37,800
81. Sen. Judd Gregg, R NH		17,139	20,500	37,639
82. Rep. Benjamin L. Cardin, D MD			37,449	37,449
83. Rep. Joe Skeen, R NM		17,480	19,750	37,230
84. Rep. Christopher H. Smith, R NJ			37,215	37,215
85. Rep. Ron Packard, R CA			37,100	37,100
86. Rep. Marge Roukema, R NJ	2,000		34,290	36,290
87. Rep. John Lewis, D GA	2,000		34,000	36,000
88. Rep. Larry Combest, R TX			35,605	35,605
89. Rep. Robert G. Torricelli, D NJ			35,550	35,550
90. Rep. William O. Lipinski, D IL			35,334	35,334
91. Rep. Frank Pallone, D NJ			35,130	35,130
92. Rep. Susan Molinari, R NY			35,000	35,000
93. Rep. Richard A. Gephardt, D MO			34,975	34,975
94. Sen. Craig Thomas, R WY		5,164	29,700	34,864
95. Rep. Robert E. Cramer, D AL			34,700	34,700
96. Sen. Bob Dole, R KS			34,500	34,500
97. Rep. Nita M. Lowey, D NY			34,500	34,500
98. Sen. Connie Mack, R FL			34,500	34,500
99. Rep. Bud Shuster, R PA			34,300	34,300
100. Rep. Eliot L. Engel, D NY			34,137	34,137
101. Rep. Richard H. Baker, R LA	2,000	2,000	29,999	33,999
102. Rep. Bill Paxon, R NY			33,889	33,889
103. Rep. Nancy Pelosi, D CA			33,850	33,850
104. Rep. Steven H. Schiff, R NM			33,850	33,850
105. Rep. Peter A. DeFazio, D OR	1,000		32,837	33,837
106. Rep. James T. Walsh, R NY			33,450	33,450
107. Rep. David R. Obey, D WI	3,000		30,250	33,250
108. Rep. Gary L. Ackerman, D NY			32,950	32,950
109. Rep. Thomas M. Foglietta, D PA			32,750	32,750

NAME	HONORARIA	INDEPENDENT EXPEND.	DIRECT CONTRIB.	TOTAL
110. Rep. Harris W. Fawell, R IL			32,700	32,700
111. Rep. Duncan Hunter, R CA		16,010	16,500	32,510
112. Rep. John T. Myers, R IN			32,427	32,427
113. Rep. David Dreier, R CA	1,000		31,300	32,300
114. Rep. Glenn English, D OK			32,287	32,287
115. Sen. Slade Gorton, R WA			32,237	32,237
116. Rep. Tom Petri, R WI			32,057	32,057
117. Sen. Richard G. Lugar, R IN		2,000	29,650	31,650
118. Rep. Lamar Smith, R TX			31,167	31,167
119. Rep. Jim McCrery, R LA			31,000	31,000
120. Rep. Tony P. Hall, D OH	2,000		28,750	30,750
121. Rep. H. James Saxton, R NJ			30,650	30,650
122. Rep. Michael G. Oxley, R OH			30,400	30,400
123. Rep. Lewis F. Payne, D VA			30,100	30,100
124. Sen. Wendell H. Ford, D KY		2,000	28,000	30,000
125. Sen. Howell Heflin, D AL			30,000	30,000
126. Sen. Robert C. Smith, R NH			30,000	30,000
127. Rep. Bill Zeliff, R NH			30,000	30,000
128. Rep. Bill K. Brewster, D OK			29,974	29,974
129. Rep. John M. Spratt, D SC		750	29,136	29,886
130. Rep. Julian C. Dixon, D CA	1,000		28,800	29,800
131. Rep. Gene Taylor, D MS			29,528	29,528
132. Sen. William V. Roth, R DE	1,000		28,500	29,500
133. Rep. Bart Gordon, D TN			29,162	29,162
134. Sen. Jeff Bingaman, D NM			29,000	29,000
135. Rep. Richard J. Durbin, D IL	1,000		27,770	28,770
136. Rep. Jack Reed, D RI			28,620	28,620
137. Rep. Charles B. Rangel, D NY			28,550	28,550
138. Rep. Elton Gallegly, R CA			28,500	28,500
139. Sen. John W. Warner, R VA		5,000	23,500	28,500
140. Rep. Robert A. Borski, D PA			28,100	28,100
141. Rep. Paul E. Kanjorski, D PA			27,950	27,950
142. Rep. Paul B. Henry, R MI			27,750	27,750
143. Rep. Bill Richardson, D NM	1,000		26,682	27,682
144. Rep. Thomas W. Ewing, R IL			27,500	27,500
145. Sen. Ben Nighthorse Campbell, D CO			27,499	27,499
146. Rep. Toby Roth, R WI			27,467	27,467
147. Rep. Bob Clement, D TN			27,450	27,450
148. Sen. John McCain, R AZ			27,450	27,450
149. Rep. Benjamin A. Gilman, R NY			27,400	27,400
150. Rep. Dana Rohrabacher, R CA			27,350	27,350
151. Sen. Larry Pressler, R SD			27,250	27,250

NAME	HONORARIA	INDEPENDENT EXPEND.	DIRECT CONTRIB.	TOTAL
152. Rep. Cliff Stearns, R FL			27,200	27,200
153. Rep. Howard Coble, R NC			27,109	27,109
154. Rep. George W. Gekas, R PA			26,900	26,900
155. Rep. Charles H. Taylor, R NC			26,896	26,896
156. Rep. Jim Ramstad, R MN			26,780	26,780
157. Rep. Greg Laughlin, D TX			26,625	26,625
158. Rep. Ileana Ros-Lehtinen, R FL			26,600	26,600
159. Sen. John H. Chafee, R RI			26,500	26,500
160. Rep. Peter J. Visclosky, D IN			26,050	26,050
161. Rep. Amo Houghton, R NY			25,850	25,850
162. Rep. Tom Sawyer, D OH			25,699	25,699
163. Sen. Thad Cochran, R MS			25,669	25,669
164. Rep. David L. Hobson, R OH			25,550	25,550
165. Rep. Sam M. Gibbons, D FL			25,450	25,450
166. Rep. Joel Hefley, R CO	1,000		24,334	25,334
167. Rep. Sherwood Boehlert, R NY			25,150	25,150
168. Rep. Fred Upton, R MI	1,000		24,099	25,099
169. Sen. Jesse Helms, R NC			25,000	25,000
170. Rep. Harry Johnston, D FL			25,000	25,000
171. Rep. Jose E. Serrano, D NY			25,000	25,000
172. Rep. Tom Lantos, D CA			24,950	24,950
173. Rep. Nathan Deal, D GA			24,700	24,700
174. Rep. Pete Geren, D TX			24,700	24,700
175. Rep. Paul E. Gillmor, R OH			24,650	24,650
176. Sen. William S. Cohen, R ME		2,000	22,500	24,500
177. Rep. Michael R. McNulty, D NY			24,500	24,500
178. Rep. C. Christophe Cox, R CA			24,450	24,450
179. Rep. Jerry F. Costello, D IL			23,850	23,850
180. Rep. Robert L. Livingston, R LA			23,625	23,625
181. Rep. E. de la Garza, D TX			23,467	23,467
182. Sen. Don Nickles, R OK			23,100	23,100
183. Rep. Porter J. Goss, R FL			23,000	23,000
184. Rep. Wayne Allard, R CO			22,994	22,994
185. Rep. Major R. Owens, D NY			22,950	22,950
186. Rep. John A. Boehner, R OH			22,900	22,900
187. Rep. F. James Sensenbrenner, R WI			22,700	22,700
188. Sen. Sam Nunn, D GA	5,470		17,000	22,470
189. Rep. Mel Hancock, R MO			22,350	22,350
190. Sen. Strom Thurmond, R SC			22,100	22,100
191. Rep. Joseph M. McDade, R PA			22,075	22,075
192. Sen. Jim Exon, D NE			22,000	22,000
193. Sen. Ernest F. Hollings, D SC			22,000	22,000

NAME	HONORARIA	INDEPENDENT EXPEND.	DIRECT CONTRIB.	TOTAL
194. Rep. Dick Zimmer, R NJ			21,645	21,645
195. Rep. Jimmy Hayes, D LA	1,000		20,600	21,600
196. Rep. Solomon P. Ortiz, D TX			21,300	21,300
197. Sen. David Pryor, D AR			21,100	21,100
198. Rep. Owen B. Pickett, D VA			21,050	21,050
199. Rep. John Linder, R GA			20,800	20,800
200. Rep. Dave Camp, R MI			20,700	20,700
201. Rep. Dale E. Kildee, D MI			20,675	20,675
202. Sen. Daniel Patrick Moynihan, D NY			20,500	20,500
203. Rep. Wally Herger, R CA			20,100	20,100
204. Rep. James A. Barcia, D MI			20,000	20,000
205. Sen. Christopher S. Bond, R MO			20,000	20,000
206. Sen. Pete V. Domenici, R NM			20,000	20,000
207. Sen. Dianne Feinstein, D CA			20,000	20,000
208. Rep. John L. Mica, R FL			20,000	20,000
209. Rep. Jack Kingston, R GA			19,700	19,700
210. Rep. Norm Dicks, D WA			19,575	19,575
211. Rep. W.J. Tauzin, D LA			18,950	18,950
212. Rep. Jim Nussle, R IA			18,500	18,500
213. Rep. John T. Doolittle, R CA			18,450	18,450
214. Rep. G.V. Montgomery, D MS		2,000	16,300	18,300
215. Rep. Robert E. Andrews, D NJ			18,150	18,150
216. Sen. Arlen Specter, R PA			18,000	18,000
217. Rep. William L. Clay, D MO			17,950	17,950
218. Rep. Rick Boucher, D VA			17 850	17 850
219. Rep. John Tanner, D TN			17,700	17,700
220. Rep. Bill Baker, R CA			17,500	17,500
221. Sen. Mark O. Hatfield, R OR			17,500	17,500
222. Rep. Gerald D. Kleczka, D WI			17,150	17,150
223. Rep. Richard E. Neal, D MA			17,150	17,150
224. Rep. Michael D. Crapo, R ID			17,046	17,046
225. Rep. Anna G. Eshoo, D CA			16,500	16,500
226. Rep. Gene Green, D TX			16,500	16,500
227. Sen. James M. Jeffords, R VT		2,100	14,050	16,150
228. Rep. Howard L. Berman, D CA			16,100	16,100
229. Rep. Glen Browder, D AL			16,000	16,000
230. Sen. Alan K. Simpson, R WY			16,000	16,000
231. Sen. Alfonse M. D'Amato, R NY			15,940	15,940
232. Rep. Ed Pastor, D AZ			15,850	15,850
233. Rep. Bill Barrett, R NE			15,550	15,550
234. Rep. Pete Peterson, D FL			15,500	15,500
235. Rep. John J. Duncan, R TN			15,450	15,450

NAME	HONORARIA	INDEPENDENT EXPEND.	DIRECT CONTRIB.	TOTAL
236. Sen. Rick Santorum, R PA			15,385	15,385
237. Sen. Kay Bailey Hutchison, R TX			15,350	15,350
238. Rep. Bill Orton, D UT			15,300	15,300
239. Rep. Floyd H. Flake, D NY			15,250	15,250
240. Rep. Joe Moakley, D MA			15,100	15,100
241. Sen. Bill Bradley, D NJ			15,050	15,050
242. Sen. Dale Bumpers, D AR	2,000	2,000	11,000	15,000
243. Rep. Peter T. King, R NY			15,000	15,000
244. Rep. Deborah Pryce, R OH			15,000	15,000
245. Sen. Frank H. Murkowski, R AK			14,825	14,825
246. Rep. Thomas M. Barrett, D WI			14,700	14,700
247. Rep. Mac Collins, R GA			14,700	14,700
248. Rep. Pat Danner, D MO			14,700	14,700
249. Rep. Tom Bevill, D AL			14,650	14,650
250. Rep. Sander M. Levin, D MI			14,625	14,625
251. Rep. Kweisi Mfume, D MD			14,600	14,600
252. Rep. Jennifer Dunn, R WA			14,350	14,350
253. Rep. Bob Filner, D CA			14,350	14,350
254. Rep. Tim Hutchinson, R AR			14,350	14,350
255. Sen. Tom Daschle, D SD			14,250	14,250
256. Rep. Alan B. Mollohan, D WV			14,150	14,150
257. Rep. Cass Ballenger, R NC			14,100	14,100
258. Rep. Howard P. McKeon, R CA			14,000	14,000
259. Rep. Martin Olav Sabo, D MN			13,900	13,900
260. Rep. Tim Roemer, D IN			13,700	13,700
261. Sen. Christopher J. Dodd, D CT			13,500	13,500
262. Rep. Chet Edwards, D TX			13,500	13,500
263. Sen. Paul Coverdell, R GA			13,400	13,400
264. Rep. Norman Sisisky, D VA			13,300	13,300
265. Sen. Mitch McConnell, R KY			13,200	13,200
266. Rep. Matthew G. Martinez, D CA			13,100	13,100
267. Rep. Charles E. Schumer, D NY			13,100	13,100
268. Rep. Gary A. Condit, D CA			13,050	13,050
269. Rep. Rick A. Lazio, R NY			13,000	13,000
270. Sen. Harry Reid, D NV			13,000	13,000
271. Rep. Frank Tejeda, D TX			12,999	12,999
272. Rep. George Miller, D CA			12,950	12,950
273. Rep. Ray Thornton, D AR			12,850	12,850
274. Rep. James P. Moran, D VA			12,700	12,700
275. Sen. Ted Stevens, R AK			12,500	12,500
276. Rep. James M. Talent, R MO			12,500	12,500
277. Rep. Jay C. Kim, R CA			12,350	12,350

NAME	HONORARIA	INDEPENDENT EXPEND.	DIRECT CONTRIB.	TOTAL
278. Rep. Ed Royce, R CA			12,350	12,350
279. Rep. William J. Coyne, D PA			12,225	12,225
280. Rep. Lee H. Hamilton, D IN			12,050	12,050
281. Rep. Carolyn B. Maloney, D NY			12,000	12,000
282. Rep. Maxine Waters, D CA			12,000	12,000
283. Rep. Sam Johnson, R TX			11,984	11,984
284. Rep. John D. Dingell, D MI			11,950	11,950
285. Rep. Jim McDermott, D WA			11,750	11,750
286. Rep. Esteban E. Torres, D CA			11,750	11,750
287. Sen. Joseph R. Biden, D DE			11,500	11,500
288. Sen. John B. Breaux, D LA		607	10,550	11,157
289. Sen. J. Bennett Johnston, D LA			11,100	11,100
290. Rep. Dan Miller, R FL			11,000	11,000
291. Rep. David Minge, D MN			11,000	11,000
292. Rep. Donald Manzullo, R IL			10,950	10,950
293. Sen. Bob Graham, D FL			10,949	10,949
294. Rep. Bob Franks, R NJ			10,500	10,500
295. Rep. Richard W. Pombo, R CA			10,400	10,400
296. Rep. James L. Oberstar, D MN			10,350	10,350
297. Rep. Harold E. Ford, D TN			10,250	10,250
298. Rep. John M. McHugh, R NY			10,245	10,245
299. Rep. Spencer Bachus, R AL			10,200	10,200
300. Sen. Barbara A. Mikulski, D MD			10,150	10,150
301. Rep. John Baldacci, D ME			10,000	10,000
302. Rep. Roscoe G. Bartlett, R MD			10,000	10,000
303. Sen. Robert F. Bennett, R UT			10,000	10,000
304. Rep. Sam Brownback, R KS			10,000	10,000
305. Rep. Richard M. Burr, R NC			10,000	10,000
306. Rep. Steve Buyer, R IN			10,000	10,000
307. Rep. Charles T. Canady, R FL			10,000	10,000
308. Rep. Helen Chenoweth, R ID			10,000	10,000
309. Rep. Tom Coburn, R OK			10,000	10,000
310. Rep. Thomas M. III Davis, R VA			10,000	10,000
311. Sen. Mike DeWine, R OH			10,000	10,000
312. Rep. John Ensign, R NV			10,000	10,000
313. Rep. Sam Farr, D CA			10,000	10,000
314. Rep. Chaka Fattah, D PA			10,000	10,000
315. Rep. Jon D. Fox, R PA			10,000	10,000
316. Sen. Bill Frist, R TN			10,000	10,000
317. Rep. Gil Gutknecht, R MN			10,000	10,000
318. Rep. Joe Knollenberg, R MI			10,000	10,000
319. Sen. Joseph I. Lieberman, D CT			10,000	10,000

NAME	HONORARIA	INDEPENDENT EXPEND.	DIRECT CONTRIB.	TOTAL
320. Rep. Frank A. LoBiondo, R NJ			10,000	10,000
321. Rep. William P. "Bill" Luther, D MN			10,000	10,000
322. Rep. Mel Reynolds, D IL			10,000	10,000
323. Rep. Matt Salmon, R AZ			10,000	10,000
324. Rep. John Shadegg, R AZ			10,000	10,000
325. Rep. Jerry Weller, R IL			10,000	10,000
326. Rep. Roger Wicker, R MS			10,000	10,000
327. Sen. Lauch Faircloth, R NC			9,982	9,982
328. Sen. Hank Brown, R CO			9,972	9,972
329. Rep. Mark Foley, R FL			9,700	9,700
330. Rep. Enid Greene Waldholtz, R UT			9,700	9,700
331. Rep. Pete Stark, D CA			9,600	9,600
332. Rep. Tillie Fowler, R FL			9,500	9,500
333. Rep. Ernest Jim Istook, R OK			9,500	9,500
334. Rep. Dave Weldon, R FL			9,500	9,500
335. Rep. James E. Clyburn, D SC			9,450	9,450
336. Rep. Henry Bonilla, R TX			9,350	9,350
337. Rep. Albert R. Wynn, D MD			9,350	9,350
338. Rep. Barbara Cubin, R WY			9,000	9,000
339. Sen. Charles S. Robb, D VA			9,000	9,000
340. Rep. Cardiss Collins, D IL			8,725	8,725
341. Rep. Pat Williams, D MT			8,600	8,600
342. Rep. Collin C. Peterson, D MN			8,550	8,550
343. Rep. Karen L. Thurman, D FL			8,500	8,500
344. Rep. Donald M. Payne, D NJ			8,450	8,450
345. Rep. John W. Olver, D MA			8,350	8,350
346. Rep. Lucille Roybal-Allard, D CA			8,350	8,350
347. Sen. Conrad Burns, R MT			8,139	8,139
348. Rep. Sherrod Brown, D OH			8,000	8,000
349. Rep. Eddie Bernice Johnson, D TX			7,700	7,700
350. Sen. Donald W. Riegle, D MI			7,600	7,600
351. Sen. Nancy Landon Kassebaum, R KS			7,500	7,500
352. Rep. Tim Holden, D PA			7,350	7,350
353. Rep. Bobby L. Rush, D IL			7,350	7,350
354. Rep. John J. LaFalce, D NY			7,200	7,200
355. Sen. John D. Rockefeller, D WV			7,000	7,000
356. Rep. Craig Washington, D TX			7,000	7,000
357. Rep. Cal Dooley, D CA			6,850	6,850
358. Rep. Bob Wise, D WV			6,850	6,850
359. Rep. Randy Cunningham, R CA			6,700	6,700
360. Rep. Robert W. Goodlatte, R VA			6,606	6,606
361. Rep. Ken Calvert, R CA			6,600	6,600

NAME	HONORARIA	INDEPENDENT EXPEND.	DIRECT CONTRIB.	TOTAL
362. Sen. Trent Lott, R MS			6,515	6,515
363. Sen. Frank R. Lautenberg, D NJ			6,500	6,500
364. Sen. Rod Grams, R MN			6,350	6,350
365. Sen. Tom Harkin, D IA			6,350	6,350
366. Rep. Eva Clayton, D NC			6,100	6,100
367. Rep. Gerry E. Studds, D MA			6,000	6,000
368. Rep. Nydia M. Velazquez, D NY			6,000	6,000
369. Rep. Melvin Watt, D NC			6,000	6,000
370. Rep. J.C. Watts, R OK			6,000	6,000
371. Rep. Joseph P. Kennedy, D MA			5,850	5,850
372. Rep. Walter R. Tucker, D CA			5,850	5,850
373. Rep. George E. Brown, D CA			5,810	5,810
374. Rep. Robert S. Walker, R PA			5,750	5,750
375. Rep. Bruce F. Vento, D MN			5,725	5,725
376. Rep. Ron Klink, D PA			5,556	5,556
377. Sen. Robert C. Byrd, D WV			5,550	5,550
378. Rep. Blanche Lambert, D AR			5,500	5,500
379. Rep. Karen McCarthy, D MO			5,500	5,500
380. Rep. Frank Riggs, R CA			5,350	5,350
381. Rep. Christopher Shays, R CT			5,300	5,300
382. Sen. Paul Simon, D IL			5,100	5,100
383. Sen. John Ashcroft, R MO			5,000	5,000
384. Rep. Scotty Baesler, D KY			5,000	5,000
385. Rep. Sanford D. Bishop, D GA			5,000	5,000
386. Rep. Ed Bryant, R TN			5,000	5,000
387. Rep. Saxby Chambliss, R GA			5,000	5,000
388. Rep. Dick Chrysler, R MI			5,000	5,000
389. Rep. Wes Cooley, R OR			5,000	5,000
390. Rep. Philip M. Crane, R IL			5,000	5,000
391. Rep. Frank A. Cremeans, R OH			5,000	5,000
392. Rep. Phil English, R PA			5,000	5,000
393. Rep. Rodney Frelinghuysen, R NJ			5,000	5,000
394. Rep. Daniel Frisa, R NY			5,000	5,000
395. Rep. Greg Ganske, R IA			5,000	5,000
396. Rep. Lindsey Graham, R SC			5,000	5,000
397. Rep. J.D. Hayworth, R AZ			5,000	5,000
398. Rep. Sue W. Kelly, R NY			5,000	5,000
399. Rep. Ray LaHood, R IL			5,000	5,000
400. Rep. Steve Largent, R OK			5,000	5,000
401. Rep. Zoe Lofgren, D CA			5,000	5,000
402. Rep. David M. McIntosh, R IN			5,000	5,000
403. Rep. Cynthia A. McKinney, D GA			5,000	5,000

NAME	HONORARIA	INDEPENDENT EXPEND.	DIRECT CONTRIB.	TOTAL
404. Rep. Sue Myrick, R NC			5,000	5,000
405. Rep. Jerrold Nadler, D NY			5,000	5,000
406. Rep. George Nethercutt, R WA			5,000	5,000
407. Rep. Mark W. Neumann, R WI			5,000	5,000
408. Rep. Jack Quinn, R NY			5,000	5,000
409. Rep. Steve Stockman, R TX			5,000	5,000
410. Sen. Fred Thompson, R TN			5,000	5,000
411. Rep. Nick J. Rahall, D WV			4,900	4,900
412. Rep. Luis V. Gutierrez, D IL			4,850	4,850
413. Rep. Richard "Doc" Hastings, R WA			4,800	4,800
414. Rep. Barney Frank, D MA			4,700	4,700
415. Rep. Xavier Becerra, D CA			4,500	4,500
416. Rep. David E. Bonior, D MI	2,000		2,350	4,350
417. Rep. Sam Gejdenson, D CT			4,150	4,150
418. Rep. Ronald V. Dellums, D CA			4,000	4,000
419. Rep. James A. Traficant, D OH			4,000	4,000
420. Rep. Rosa DeLauro, D CT			3,700	3,700
421. Rep. Mark E. Souder, R IN			3,570	3,570
422. Rep. Corrine Brown, D FL			3,500	3,500
423. Rep. William J. Jefferson, D LA			3,500	3,500
424. Rep. Michael N. Castle, R DE			3,450	3,450
425. Rep. Louis Stokes, D OH			3,375	3,375
426. Rep. Ron Wyden, D OR	1,000		2,225	3,225
427. Rep. James C. Greenwood, R PA			3,000	3,000
428. Rep. Frank R. Mascara, D PA			3,000	3,000
429. Rep. Paul McHale, D PA			3,000	3,000
430. Rep. Peter Deutsch, D FL			2,850	2,850
431. Rep. Jane Harman, D CA			2,850	2,850
432. Rep. Carrie Meek, D FL			2,850	2,850
433. Rep. Bob Barr, R GA			2,500	2,500
434. Rep. Cleo Fields, D LA			2,500	2,500
435. Rep. Bill Martini, R NJ			2,500	2,500
436. Rep. Peter I. Blute, R MA			2,000	2,000
437. Rep. Lincoln Diaz-Balart, R FL			2,000	2,000
438. Sen. Daniel K. Inouye, D HI			2,000	2,000
439. Rep. Randy Tate, R WA			2,000	2,000
440. Rep. Bennie Thompson, D MS			2,000	2,000
441. Rep. Lynn Woolsey, D CA			2,000	2,000
442. Rep. Edward J. Markey, D MA			1,950	1,950
443. Sen. Kent Conrad, D ND			1,859	1,859
444. Rep. Robert Menendez, D NJ			1,850	1,850
445. Sen. John Glenn, D OH			1,650	1,650

NAME	HONORARIA	INDEPENDENT EXPEND.	DIRECT CONTRIB.	TOTAL
446. Rep. Lane Evans, D IL			1,350	1,350
447. Rep. Earl F. Hilliard, D AL			1,350	1,350
448. Sen. Paul S. Sarbanes, D MD			1,025	1,025
449. Rep. Charles Bass, R NH			1,000	1,000
450. Rep. Sonny Bono, R CA			1,000	1,000
451. Sen. Richard H. Bryan, D NV			1,000	1,000
452. Rep. Alcee L. Hastings, D FL			1,000	1,000
453. Rep. Glenn Poshard, D IL			1,000	1,000
454. Rep. Andrea Seastrand, R CA			1,000	1,000
455. Rep. Patricia Schroeder, D CO			925	925
456. Rep. Wayne T. Gilchrest, R MD			850	850
457. Rep. Tom Latham, R IA			500	500
458. Sen. Patrick J. Leahy, D VT			500	500
459. Rep. Neil Abercrombie, D HI			350	350
460. Rep. Terry Everett, R AL			350	350
461. Rep. Earl Pomeroy, D ND			350	350
462. Rep. Bart Stupak, D MI			350	350
463. Rep. John Conyers, D MI			300	300
464. Rep. Bob Ney, R OH			300	300
465. Sen. Daniel K. Akaka, D HI			0	0
466. Rep. Bill Archer, R TX			0	0
467. Rep. Anthony C. Beilenson, D CA			0	0
468. Rep. Ken Bentsen, D TX			0	0
469. Rep. Brian P. Bilbray, R CA			0	0
470. Sen. Barbara Boxer, D CA			0	0
471. Rep. Jim Bunn, R OR			0	0
472. Rep. Steve Chabot, R OH			0	0
473. Rep. Jon Christensen, R NE			0	0
474. Rep. Barbara-Rose Collins, D MI			0	0
475. Rep. Jay Dickey, R AR			0	0
476. Rep. Lloyd Doggett, D TX			0	0
477. Sen. Byron L. Dorgan, D ND			0	0
478. Rep. Mike Doyle, D PA			0	0
479. Rep. Robert L. Jr. Erlich, R MD			0	0
480. Sen. Russell D. Feingold, D WI			0	0
481. Rep. Michael Patrick Flanagan, R IL			0	0
482. Rep. Michael P. Forbes, R NY			0	0
483. Rep. David Funderbunk, R NC			0	0
484. Rep. Elizabeth Furse, D OR			0	0
485. Rep. Henry B. Gonzalez, D TX			0	0
486. Rep. Bill Goodling, R PA			0	0
487. Rep. Fred Heineman, R NC			0	0

NAME	HONORARIA	INDEPENDENT EXPEND.	DIRECT CONTRIB.	TOTAL
488. Rep. Van Hilleary, R TN			0	0
489. Rep. Maurice D. Hinchey, D NY			0	0
490. Rep. Peter Hoekstra, R MI			0	0
491. Rep. Martin R. Hoke, R OH			0	0
492. Rep. Steve Horn, R CA			0	0
493. Rep. John Hostettler, R IN			0	0
494. Rep. Bob Inglis, R SC			0	0
495. Rep. Sheila Jackson-Lee, D TX			0	0
496. Rep. Andrew Jacobs, D IN			0	0
497. Rep. Walter B. Jr. Jones, R NC			0	0
498. Rep. Marcy Kaptur, D OH			0	0
499. Sen. Dirk Kempthorne, R ID			0	0
500. Rep. Patrick J. Kennedy, D RI			0	0
501. Sen. Edward M. Kennedy, D MA			0	0
502. Sen. Bob Kerrey, D NE			0	0
503. Sen. John Kerry, D MA			0	0
504. Sen. Herb Kohl, D WI			0	0
505. Rep. Steven C. LaTourette, R OH			0	0
506. Rep. Jim Leach, R IA			0	0
507. Sen. Carl Levin, D MI			0	0
508. Rep. James B. Jr. Longley, R ME			0	0
509. Rep. Martin T. Meehan, D MA			0	0
510. Rep. Jack Metcalf, R WA			0	0
511. Rep. Patsy T. Mink, D HI			0	0
512. Sen. Carol Moseley-Braun, D IL			0	0
513. Sen. Patty Murray, D WA			0	0
514. Rep. William H. Natcher, D KY			0	0
515. Rep. Charlie Norwood, R GA			0	0
516. Sen. Claiborne Pell, D RI			0	0
517. Rep. Rob Portman, R OH			0	0
518. Rep. George P. Radanovich, R CA			0	0
519. Rep. Ralph Regula, R OH			0	0
520. Rep. Lynn Rivers, D MI			0	0
521. Rep. Bernard Sanders, I VT			0	0
522. Rep. Mark Sanford, R SC			0	0
523. Rep. Joe Scarborough, R FL			0	0
524. Rep. Robert C. Scott, D VA			0	0
525. Rep. Linda Smith, R WA			0	0
526. Rep. Nick Smith, R MI			0	0
527. Rep. William M. "Mac" Thornberry, R TX			0	0
528. Rep. Todd Tiahart, R KS			0	0
529. Rep. Peter G. Torkildsen, R MA			0	0

NAME	HONORARIA	INDEPENDENT EXPEND.	DIRECT CONTRIB.	TOTAL
530. Rep. Zach Wamp, R TN			0	0
531. Rep. Mike Ward, D KY			0	0
532. Sen. Paul Wellstone, D MN			0	0
533. Rep. Rick White, R WA			0	0
534. Rep. Edward Whitfield, R KY			0	0
535. Rep. Sidney R. Yates, D IL			0	0

Notes

PREFACE

Sources on the mythology of Asklepios and Mercury include Jean Shinoda Bolen, *Gods in Everyman* (New York: Harper & Row, 1989); George M. Fister and Thomas A. Hendricks, "The Emblem of the American Medical Association," *JAMA*, 4 April 1959, 1630–1631; Walter J. Friedlander, *The Golden Wand of Medicine: A History of the Caduceus Symbol in Medicine* (New York: Greenwood Press, 1992); Robert K. King, "The Asklepian Connection: Toward an Archetypal Foundation for Healing," *Massage Therapy Journal*, Summer 1991, 80–86; and Robert E. Rakel, "One Snake or Two?" *JAMA*, 26 April 1985, 2369.

CHAPTER 1: THE AMERICAN DOCTORS' ASSOCIATION

1. George D. Lundberg, "The Increasing Representativeness of AMA Leaders," *JAMA*, 5 September 1990, 1153–1154;   **2.** James Stacey, "How the AMA Develops Policy," *JAMA*, 16 September 1983, 1426–1427;   **3.** AMA Council on Long Range Planning and Development, "Demographic Analyses of AMA Leadership," annual meeting, 1993, 12. See also Lundberg;   **4.** Robert J. Blendon, "The Public's View of the Future of Health Care," *JAMA*, 24 June 1988, 3591. And more generally, 3587–3593;   **5.** Lynn K. Harvey, "Public Opinion on Health Care Issues," May 1993, American Medical Association. Also Lynn K. Harvey, "Physician and Public Opinion on Health Care Issues," May 1992, American Medical Association;   **6.** "Doctors Do a Good Job, Public Diagnosis Finds," *New York Times*, 8 February 1956, 35;   **7.** Natalie Angier, "From Dr. Welby to Dr. Giggles, a Steep Slide," *New York Times*, 22 August 1993, 9, 14–15;   **8.** Harry Schwartz, "Where Are MDs Who Make $600,000 a year?" *American Medical News*, 17 February 1989, 29–30, and "New Survey Shows Americans Believe Medical Specialists, Health Execs 'Grossly Overpaid,'" Families USA Foundation, Press Release, 30 March 1993;   **9.** James Stacey, *Inside the New Temple: The High Cost of Mistaking Medicine for Religion* (Winnetka, Ill.: Conversation Press, Inc., 1993), 1–3;   **10.** Dennis L. Breo, "Arnold Relman—The Last Angry Doctor," *JAMA*, 5 June 1991, 2865;   **11.** George D. Lundberg, "Medicine—A Profession in Trouble?" *JAMA*, 17 May 1985, 2880;   **12.** Richard Knox, "AMA Opposition Dismissed as Maybe Not 'That Influential,'" *Boston Globe*, 8 December 1993, 20, and Jeffrey H. Birnbaum and Michael K. Frisby, "Clinton, in Interview, Shrugs Off Russian Vote for Ultranationalists and Frets Over AMA Policy," *Wall Street Journal*, 16 December 1993, A20.

Chapter 2: Fighting "The Inevitable"

In addition to the other sources listed, interviews were conducted with Virginia Trotter Betts, president of the American Nurses Association; Douglas Fraser, former United Auto Workers president and board member of the Committee for National Health Insurance; Melvin Glasser, executive director of the Committee for National Health Insurance; Dr. Philip Lee, former chairman of the Physician Payment Review Commission, currently Assistant Secretary for Health at the Department of Health and Human Services; Ronald Pollack, executive director of Families USA; Uwe E. Reinhardt, James Madison Professor of Political Economy, Princeton; Senator Paul Wellstone (D-Minn.); and Gail Wilensky, former health adviser to President George Bush. The AMA declined to make an official available for an interview on this topic.

1. Estimates by Congressional Budget Office, October 1992;   **2.** Ronald L. Numbers, *Almost Persuaded: American Physicians and Compulsory Health Insurance, 1912–1920* (Baltimore: The Johns Hopkins University Press, 1978), 34. The section on the First Battle is primarily based on Numbers' book;   **3.** Ibid., 52;   **4.** James G. Burrow, *AMA: Voice of American Medicine* (Baltimore: The Johns Hopkins Press, 1963), 97;   **5.** Numbers, 32;   **6.** Burrow, 145;   **7.** Numbers, 97;   **8.** "The Committee on the Costs of Medical Care," 99 JAMA, 3 Dec. 1932, 1950–1951. The section on the Second Battle is primarily based on Burrow and Paul Starr, *The Social Transformation of American Medicine* (New York: Basic Books, 1982), and Peter A. Corning, *The Evolution of Medicare* (Washington: Government Printing Office: Department of Health, Education and Welfare, Office of Research and Statistics, Research Report No. 29, 1969);   **9.** Starr, 265;   **10.** Frank D. Campion, *The AMA and U.S. Health Policy Since 1940* (Chicago: Chicago Review Press, 1984), 268;   **11.** For an expanded version of this story, see James Rorty, *American Medicine Mobilizes* (New York: W. W. Norton, 1939);   **12.** Starr, 305–306;   **13.** Burrow, 213–215;   **14.** Starr, 275–279;   **15.** Monte M. Poen, *Harry S Truman Versus the Medical Lobby: The Genesis of Medicare* (Columbia: University of Missouri Press, 1979), 130. The section on the Third Battle is primarily based on Poen's book, but also relied on Burrow, Campion, and Starr;   **16.** Burrow, 344;   **17.** Campion, 175;   **18.** Burrow, 347–348. For a discussion of the AMA's evolving views on private health insurance, see "The Voluntary Health Insurance Issue," 228–251, in Burrow;   **19.** Campion, 158. Campion lists the spending by year: $1.6 million in 1949, $2.6 million in 1950, $530,000 in 1951, and $225,000 in 1952. Total: $4,985,000;   **20.** Burrow, 343, 345;   **21.** Campion, 161;   **22.** The section on the Fourth Battle is based primarily on Richard Harris, *A Sacred Trust* (New York: New American Library, 1966), Burrow, Campion, and Starr;   **23.** Campion, 259. From 1960 through 1965, the AMA reported it spent $1,605,022 on lobbying, and the AFL-CIO reported it spent $925,952;   **24.** Harris, 139;   **25.** Campion, 264. See also Harris for descriptions of this event;   **26.** "Medical Care for the Aged," Executive Hearings, Committee on Ways and Means, January–February 1965, 742;   **27.** Ibid.;   **28.** Harris, 187;   **29.** The section on the Fifth Battle is based primarily on the annual editions of the *Congressional Quarterly Almanac* for 1969 through 1980 and *Congress and the Nation, vols. III, IV, and V* (Washington: Congressional Quarterly Service, various years), as well as Campion and Starr;   **30.** Author's calculation, based on list of congressional sponsors published in *American Medical News,* 8 March 1971, 11, and Federal Election Commission list of candidates supported by AMPAC in 1973 and 1974 as listed on committee microfilm numbers 73/407 and 74/955;   **31.** Campion, 310;   **32.** "Health Insurance: Hearings on New Proposals," *Congressional Quarterly Almanac, 1971,* 541–554;   **33.** "Health Insurance: No Action in 1974," *Congressional Quarterly Almanac, 1974,* 386–394. This section is based primarily on this article;   **34.** Ibid., 391;   **35.** Federal Election Commission on records: "Congressmen Supporting AMA's Medicredit Listed," *American Medical News,* 8 March 1971, 11;   **36.** "Health Insurance: No Action in 1974," *Congressional Quarterly Almanac, 1974,* 392–393;   **37.** Ibid., 394;   **38.** Harry Nelson, "AMA Health Insurance Views— They've Come a Long Way," *Chicago Sun-Times,* 10 December 1974, 18;   **39.** "National Health Insurance," 635–639, and "Health Care for Unemployed," 627–635, *Congressional*

Quarterly Almanac, 1975; **40.** This subsection is primarily based on "Limited Experimental Health Care Bill Enacted," *Congressional Quarterly Almanac, 1973,* 499–507, and "House Bill Eases HMO Requirements," 1975, *CQA, 1975,* 607–611; **41.** Starr, 394–396; **42.** This subsection is primarily based on "Chronology of Action on Health Programs," *Congress and the Nation, vol. V,* with particular reference to 636–640; **43.** "17 Points," editorial in *American Medical News,* 2 January 1978, 4; **44.** William C. Felch statement to Department of Health, Education and Welfare, 4 October 1977, 4; **45.** David U. Himmelstein and Steffie Woolhandler, "A National Health Program for the United States: A Physicians' Proposal," *New England Journal of Medicine,* 12 January 1989, 102–108; **46.** Wolinsky, "Americans Green with Envy over Canadian Medicine," *The Medical Post,* 7 March 1989, 11; **47.** Arnold S. Relman, "Universal Health Insurance: Its Time Has Come," *New England Journal of Medicine,* 12 January 1989, 117–118; **48.** "Strengthening the U.S. Health Care System," Board of Trustees Report AAA, American Medical Association, June 1989, found in *American Medical Association Notebook for "Health Access America,"* March 1990; **49.** "Study of the Canadian Health Care System," Board of Trustees Report V, June 1989, Policy No. 165.982, *Policy Compendium* (Chicago: American Medical Association, 1993), 152. See policy condemning "socialism" in "Opposition to Nationalized Health Care," Board of Trustees Report U, Interim Meeting, December 1988, Policy No. 165.985, 152, and "Failure of Socialized Medicine," Reaffirmed Council on Long Range Planning and Development Report F, Interim Meeting, December 1991, Policy No. 160.992, in 1993 *Policy Compendium,* 138; **50.** Janice Perrone, "Plan Focuses on Bolstering Health System," *American Medical News,* 7 July 1989, 6; **51.** James S. Todd, "It Is Time for Universal Access, Not Universal Insurance," *New England Journal of Medicine,* 6 July 1989, 46–47; **52.** Linda C. Higgins, "House Balks at 'Bill of Rights,'" *Medical World News,* 8 January 1990, 38; **53.** Charles D. Bankhead, "AMA Wrestles Issues to the Mat," *Medical World News,* July 1990, 38; **54.** "Promotion of an AMA Health Plan," Substitute Resolution 103, Interim Meeting, December 1989, Policy 165.977, 1993 *Policy Compendium,* 151; **55.** Janice Perrone, "Proposals Target Uninsured; AMA's 'Health Access America' Would Cut Costs, Cover All," *American Medical News,* 16 March 1990, 1, and AMA press kit handed out for announcement, specifically, copy of the statement delivered by Alan R. Nelson, "Assuring Access to Health Care for All Americans"; **56.** Leigh Page, "ACP's Access Proposal Signals Split; Group Is Considering Unified Insurance Plan," *American Medical News,* 11 May 1990, 3; **57.** Wolinsky, "Americans Shy Away from Canadian-Style Health Care," *The Medical Post,* 9 April 1991, 37; **58.** "Health Care System Reform—Now: Special *JAMA* Issue Proposes Range of Approaches," *American Medical News,* 27 May 1991, 3, 24–25; **59.** "Building Consensus on Health Reform: Dr. Todd Sees New Openness Among Key Players," *American Medical News,* 1 July 1991, 5; **60.** Federal Election Commission records show the American Medical Political Action Committee contributed $4,000 to the Republican candidate for Senate in Pennsylvania, Dick Thornburgh; **61.** George D. Lundberg, "National Health Care Reform: The Aura of Inevitability Intensifies," *JAMA,* 13 May 1992, 2521–2524; **62.** Michael Abramowitz, "An About-Face for the AMA: Praise for HMOs Comes at Last," *Washington Post,* Health Section, 9 June 1992, 8; **63.** "American College of Physicians Plan for Health Reform," 14 September 1992, and "Doctors Take on Medical Costs to U.S. Health Care System," press release, American College of Physicians, same date; **64.** "American College of Physicians Disheartened by AMA Rejection of Serious Cost Control in Health Care Reform," press release, American College of Physicians, 8 December 1992; **65.** "Providers: AMA v. ACP—Showdown at the M.D. Corral," *American Health Line,* vol. 1, no. 176, 10 December 1992, 8–9; **66.** George D. Lundberg, "American Health Care System Management Objectives: The Aura of Inevitability Becomes Incarnate," *JAMA,* 19 May 1993, 2554; **67.** Figures supplied by the AMA; **68.** "AMA Strategy: Work for Peace, Plan for War," *American Medical News,* 17 May 1993, 7–8; **69.** Robert Pear, "First Lady Angers Doctors on Cost," *New York Times,* 28 May 1993, 11; **70.** Pear, "AMA Urges Alternative to Insurance Requirement," *New York Times,* 8 December 1993, C20; **71.** Harris Meyer, "Support for Employer Mandate Softened," *American Medical News,* 20 December 1993, 1, 21; **72.** American College of Surgeons, Statement, 10 February 1994; **73.** Robert E. McAfee, AMA president-elect, "American Medical Association Opinion of Single-Payer System," 10 February 1994;

74. Pear, "10 Doctors' Groups Endorse Clinton's Health Plan," *New York Times*, 17 December 1993, A10; Meyer, "Reform Passage Seen This Year," *American Medical News*, 3 January 1994, 7, 29.

CHAPTER 3: LICENSE TO MAKE MONEY

In addition to the sources otherwise mentioned, interviews were conducted with Karen Davis, member of the Physician Payment Review Commission; Paul B. Ginsburg, executive director, Physician Payment Review Commission; Carron Maxwell, Blue Cross/Blue Shield; Lawrence Morris, retired vice president, Blue Cross/Blue Shield; Dr. Thomas E. Reardon, AMA Board trustee and member of the Physician Payment Review Commission; and Uwe E. Reinhardt, professor, Princeton and member of the Physicians Payment Review Commission. The AMA declined to make an official spokesperson available for an interview about the topic covered in this chapter.

1. Interview with Reinhardt;   2. Gregory C. Pope and John E. Schneider, "Trends in Physician Income," *Health Affairs*, Spring 1992, vol. 11, no. 1, 185;   3. Paul Starr, *The Social Transformation of American Medicine* (New York: Basic Books, 1982). Much of this section relies on Starr;   4. Lester S. King, "Medical Practice: Making a Living," *JAMA*, 13 April 1984;   5. Kenneth Warren Hamstra, "The American Medical Association Code of Medical Ethics of 1847," dissertation for Doctor of Philosophy, University of Texas, May 1987, 48–49;   6. Starr, passim;   7. Starr, 354;   8. "Income of Doctors up 11 pct.," *Chicago Daily News*, 2 January 1968, 18;   9. This section is primarily based on Frank Campion, *The AMA and U.S. Health Policy Since 1940* (Chicago: Chicago Review Press, 1984); Richard Harris, *A Sacred Trust* (New York: New American Library, 1966), and Starr, *Social Transformation*. Several other books, articles, and newspaper clips also were reviewed;   10. See note 8;   11. Dennis L. Breo, "I've Been in on the Whole Show," *American Medical News*, Impact, 22 June 1979, 7;   12. Resolutions 8, 42, and 53 regarding direct billing of patients adopted by House of Delegates, June 1966. Policy Compendium of the AMA, 1959–1968;   13. "Medicare and Medicaid—Problems, Issues, and Alternatives," Report of the Staff to the Committee on Finance, United States Senate, 9 February 1970. This section is based on the report;   14. Hearing by Subcommittee on Medicare and Medicaid of the Senate Committee on Finance, 15 June 1970, for the comments of Anderson, Dorman, and Long;   15. Linda H. Aiken and Karl D. Bays, "The Medicare Debate—Round One," *New England Journal of Medicine*, 1 November 1984, 1197, 1198;   16. Analysis of annual "Statements of the American Medical Association" from 1981 through 1990. In 1981–82, 24 percent of the statements related to Medicare. In 1989–90, 52 percent did;   17. Interview with Findlay. Steven Findlay, "AMA to Urge Fee Freeze on Doctors' Fees," *USA Today*, 23 February 1984, 1;   18. "Freeze Fees for a Year, AMA Urges MDs," *American Medical News*, 9 March 1984, 1, 10;   19. "Reagan Lauds Quality, But Hits Care Costs," *American Medical News*, 1/8 July 1983, 1, 20;   20. "Congress Rejects Medicare Mandatory Assignment Plan," *American Medical News*, 27 April 1984, 20;   21. Ibid. Also interview with Jacobs;   22. "MDs' Cost-Control Efforts Bring Results in Congress," *American Medical News*, 27 April 1984, 4;   23. Interview with Jacobs;   24. Interview with Jacobs;   25. Wolinsky, "Doctor Fees up 5.5% Despite AMA 'Freeze,'" *Chicago Sun-Times*, 28 April 1985, 3;   26. Ibid.;   27. Janet B. Mitchell, Gerard Wedig, and Jerry Cromwell, "The Medicare Physician Fee Freeze: What Really Happened?" *Health Affairs*, Spring 1989, 21–33;   28. Ellen Hume, "New Regimen: The AMA Is Laboring to Regain Dominance Over Nation's Doctors," *Wall Street Journal*, 13 June 1986. According to Webster's Unabridged Dictionary, "Greed implies inordinate desire as a controlling passion and usually connotes both meanness and covetousness." And it adds, "Avarice stresses both greed and miserliness";   29. *Medicare Physician Payment: An Agenda for Reform*, Physician Payment Review Commission, 1 March 1987, ix–x, 26–30;   30. Ibid. 31–45;   31. William C. Hsiao, Peter Braun, Douwe Yntema, and Edmund R. Becker, "Estimating Physicians' Work for a Resource-Based Relative-Value Scale," *New England Journal of Medicine*, 29 September 1988, 835–841. William C. Hsiao, Peter Braun, Daniel Dunn, and Edmund R. Becker,

"Resource-Based Relative Values," *JAMA,* 28 October 1988, 2347–2353. *JAMA* also carried seven other explanatory articles by Hsiao and his team as well as three assessments of the scale;   **32.** James S. Todd, "At Last, a Rational Way to Pay for Physicians' Services?" *JAMA,* 28 October 1988, 2439–2441. And "RBRVS Needs Modification Prior to Implementation: Editorials," AMA news release, same date;   **33.** "Resource-Based Relative Value Scale: An Rx for Medicare Ills?" AMA news release, 28 October 1988;   **34.** Fran Pollner, "Hot Harvard RVS Study Draws a Cool Collection of Responses," *Medical World News,* 24 October 1988, 10–11;   **35.** Interview with Reardon;   **36.** "Expenditure Targets," *Annual Report to Congress,* Physician Payment Review Commission, 31 March 1988;   **37.** "Summary and Recommendations," *Annual Report to Congress,* Physician Payment Review Commission, April 1989;   **38.** Interviews with Paul B. Ginsburg, executive director, and Karen Davis, member, Physician Payment Review Commission, and Reardon;   **39.** "ACS Announces Comprehensive New Proposals for Physician Payment Reform," American College of Surgeons, press release, 7 February 1989;   **40.** Chuck Alston, "Belt-Tightening in Medicare Pits Doctor vs. Doctor," *Congressional Quarterly,* 7 October 1989, 2605–2609;   **41.** Hearing by the Health Subcommittee of the House Ways and Means Committee, 21 March 1989;   **42.** *Annual Report to Congress,* Physician Payment Review Commission, 31 March 1988, 29–30;   **43.** Hearing by the Health Subcommittee of the House Ways and Means Committee, 21 March 1989;   **44.** Ibid.;   **45.** See note 40;   **46.** Jon Hamilton and Mark Bloom, "AMA Fights for Doctors' Pay; It's 'All-Out War' Against Medicare Fee Plan," *Washington Post,* 20 June 1989, Z8;   **47.** Ibid.; **48.** "Dr. Nelson Urges MDs: Voice Opposition to ETs," *American Medical News,* 7 July 1989, 1, 13;   **49.** For examples, see "Expenditure Targets Threaten Access to Health Care," "Medicare Expenditure Targets," and "Medical Service Rationed Under Medicare," *Congressional Record—House,* 15 June 1989, H 2599 and HF 2600;   **50.** Leigh Page, "AMA Launches Drive to Defeat Proposed Expenditure Ceilings," *American Medical News,* 7 July 1989, 1, 13. See also Alston, "Belt-Tightening";   **51.** Nancy Benac, "Seniors Groups Say AMA Looks Out for Doctors, Not Elderly," Associated Press, 21 July 1989;   **52.** Julie Rovner, "Ways and Means OKs Overhaul of Medicare Payment Plan," *Congressional Quarterly,* 1 July 1989, 1626–1628;   **53.** Deborah Mesce, "HHS Secretary Says Medicare Reform Opponents Deceive Public," Associated Press, 23 June 1989;   **54.** See note 52; **55.** "AMA Honors Public Officials for Health Care Contributions, *American Medical News,* 13 October 1989, 8. AMPAC reports for 1989, Federal Election Commission;   **56.** See note 52;   **57.** AMPAC filings with the Federal Election Commission;   **58.** James H. Sammons, "Playing Hardball," *Inside Medical Washington* (Knoxville: The Grand Rounds Press, 1991), 43–44;   **59.** AMPAC filings with the Federal Election Commission;   **60.** Julie Rovner, "Congress Agrees to Overhaul Medicare's Doctor Payments," *Congressional Quarterly,* 25 November 1989, 3240–3241; Sharon McIlrath, "New Era of Medicare Payment to Be Accompanied by MVPS," *American Medical News,* 8 December 1989, 1, 40, 42–43; and note 40;   **61.** Richard A. Knox, "Doctors Get a Message: Limit Thyself: Excessive Services Will Come Back to Cost Them," *Boston Globe,* 26 November 1989, A37;   **62.** Department of Health and Human Services, news release, July 27, 1993. In the first three months of 1993, 93.2 percent of Medicare dollars paid for bills taken by doctors on assignment; **63.** Department of Health and Human Services, news release, May 7, 1993. The surgeons' target was 6.5 percent growth in 1992, but Medicare spending dropped 3.3 percent. The nonsurgical target was 11.2 percent, but the expenditure growth was 7 percent;   **64.** Congressional Budget Office, *Projections of National Health Expenditures,* October 1992, 29.

CHAPTER 4: DEEP POCKETS

In addition to other sources listed, interviews were conducted with Herbert E. Alexander, professor, University of Southern California; Lee Ann Elliott, commissioner of the Federal Election Commission; Brooks Jackson, reporter, CNN; William B. Jenkins, former director of the Washington regional office of the General Services Administration; author Larry Sabato; John C. Surina, staff director of the Federal Election Commission; and Representative Fortney "Pete" Stark (D-Calif.). Art Golab helped research parts of this chapter. The AMA and AMPAC declined to make an official spokesperson available for this topic.

1. The AMA declined to divulge a total for its political activities, so the $100 million figure is a conservative estimate derived through the following method. AMA financial statements for 1970–73 show expenses of $3.7 million ($982,000 in 1973 alone) for its Washington office. Statements for 1974 forward omit the amount, so we estimated $1 million a year for 1974 through 1983, or $10 million. AMA budgets for 1984–90 earmarked $55.1 million for federal and state legislation, Washington, D.C., activities, and political education. The budgets for 1991 forward do not detail political activities, but the AMA says it spent $8.7 million on its Washington office alone in 1993. So we estimated $10 million a year for 1991–93, or $30 million. Altogether, the estimate totals $98.8 million;   **2.** Federal Election Commission press releases and records;   **3.** James G. Burrow, "The Political Machinery of the AMA, 1901–1921," *AMA: Voice of American Medicine* (Baltimore: The Johns Hopkins Press, 1963), 58, and more generally, 54–66;   **4.** Monte M. Poen, *Harry S Truman Versus the Medical Lobby: The Genesis of Medicare* (Columbia: University of Missouri Press, 1979), 46–47, 85–86, 142–143;   **5.** "CQ Listing of Lobby Financial Reports," *Congressional Quarterly Almanac, 1949,* 866;   **6.** Ibid. For campaign total, see Frank D. Campion, *The AMA and U.S. Health Policy Since 1940* (Chicago: Chicago Review Press, 1984), 158. Inflation figured with Department of Labor index;   **7.** Poen, 180–181;   **8.** Richard Harris, *A Sacred Trust* (New York: New American Library, 1966), 65;   **9.** See note 5 and *CQ Almanacs* for 1950–66;   **10.** For AMA's 1954 reported lobby expense, see "Lobby Spending Goes up in 1955," *Congressional Quarterly Almanac, 1956,* 657. For AMA's Washington office expense, see "Treasurer's Report," *JAMA,* 7 May 1955, 52;   **11.** "Legislative Goals of Top Spenders," *Congressional Quarterly Almanac, 1966,* 1347;   **12.** The description of the founding of AMPAC is based primarily on Campion, "A Careful Plunge into Political Action," in *The AMA and U.S. Health Policy Since 1940,* 209–231;   **13.** Joseph E. Cantor, *Political Action Committees: Their Evolution, Growth and Implications for the Poltical System* (Washington: Congressional Research Service, 1984), 25;   **14.** Campion, 218, 220;   **15.** Campion, 220. See also Stuart Auerbach, "Drug Firms' Gifts to AMA Revealed," *Chicago Sun-Times,* 1 July 1975, 8;   **16.** The section on Knowles is primarily based on newspaper accounts of the time. See Robert Gruenberg and William J. Eaton, "Fund-raisers Prevail: Doctors' Dollars Key to Knowles Rejection," *Chicago Daily News,* 28 June 1969, 1, 8;   **17.** "The Pragmatists Come to Power," in Campion, 290, 287, and more generally 285–296;   **18.** FEC press releases listing top PACs from 1972, 1974, and 1976;   **19.** "Affect Legislation, Auxiliary Urged," *American Medical News,* 25 October 1971, 16;   **20.** "AMPAC's $1 million Aided 245 Candidates," *American Medical News,* 11 November 1974, 5;   **21.** FEC records for the American Political Action Committee and its affiliates;   **22.** William Hines, "New AMA Memos Show the Greening of Capitol Hill," *Chicago Sun-Times,* 12 August 1975, 12;   **23.** Stuart Auerbach, "FEC Eyeing AMA Contribution Data," *Chicago Sun-Times,* 28 August 1975, 48;   **24.** FEC Matter Under Review 026, Termination Report, Compliance Action CA-026-75, 8 October 1975;   **25.** "Medical Political Action: Increased Importance in Critical Times," *Across the Boards, the AMPAC Bulletin for PAC leaders,* 17 December 1974, 4–5;   **26.** Common Cause press release, 3 October 1976;   **27.** FEC Matter Under Review, 270;   **28.** FEC Matter Under Review, 253, 253A, 289, 302, 369, and 618;   **29.** Carter remarks at Town Hall meeting in Spokane, 5 May 1978;   **30.** "Hospital Cost Control," *Congress and the Nation, Vol. 5,* 630–632;   **31.** Joseph A. Califano, Jr., *America's Health Care Revolution* (New York: Simon & Schuster, 1986) 147;   **32.** Philip M. Stern, *The Best Congress Money Can Buy* (New York: Pantheon Books, 1988) 141–142;   **33.** Common Cause press release, 18 December 1979;   **34.** Lee Anne Elliott interview;   **35.** "Common Cause Report on Contributions Called Misleading," *American Medical News,* 4 January 1980;   **36.** Dennis L. Breo, "AMA's Washington Office—Its Legend and Its Legacy," *American Medical News,* 18 June 1982, 38;   **37.** John R. Wright, "PACS, Contributions, and Roll Calls: Evidence From Five National Associations" (Doctoral thesis, University of Rochester, 1983) 97–103;   **38.** See note 33;   **39.** See the ad, "Rx for a Healthier America: Elect Reagan-Bush!" on page 23, and the editorial, "Political Ads," on the editorial page, *American Medical News,* 31 October 1980;   **40.** Senate Executive Report No. 97–56, 1 July 1982;   **41.** The AMA cited a University of Chicago Sociology Department survey in "AMA Insights," *JAMA,* 15 July 1983, 355;   **42.** See the organizational materials and financial statements in *JAMA,* 18 December 1981, 2810; 3 December 1982, 2845; 25 January 1985, 489;   **43.** "AMPAC sponsors campaign surveys," *American Medical News,* 22/29 October 1982, 2;   **44.** Herbert E. Alexander, *Financing Politics: Money, Elections, & Political Reform* (Washington: CQ Press, 1992) 32–35;   **45.** This section is primarily based on Michael Pertschuk, "Who Shot the AMA?" *Giant Killers* (New York: W. W. Norton, 1986), 82–114, but also relied on contemporary newspaper accounts and reports by *Congressional Quarterly*;   **46.** Cited in Larry Sabato, *PAC Power, Inside the World of Political Action Committees* (New York: W. W. Norton, 198), 134–135;   **47.** This section is based on Washington real estate records, AMA financial reports, hundreds of pages of FEC documents released in response to a Freedom of Information Act request, and interviews with officials of the FEC, GSA, and the agent for the former owners of the PEPCO building;   **48.** "Update Report on the Search for New Quarters," memorandum from John C. Surina, staff director, to the commission, 27 September 1984;   **49.** Letter from Surina to Jenkins, 30 July 1985;   **50.** This section is based on contemporary newspaper and magazine accounts, FEC campaign contribution records, FEC Matter Under Review 2272, congressional testimony, and interviews with Stark, Elliott, and Jacobs;   **51.** Alexander interview;   **52.** Duncan interview; **53.** Analysis of FEC data supplied by the National Library on Money and Politics; **54.** "Hazardous to Your Health," Common Cause, September 1993;   **55.** See the AMA's investment in members of Congress in the appendix;   **56.** Timothy Noah, "AMA Lavishly Courts Congressional Staffers Who Will Affect Outcome of Clinton's Health Plan," *Wall Street Journal*, 30 June 1993, A16.

CHAPTER 5: PRINCIPLES FOR PROFITS

In addition to other sources listed, interviews were conducted with Arthur Caplan, executive director of the Center for Biomedical Ethics at the University of Minnesota; Dr. Russel H. Patterson, former chairman of the AMA's Council on Ethics and Judicial Affairs; Dr. Arnold S. Relman, editor emeritus of the *New England Journal of Medicine*; Representative Fortney "Pete" Stark (D-Calif.); and Robert Veatch, ethicist at Georgetown University. The AMA declined to make an official spokesperson available for the subject covered in this chapter.

1. Kenneth Warren Hamstra, "The American Medical Association Code of Medical Ethics of 1847," doctoral dissertation, University of Texas at Austin, May 1987. The dissertation included the 1847 code in an appendix;   **2.** Marc A. Rodwin, *Medicine Money & Morals, Physicians' Conflicts of Interest* (New York: Oxford University Press, 1993) 22;   **3.** *JAMA*, 21 June 1902, 1661. See also Rodwin, 27;   **4.** Ibid., 28–29;   **5.** See Rodwin and Loyal Davis, *Fellowship of Surgeons, A History of the American College of Surgeons* (Chicago: American College of Surgeons, 1981), 414–436;   **6.** Judicial Council report, June 1947, 39–41. AMA compendium of policies through 1958;   **7.** "Report of the Judicial Council," *JAMA*, 25 June 1949, 701;   **8.** "Resolution on Proposed Amendment to Principles of Medical Ethics," *JAMA*, 23 December 1950, 1481;   **9.** Edwin B. Dunphy, "Responsibility of Ophthalmologists in an Era of Social Revolution," *JAMA*, 20 September 1952, 169–171; **10.** "Drug Store Sales Rise," *New York Times*, 7 January 1956, 26;   **11.** "Ownership of Drugstores," *JAMA*, 30 October 1954, 837;   **12.** "Proceedings of the Atlantic City Meeting," *JAMA*, 9 July 1955, 841–855;   **13.** Homer L. Pearson, "Supplementary Report of Judicial Council," Proceedings of the Boston Clinical Meeting, *JAMA*, 31 December 1955, 1748–1749;   **14.** "Principles of Medical Ethics," *JAMA*, 27 July 1957, 1484;   **15.** Ed Rosenthal, "M.D. Ownership Called Unethical in AMA Judicial Council Report," *Drug News Weekly*, 28 November 1962, cited in *Physician Ownership in Pharmacies and Drug Companies*, hearings before the Subcommittee on Antitrust and Monopoly of the Committee on the Judiciary of the United States Senate, 4, 5, 6, 11, 12, and 14 August 1964, 263; **16.** James H. Sammons, "The Ethical Considerations of Physician Ownership of Pharmacies and Drug Companies," address to the AMA Institute, 31 August 1962, cited in *Physician Ownership*, 247–250;   **17.** Robert Reinhold, "A.M.A., Facing Legal Pressures, Adopts Less Rigid Code for Doctors," *New York Times*, 23 July 1980, 1;   **18.** "Changing times for the AMA," *American Medical News*, 1/8 August 1980, 4;   **19.** Arnold S. Relman, "The New Medical-Industrial Complex," *New England Journal of Medicine*, 23 October 1980, 963–970; **20.** "Conflict of Interest—Guidelines," Report C of Judicial Council adopted at December

1984 interim meeting of the AMA;   **21.** Statement of the AMA to the Subcommittee on Health and Subcommittee on Oversight, Committee on Ways and Means, House of Representatives, 2 March 1989;   **22.** AMA statement to Committee on Ways and Means, 2 March 1989;   **23.** Arnold S. Relman, "Dealing with Conflicts of Interest," *New England Journal of Medicine*, 19 September 1985, 749–751;   **24.** "Conflicts of Interest and the Physician Entrepreneur," letters, *New England Journal of Medicine*, 23 January 1986, 250–253;   **25.** This section relies on materials provided by the National Association of Retail Druggists, articles in *The Wall Street Journal*, other newspaper and magazine articles, congressional hearings, AMA statements, *American Medical News*, *JAMA*, and the *New England Journal of Medicine*;   **26.** AMA statement, *Physician Dispensing of Drugs*, Hearing before the Subcommittee on Health and the Environment, Committee on Energy and Commerce, U.S. House of Representatives, 22 April 1987, Serial no. 100-36, 12–36; **27.** Examples from *Physician Drug Sales for Profit, A Guide for Pharmacists*, National Association of Retail Druggists, 1987;   **28.** AMA statement, *Physician Dispensing of Drugs*; **29.** Diane M. Gianelli, "House Panel Nixes Amendment to Limit MD Drug Dispensing," *American Medical News*, 24 April 1987, 1, 52;   **30.** AMA statement, *Physician Dispensing of Drugs*;   **31.** Linda Bosy, "AMA lends support to MD drug dispensing," *American Medical News*, 3/10 July 1987, 10. See also AMA Policy No. 120.990, "Physician Dispensing," *Policy Compendium* (Chicago: American Medical Association, 1993), 92;   **32.** Relman interview;   **33.** Arnold S. Relman, "Doctors and the Dispensing of Drugs," *New England Journal of Medicine*, 30 July 1987, 311–312;   **34.** Walt Bogdanich and Michael Waldholz, "Hospitals That Need Patients Pay Bounties for Doctors' Referrals," and "Doctor-Owned Labs Earn Lavish Profits in a Captive Market," *Wall Street Journal*, 27 February 1989, 1, A4, and 1 March 1989, 1, A6;   **35.** *Issues Related to Physician Self-Referrals*, Hearings before the Subcommittee on Health and the Subcommittee on Oversight of the House Ways and Means Committee, 2 March 1989 and 1 June 1989, Serial no. 101–58;   **36.** Ibid., 64; **37.** Ibid., 88–89;   **38.** Ibid., 104;   **39.** Richard P. Kusserow, Inspector General, Department of Health and Human Services, *Financial Arrangements Between Physicians and Health Care Business*, May 1989;   **40.** Laurie Jones, "AMA: U.S. Report on Self-Referrals Proves Nothing," *American Medical News*, 12 May 1989, 1, 46–48;   **41.** "Statement of the General Accounting Office," *Medicare and Medicaid Initiatives*, Hearing before the Subcommittee on Health and the Environment, House Committee on Energy and Commerce, 8 June 1989, Serial no. 101–46, 376–390;   **42.** AMA statement, *Medicare and Medicaid Initiatives*, 391;   **43.** John K. Iglehart, "Health Policy Report: Efforts to Address the Problem of Physician Self-Referral," *New England Journal of Medicine*, 19 December 1991, 1820–1824;   **44.** John J. Ring, "The Right Road for Medicine: Professionalism and the New AMA," inaugural address, 26 June 1991;   **45.** Dennis L. Breo, "Arnold Relman—the Last Angry Doctor," *JAMA*, 5 June 1991, 2864–2865, 2869;   **46.** Arnold S. Relman, "'Self-Referral'—What's at Stake," *New England Journal of Medicine*, 19 November 1992, 1522–1524;   **47.** Brian McCormick, "Most Doctor Self-referral Deemed Unethical; House Approves Guidelines," *American Medical News*, 23/20 December 1991, 1, 43; **48.** Brian McCormick, *American Medical News*, 1 June 1992, 1, 11;   **49.** Brian McCormick, "Referral Ban Softened," *American Medical News*, 6/13 July 1992, 1, 52;   **50.** See note 46; **51.** "Proposed Changes to Mandatory Programs," *Congressional Quarterly*, 20 February 1993, 411. The chart shows a projected savings of $250 million from 1994–97; **52.** Diane M. Gianelli, "Stark Seeks Stiffer Self-referral Standards," *American Medical News*, 25 January 1993, 3, 24;   **53.** AMA statement to the Subcommittee on Health, Committee on Ways and Means, Presented by Nancy W. Dickey, 20 April 1993;   **54.** Relman interview.

CHAPTER 6: MEDICAL MONOPOLY

In addition to other sources listed, interviews were conducted with B. J. Anderson, special counsel, American Medical Association; Dr. Norman Gevitz, medical historian, University of Illinois at Chicago; William Hines, former Washington bureau chief, *Chicago Sun-Times*; George P. McAndrews, attorney, Chicago; Dr. Jerome McAndrews, vice president for professional affairs, American Chiropractic Association; Judith Randal, medical writer, formerly of the New York *Daily News;* Dr. James S. Todd, executive vice president of the AMA; Dr. Walter Wardwell, emeritus professor of sociology, University of Connecticut; Dr. Chester Wilk, chiropractic physician, Park Ridge, Ill.; Dr. Sidney Wolfe, executive director, Public Citizen Health Research Group.

1. David M. Eisenberg et al., "Unconventional Medicine in the United States," 3 *New England Journal of Medicine,* 28 January 1993, 246. See also Paul Starr, *The Social Transformation of Medicine* (New York: Basic Books, 1982), 107;   **2.** Norman Gevitz, "Osteopathic Medicine: From Deviance to Difference," in *Other Healers: Unorthodox Medicine in America,* 124–156; Gevitz, "The Chiropractors and the AMA: Reflections on the History of the Consultation Clause," *Perspectives in Biology and Medicine,* Winter 1989, 290; Gevitz, *The D.O.'s: Osteopathic Medicine in America* (Baltimore: The Johns Hopkins University Press, 1982);   **3.** Walter I. Wardwell, "Chiropractors: Evolution to Acceptance," in *Other Healers: Unorthodox Medicine in America;*   **4.** Morris Fishbein, *The Medical Follies* (New York: Boni & Liveright, 1925), 61;   **5.** Ibid, 98;   **6.** Developments relating to the efforts to suppress chiropractic in Iowa and subsequently by the AMA are based on the Throckmorton deposition and other documents from the *Wilk et al. v. AMA et al.* trial;   **7.** Robert B. Throckmorton, legal counsel, Iowa Medical Society, "The Menace of Chiropractic," an outline of remarks given to the North Central Medical Conference, Minneapolis, 11 November 1962, plaintiff's exhibit 172, *Wilk,* 6;   **8.** Ibid., 6;   **9.** Ibid., 9;   **10.** Deposition of Throckmorton, *Wilk et al. v. AMA et al.,* 11 July 1978, 35. The Department of Investigation was formed in 1906 as an outgrowth of efforts by *JAMA* to attack health fraud and quackery. In 1913 the AMA formed the Propaganda Department to gather and disseminate information about quackery. The agency's name was changed to the Bureau of Investigation in 1925 and then to the Department of Investigation in 1958. Arthur W. Hafner et al., *Guide to the American Medical Association Health Fraud and Alternative Medicine Collection* (Chicago: American Medical Association, 1992), viii;   **11.** AMA Committee on Quackery, Report to the AMA Council on Long Range Planning and Development, 9 April 1971. The committee emphasized to the council: "The Committee believes that the campaign against chiropractic is an effective 'unity' mechanism for medicine at all levels and physicians must be made aware of this extremely beneficial side effect, particularly at this time." Plaintiff's exhibit 466, *Wilk;*   **12.** Memo from Robert Youngerman to Robert Thockmorton, 24 September 1963, plaintiff's exhibit 173, *Wilk;*   **13.** Throckmorton, a veteran of the Iowa wars against chiropractic, was shocked by the board's decision to use the word "quackery." In his deposition, 11 July 1978, 41, he described this as "an unnecessary affront";   **14.** The Committee on Quackery stated in a memo that "since its formation in 1964 [the Committee] has considered its mission to be, first the containment of chiropractic, and, ultimately, the elimination of chiropractic as a recognized health-care provider";   **15.** Material relating to H. Doyl Taylor is based on a deposition in the case of *Wilk et al. v. AMA et al.,* on 28 April 1987, in Phoenix, 15;   **16.** In an interview Dr. Chester A. Wilk described Taylor as Eichmann;   **17.** Susan Getzendanner, U.S. District Court Judge, Northern District of Illinois, Eastern Division, Memorandum Opinion and Order, *Wilk et al. v. AMA et al.,* No. 76 C 3777, 13;   **18.** In 1961 the House of Delegates had adopted a generic position declaring unethical any relationship between a medical doctor and a cultist. This position and the 1966 policy against chiropractic were consistent with Principle 3 of the Principles of Medical Ethics, adopted in 1955, which stated: "A physician should practice a method of healing founded on a scientific basis, and he should not voluntarily associate professionally with anyone who violates this principle";   **19.** In his deposition for the *Wilk* case, William Monaghan, a former Department of Investigation staffer, described attending under cover a meeting of the American Chiropractic Association in New York. A former journalist and not a chiropractor, he registered at the meeting as "Dr. Bob Meier, D.C.," assuming the name of another AMA staffer. Deposition in *Wilk et al. v. AMA et al.,* 21 June 1979, 32–39;   **20.** Ralph Lee Smith, *At Your Own Risk: The Case Against Chiropractic* (New York: Trident Press, 1969);   **21.** Samuel R. Sherman, letter from H. Doyl Taylor, director, AMA Department of Investigation, 20 February 1968, Plaintiff's exhibit 220, *Wilk et al. v. AMA et al.;*   **22.** Letter from Sherman to Taylor dated 1 March 1968;   **23.** In the undated memo,

Stevens said the HEW physician refused to allow the Kentucky Medical Association to pay for his meal because he saw that as a conflict of interest. "I think he needs to be watched carefully," said Stevens. The memo was Plaintiff's exhibit 332 in the *Wilk* case;   **24.** Taylor received a letter on 3 September 1968 from the American Society of Internal Medicine that included a list of panelists considered "soft" on the chiropractic;   **25.** Deposition of Mennell, in *Wilk et al. v. AMA et al.*, 75;   **26.** Mennell transcript, 99;   **27.** American Chiropractic Association, International Chiropractors Association and Council of State Chiropractic Boards Inc., "Chiropractic's 'White Paper' on Health, Education and Welfare Secretary's Report 'Independent Practitioners Under Medicare,'" May 1969;   **28.** Minutes from the "Chiropractic Workshop," Michigan State Medical Society, held in Lansing on 10 May 1973, exhibit 1283, *Wilk et al. v. AMA et al.* Sabatier said in dealing with chiropractors that medicine ought to be careful "to condemn the sin and not the sinner";   **29.** Comment on "dynamite" from letter 2 February 1971 by Marvin Reiter, of the National Association of Blue Shield Plans, in which he recounts a conversation with Taylor; **30.** "Chiropractors, AMA Swap Fraud Claims," *Chicago Sun-Times*, 9 October 1966, 51;   **31.** Memo to the AMA Board of Trustees, 4 January 1971, plaintiff's exhibit 464, *Wilk*;   **32.** William Trever, *In the Public Interest* (Los Angeles: Scriptures Unlimited, 1972). The book was dedicated to H. Doyl Taylor, director of the AMA Department of Investigation, with a quote from the Roman philosopher Seneca: "If you would wish another to keep your secret, first keep it yourself." Taylor is featured in several demeaning cartoons in the book;   **33.** Chiropractors often repeated stories of AMA plots to destroy them. For example, chiropractors attending a convention in 1930 in New York told of how AMA officials "met in a secret conclave" in Chicago in 1922 and adopted the slogan "Chiropractic must die" and gave themselves ten years to destroy chiropractic. This account ran in Louis S. Reed, *The Healing Cults* (Chicago: University of Chicago Press, 1932), 35;   **34.** Trever, 1;   **35.** Chester A. Wilk *Chiropractic Speaks Out: A Reply to Medical Propaganda, Bigotry and Ignorance* (Park Ridge, Ill.: Wilk Publishing, 1973);   **36.** The case was *England et al. v. Louisiana State Board of Medical Examiners et al.* The lower court held it was not "irrational and unreasonable" for the Louisiana legislature to require chiropractors to comply with the state medical practices act; **37.** Ron Shaffer, "Scientologists Kept Files on 'Enemies,'" *Washington Post*, 16 May 1978, A1; William Hines, "Flunked Private Eye Gets AMA Mission," *Chicago Sun-Times*, 18 August 1975, 8. The Hines article also relates the story of Thomas Spinelle, the former Secret Service agent who investigated the case for the AMA. Hines found that Spinelle had failed his private-investigator exam twice in 1975;   **38.** This account is based on interviews with B. J. Anderson, AMA special counsel, and some former AMA leaders who wished to remain anonymous. In trying to dig out the infiltrators, the AMA ran lie-detector tests on employees in Chicago and Washington. According to the *Los Angeles Times*, a secretary who worked for the AMA's chief executive turned out to be among the Scientology moles. It had been learned that she had spent several weekends at the Chicago headquarters without specific assignments, and confidential documents were found in her desk. Robert Rawitch and Robert Gillette, "Church Wages Propaganda on a Wide Scale," *Los Angeles Times*, 27 August 1978;   **39.** Ralph Lee Smith, "Scientology—Menace to Mental Health," *Today's Health*, December 1968, 34–39;   **40.** The "doom program" is cited in "Dianetic Sect Said to Spy on A.M.A.," *New York Times*, 2 November 1979, 19. Also, Hubbard wrote in a memo in 1963: "Certain vested interests, mainly the American Medical Association, a private healing monopoly, wish to do all possible harm to the Scientology movement over the world in order to protect their huge medical-psychiatric income and desired monopoly, which runs into tens of billions annually" (Rawitch and Gillette, "Church Wages Propaganda on a Wide Scale"); **41.** In 1977 FBI agents, armed with sledgehammers, buzz saws, crowbars, and search warrants, raided Scientology's Guardian Offices in Washington and Los Angeles. Seeking to recover stolen government documents, the FBI turned up AMA materials, which AMA officials tied to Sore Throat. The church leadership admitted that the people implicated in the AMA invasion were church members, but said they had acted alone without the knowledge of the church leadership. In addition to AMA material, the FBI found copies of the tax returns of Los Angeles mayor Tom Bradley and singer Frank Sinatra and confidental material from the FBI and IRS; Interview with B. J. Anderson, special counsel to the AMA; Anthony Marro, "Federal Agents Raid Scientology Church," *New York Times*, 9 July 1977, 1;

"Dianetic Sect Said to Spy on A.M.A.," *New York Times*, 2 November 1979, 19;   **42.** David Burnham, "A.M.A. Criticized on Chiropractic. House Unit Poses Question of Antitrust Aspects," *New York Times*, 29 October 1975, 81;   **43.** Since the 1960s, the once-outcast osteopathic physicians had become part of the establishment, offering the medical and surgical services like allopaths as well as manipulation like chiropractic physicians. The AMA said it was up to each state medical society to set its own policy on osteopathy. In 1989 the AMA gave full recognition to osteopaths as physicians. In 1993 about 5,000 DOs were AMA members;   **44.** From the deposition of Ralph Marshall, executive director of the New Mexico Medical Society, 22 February 1979, 55–66. Marshall said that Whalen Strobhar, assistant AMA vice president, told the executives that the AMA counsel had recommended destruction of files because the Federal Trade Commission was subpoenaing materials related to election and Political Action Committee activities. When asked if he had destroyed any files from the Committee on Quackery, Marshall said, "If they were in there, they were purged," 57;   **45.** Richard Lewis, "AMA Revamps Stand On Chiropractic," *American Medical News*, 3/10 August 1979, 1;   **46.** James E. Doyle, Senior Judge, U.S. Court of Appeals for the Seventh Circuit, *Wilk et al. v. AMA et al.*, 19 September 1983, 13; **47.** Testimony of Dr. Chester A. Wilk in Transcript of the Proceedings, *Wilk et al. v. AMA et al.*, 21 May 1987, 1014;   **48.** Transcript of Proceedings, *Wilk*, 26 May 1987, 1266; **49.** Ibid., 3132;   **50.** *Wilk et al. v. AMA et al.*, Transcript of Proceedings, 2 July 1987, 3396; **51.** Getzendanner, Memorandum Opinion and Order, 5;   **52.** Ibid., 23;   **53.** Ibid., 17; **54.** Ibid., 35;   **55.** Ibid, 49;   **56.** Ibid., 48;   **57.** Michael Briggs, "Chiropractors' Victory Over AMA Ban Is Upheld," *Chicago Sun-Times*, 27 November 1990, 6. Kirk B. Johnson, AMA general counsel, said the ruling would have little impact on the AMA or doctor-patient relations because the AMA had considered it ethical since 1980 for physicians to refer patients to "limited practitioners" such as chiropractors;   **58.** Settlement figures come from AMA financial statements. Wolinsky, "After 15-Year Fight, AMA Gives OK to Chiropractors," *Chicago Sun-Times*, 9 January 1992, 3;   **59.** Natalie Angier, "Where the Unorthodox Gets a Hearing at N.I.H.," *New York Times*, 16 March 1993, B5;   **60.** The holdings are described in Hafner, *Guide to the American Medical Association Health Fraud and Alternative Medicine Collection* (Chicago: American Medical Association, 1992). Scholars and researchers can use the collection, which includes information on more than 3,500 fraudulent or alternative-health practitioners, products, and projects that were the subject of inquiries or investigations by the Department of Investigation;   **61.** Barbara Ehrenreich and Deirdre English, *Witches, Midwives, and Nurses: A History of Women Healers* (Old Westbury, N.Y.: The Feminist Press, 1973), 35;   **62.** Ibid., 37–38;   **63.** American Nurses Association, "American Nurses Association Asks Congress to End Medical Monopoly of Health-Care System," 17 May 1993;   **64.** Michael Weisskopf, "In Health Debate, Nurses Exerting Power of Numbers and Purses," *Washington Post*, 16 May 1993. A1;   **65.** Joe Neel, "Extending the Extenders: Clinton Plan Carves Out Bigger Role for Them—But Not Big Enough for Nurses," *Physician's Weekly*, 27 December 1993;   **66.** American Medical Association Report of the Board of Trustees, "Economic and Quality of Care Issues with Implications on Scopes of Practice—Physicians and Nurses," December 1993; **67.** American Nurses Association, "American Nurses Association Expresses Disappointment at AMA Opposition to an Expanded Role for Nurses," news release, 9 December 1993.

Chapter 7: Smoking Gun

In addition to other sources listed, interviews were conducted with Kim Koontz-Bayliss, former legislative aide on health to Representative Mike Synar (D-Okla.); Dr. Alan Blum, founder of DOC (Doctors Ought to Care); Dr. Daniel T. Cloud, former AMA president; Richard Daynard, chairman, Tobacco Products Liability Project; Dr. Ronald M. Davis, former AMA Board member; Clifford E. Douglas, manager of government relations, Tobacco Tax Policy Project, American Cancer Society; Dr. F. William Dowda, former AMA Board member; Dr. Joel S. Dunnington, delegate to the AMA's Hospital Medical Staff Section; Representative Richard J. Durbin (D-Ill.); Horace K. Kornegay, former head of the Tobacco Institute; former U.S. senator Maurine Neuberger (D-Ore.); Dan Greenfield, press spokesman for Synar; Dr. Harrison L. Rogers, former AMA president; Representative Roy J. Rowland (D-Ga.); Dr. Mona Sarfaty, former senior health-policy adviser, U.S. Senate; and Congressman Henry A. Waxman (D-Calif.).

1. There is a range of estimates for annual tobacco-related deaths in the United States, running from 419,000 to in excess of 500,000. Dr. R. T. Ravenholt, "Tobacco Industry Trepidations," *Priorities,* Summer 1993, 15; Spencer Rich, "U.S. Sees 1st Drop in Smoking Deaths," *Chicago Sun-Times,* 27 August 1993, 3; Roger Herdman, "Smoking-Related Deaths and Financial Costs: Office of Technology Assessment Estimates for 1990," Senate Special Committee on Aging, 6 May 1993;   2. Maurine B. Neuberger, *Smoke Screen: Tobacco and the Public Welfare* (Englewood Cliffs, N.J.: Prentice-Hall, 1963), 30–31;   3. Alan Blum, "When 'More Doctors Smoked Camels': Cigarette Advertising in the *Journal,*" *The Cigarette Underworld* (Secaucus, N.J.: Lyle Stuart, 1985), 110. This article, contained in a reprint of the December 1983 edition of the *New York State Journal of Medicine,* provides a history of cigarette advertising in medical journals;   4. James Rorty, "The AMA and the Cigarette Business," *American Medicine Mobilizes* (New York: W. W. Norton, 1939), 183. Rorty devotes an entire chapter to the involvement by the AMA and Dr. Morris Fishbein in the Philip Morris campaign. Much of this account relies on Rorty's research;   5. Michael G. Mulinos and Raymond L. Osborne, "Irritating Properties of Cigarette Smoke as Influenced by Hygroscopic Agents," *New York State Journal of Medicine* 35, 1 June 1935, 590–592. Another study frequently mentioned was by Frederick B. Flinn, "Some Clinical Observations on the Influence of Certain Hygroscopic Agents in Cigarettes, *Laryngoscope* 45 (1935) 149–154. In a human study, Flinn found that the combustion products of diethylene glycol were less irritating than glycerine and that diethylene glycol could help soothe irritation; 6. The campaign aimed at physicians is described in *Fortune,* March 1936, 116;   7. Rorty, 184; *Fortune,* November 1938, 152;   8. "Deaths Following Elixir of Sulfanilamide-Massengill—II," *JAMA,* 30 October 1937, 1456–1457. The 23 October 1937 issue of the journal presented a series of reports from the AMA Chemical Laboratory and others on the deaths and laboratory findings. Rorty describes this episode;   9. Ernst L. Wynder and Evarts A. Graham, "Tobacco Smoking as a Possible Etiologic Factor in Bronchogenic Carcinoma," *JAMA* May 1950, 329–338;   10. L. E. Burney, "Policy Over Politics: The First Statement on Smoking and Health by the Surgeon General of the United States Public Health Service," *The Cigarette Underground,* 12–13. He originally published his charges in *JAMA* in 1959. Burney was disappointed when Dr. John Talbott, *JAMA's* editor, attacked him in an editorial. He feared that the profession and public would view the critical comments as "the unspoken position of the AMA";   11. "'AMA Journal' Stops Taking Cigaret Ads," *Advertising Age,* 9 November 1953, 1. *Ad Age* also reported that the AMA banned alcohol advertising;   12. Dr. Walter Wolman, former director of the Chemical Laboratory of the AMA, stated in a deposition in a tobacco liability case, *Ieradi v. Lorillard,* that the study on the filters was ordered by the Advertising Committee of the AMA. The deposition was taken on 19 May 1991, 22. The filter studies appeared in *JAMA,* 4 July 1953, 917–920; 11 July 1953, 1035–1036;   13. "Cigarette Hucksterism and the A.M.A.," *JAMA,* 3 April 1954, 1180;   14. "AMA Looses Blast at Lorillard for Kent Rebuttal Ad," *Advertising Age,* 12 April 1954, 1;   15. Fishbein's retainer with Lorillard was brought up in the *Ieradi* case. Fishbein mentioned his work on the Micronite filter in *Morris Fishbein, M.D.: An Autobiography* (Garden City, N.Y.: Doubleday, 1969);   16. A letter uncovered in the Cipollone tobacco liability trial showed the industry's interest in recruiting the AMA. In a letter dated 2 September 1959, C. C. Little, scientific director of the Tobacco Industry Research Council, suggested to Bowman Gray, president R. J. Reynolds Tobacco, strategies of working with the AMA and maintaining contacts with Dr. F. J. L. Blasingame, AMA's chief executive. Before working for the tobacco industry, Little, a geneticist and cancer specialist, had headed the American Cancer Society. More about Little is contained in Elizabeth M. Whelan's *A Smoking Gun: How the Tobacco Industry Gets Away with Murder* (Philadelphia: George F. Stickley, 1984);   17. Richard Harris, *A Sacred Trust* (New York: New American Library, 1966), 159;   18. Walter Sullivan, "Cigarettes Peril Health, U.S. Report Concludes: Remedial Action Urged," *New York Times,* 12 January 1964, 1. See also Maurice Corina, *Trust in Tobacco* (New York: St. Martin's Press, 1975), 232–256;   19. "AMA Position on Cigaret Smoking

Outlined," *AMA News,* 13 April 1964, 5;   **20.** "Smoking Study Funds Donated" and "Research Group Named," *AMA News,* 17 February 1964, 1; "The AMA Tackles Smoking: 'A strong stand,'" *The Cigarette Underworld,* 123. This article examines the AMA-ERF study and follows policy developments through the sale in 1981 of cigarette stocks owned by the AMA Members Retirement Plan;   **21.** Whelan, *Smoking Gun,* 104; Joseph R. Hixon, "AMA at Last Finds Perils in Smoking," *Chicago Sun-Times,* 8 May 1964;   **22.** Harry Nelson, "AMA Admits Cigaret Smoking Is Hazard," *Chicago Sun-Times,* 25 June 1964, 5; **23.** *JAMA,*6 November 1967, 9–10;   **24.** This document came out in the discovery process in the tobacco liability case *Cipollone v. Liggett Group Inc.* In a deposition in connection with the case, Howard said the House of Delegates "did not seek to placate the tobacco industry," but, on the other hand, he said AMA lobbyists "sought whatever help we could get, from any source wherever it came";   **25.** F. J. L. Blasingame, Letter to Chief, Division of Trade Regulation Rules, Bureau of Industry Guidance, Federal Trade Commission, 28 February 1964. The letter was reprinted in "Full Text of AMA Letter of Testimony to FTC," *JAMA,* 6 April 1964, 31; Eileen Shanahan, "Ads Held as a Cause of Smoking Habit: U.S. Aide Favors Proposed Curbs at the FTC Hearing," *New York Times,* 17 March 1964, 13; **26.** "AMA View Decried in Tobacco Dispute," *New York Times,* 20 March 1964, 23; "Lawmaker Assails Charges vs AMA on Tobacco," *JAMA,* 6 April 1964, 15–16; "AMA Presents Cigaret Labeling Views to FTC," ibid., 29–31; "AMA Opposes Warning on Tobacco, Association Comes Under Sharp Criticism as It Takes Position, Shared by Industry, Against Mandatory Labeling of Cigarettes as Health Hazard," *Medical World News,* 10 April 1964, 51–53;   **27.** "AMA View Decried in Tobacco Dispute," *New York Times,* 20 March 1964, 23; "Lawmaker Assails Charges vs AMA on Tobacco," *JAMA,* 6 April 1964, 15–16; "AMA Presents Cigaret Labeling Views to FTC," ibid., 29–31; "AMA Opposes Warning on Tobacco, Association Comes Under Sharp Criticism as It Takes Position, Shared by Industry, Against Mandatory Labeling of Cigarettes as Health Hazard," *Medical World News,* 10 April 1964, 51–53;   **28.** Nelson, "AMA Admits Cigaret Smoking Is Hazard." See also Harris, *Sacred Trust,* chapter 30;   **29.** Drew Pearson and Jack Anderson, *The Case Against Congress: A Compelling Indictment of Corruption on Capitol Hill* (New York: Simon & Schuster, 1968), 329–330;   **30.** AMA-ERF Committee for Research on Tobacco and Health, *Tobacco and Health* (Chicago: American Medical Association Education and Research Foundation, 1978);   **31.** Whelan, *Smoking Gun,* 120–132;   **32.** In a press release issued on 7 August 1978, Horace R. Kornegay, president of the Tobacco Institute, attacked the AMA for trying to discredit Carter by releasing the AMA-ERF study on 4 August in "an obvious attempt to embarrass the President in tobacco country." He said the AMA-ERF project had actually ended in 1972 and that the contents of the report were a rehash of articles six to twelve years old. "The industry deplores the politics of the release of this document by the AMA," he said. In response, the AMA said it had intended to release the study in May, but because of a series of unforeseen events, the final report was not released until 24 July, with fourth-class mailing resulting in "uneven distribution";   **33.** Transcript of AMA House of Delegates meeting, June 1980, 586–588;   **34.** This is based on an interview with Cloud, but some of the same material was covered in an article by Morton Mintz, "Like Twin Serpents on the Caduceus: The Sorry History of How the American Medical Association and Cigarette Makers Doctored the Evidence on Smoking's Ills," *Legal Times,* 7 May 1990, 33. The AMA and Southern Congressmen joined together in the 1960s to oppose regulation of cigarette labels and advertising, in the 1970s to oppose FTC regulation of medical advertising, and in the late 1970s and early 1980s to support efforts to exempt doctors and other professionals from regulation by the FTC;   **35.** Dr. James H. Sammons, letter to Dr. Stephen J. Dresnick, chairman, AMA Resident Physicians Section, 11 October 1979;   **36.** "Residents Seek Bigger Vote," *American Medical News,* 1/8 August 1980, 18; "Doctor's Dilemma," *Wall Street Journal,* 12 March 1981, sec. 2, 29;   **37.** The cartoon by Wayne Stayskal appeared in the *Chicago Tribune,* 15 June 1981, Section 1, 27;   **38.** Wolinsky, "AMA Urged to Snuff Out Its Tobacco Stock," *Chicago Sun-Times,* 9 June 1981, 25; Wolinsky, "AMA Dumps $1.4 Million in Embarrassing Tobacco Stock," *Sun-Times,* 29 September 1981, 3;   **39.** Wolinsky, "AMA Burns Smoking Issue at Both Ends," *Chicago Sun-Times,* 18 June 1985, 3; Wolinsky, "AMA's Chief Edgy About Tobacco Land," *Sun-Times,* 19 June 1985, 24;   **40.** Wolinsky, "AMA's Mixed Smoke Signals," *Sun-Times,* 19 June

1985, 7; Wolinsky, "AMA Boss Sells Tobacco Farm," *Sun-Times,* 25 October 1985, 6. Rogers supplied other details in an interview in 1992;   **41.** Wolinsky, "AMA Toughens Stand on Smoking," *Sun-Times,* 21 June 1985, 28;   **42.** "Tobacco Product Liability," Report G, AMA Board of Trustees, December 1985;   **43.** Wolinsky, "Tobacco Foes Lash AMA Board Stand Against Lawsuits," *Chicago Sun-Times,* 26 November 1985, 22;   **44.** Wolinsky, "AMA Retreats From Criticism of Suits," *Sun-Times,* 12 December 1985, 8; Jon Hamilton, "AMA Attacks Tobacco, Butt Doubts Smolder," *Physician's Weekly,* 3 February 1986; **45.** Philip M. Boffey, "A.M.A. Votes to Seek Total Ban on Advertising Tobacco Products," *New York Times,* 11 December 1985, 1; Wolinsky, "AMA Panel Urges Tobacco Ad Ban," *Chicago Sun-Times,* 5 December 1985, 3; Wolinsky, "AMA Split on Tobacco War Strategy," *Sun-Times,* 15 December 1985, 6;   **46.** Interview with Durbin;   **47.** Interview with Waxman;   **48.** In fact, in earlier efforts by Waxman and Senator Orrin G. Hatch (R-Utah) to pass a stronger warning label in the early 1980s, congressional staffers said the AMA had disappointed. John K. Iglehart, reporting in "Smoking and Public Policy," *New England Journal of Medicine,* 23 February 1984, 539–544, said that there was "a perception held in some Washington quarters that although the AMA expresses support for tougher government policies against smoking, its advocacy is less than strong, perhaps as a consequence of its own attempt to balance the conflicting interests involved in this issue." U.S. Representative Richard Cheney (R-Wy.), the future Secretary of Defense, told Iglehart he had worked with the AMA on other issues, but "I don't hear from the AMA on the issue of smoking and health . . . The AMA ought to weigh in on this issue. It could do a lot to polish its own image by expressing a professional judgment that points out more actively the dangers of smoking";   **49.** House of Representatives Subcommittee on Health and the Environment, Committee on Energy and Commerce, Hearings on Tobacco Control and Health Protection Act (H.R. 401) (Washington: Government Printing Office, 1990), 420–421; **50.** Interview with Todd and article by Wolinsky, "Critics Rap AMA for Award to Ally of Tobacco Lobby," *Chicago Sun-Times,* 10 February 1992, 12;   **51.** Clifford Douglas described the vote in an interview;   **52.** "Nathan Davis Award Recipients Announced," AMA news release, 15 October 1991. Rowland was cited for "his commitment to effective health care legislation," including authoring the legislation that created the National Commission on AIDS and service on committees dealing with rural health and infant mortality; **53.** Wolinsky, "Critics Rap AMA for Award to Ally of Tobacco Lobby," *Chicago Sun-Times,* 10 February 1992, 12;   **54.** Interviews with Douglas and Sarfaty;   **55.** "AMA Can't Kick Addiction to Tobacco Subsidiaries' Money," *Physician's Weekly,* 18 January 1993; **56.** Based on interview with Dunnington;   **57.** *Washington Post,* 27 January 1993, A16; **58.** "Support From the 'Tobacco Industry,'" AMA Board of Trustees Report SS, June 1993; **59.** From Dunnington's prepared remarks to Reference Committee D, 14 June 1993; **60.** Quotes from a transcipt of the House of Delegates meeting, 17 June 1993. Regarding the medical schools, see also Malcolm Manber, "Puff Job: Medical Groups and Researchers Often Say Yes to Tobacco-Linked Funding," *Physician's Weekly,* 10 May 1993. This article points out that 66 of 126 U.S. medical schools have grants from the Council for Tobacco Research, "an industry front";   **61.** "AMA's Tobacco Activism," *American Medical News,* 9 August 1993, 12.

CHAPTER 8: A DOCTOR'S RIGHT TO CHOOSE

In addition to the sources listed below, the following people were interviewed: Ann Allen, general counsel, American College of Obstetricians and Gynecologists; Jo Blum, assistant director, Washington office of Planned Parenthood; Dr. Joseph F. Boyle, past president of the AMA; Joseph W. Dellapenna, professor of law, Villanova University; Dr. Nancy W. Dickey, member, AMA Board of Trustees; Dr. Eugene F. Diamond, Loyola University Stritch College of Medicine; U.S. Representative Henry J. Hyde (R-Ill.); Kirk B. Johnson, general counsel, AMA; Jane Larson, professor of law, Northwestern University; Rachael Pine, of the New York–based Center for Reproductive Law and Policy; Joseph M. Scheidler, executive director, Pro-Life Action League; Joseph R. Stanton, president of the Value of Life Committee; Dr. James S. Todd, executive vice president, AMA.

The following books provided background on abortion: German G. Grisez, *Abortion: The Myths, the Realities, and the Arguments* (New York: Corpus Books, 1970); Lawrence Lader, *Abortion* (Indianapolis: Bobbs-Merrill, 1966); Carl N. Flanders, *Library in a Book: Abortion* (New York: Facts on File, 1991); Frederick S. Jaffe, Barbara L. Lindheim, and Philip R. Lee, *Abortion Politics: Private Morality and Public Policy* (New York: McGraw-Hill, 1981); James C. Mohr, *Abortion in America: The Origins and Evolution of National Policy, 1800–1900* (New York: Oxford University Press, 1978); Bernard N. Nathanson, M.D., *Aborting America* (Garden City: Doubleday, 1979); Carroll Smith-Rosenberg, *Disorderly Conduct: Visions of Gender in Victorian America* (New York: Alfred A. Knopf, 1985); and Laurence H. Tribe, *Abortion: The Clash of Absolutes* (New York: W. W. Norton, 1990).

1. "Report on Criminal Abortion," *Transactions of the American Medical Association,* 1859, 75; **2.** Ibid., 76; **3.** Ibid., 27; **4.** Horatio Robinson Storer, "The Criminality and Physical Evils of Forced Abortion, Being the Prize Essay to Which the American Medical Association Awarded the Gold Medal for MDCCCLXV," *Transactions of the American Medical Association,* 1865, 709–745. The background on the entry is on 711–713. Of the essay competition, Mohr asked, "How many physicians were likely to have had a major manuscript on that subject ready to go?" in *Abortion in America,* 158; **5.** Storer, 736; **6.** Ibid., 745; **7.** Mohr, *Abortion in America,* 147–148; **8.** "Report of the Committee on Criminal Abortion," *Transactions of the American Medical Association,* 1871, 251, 246; **9.** Ibid., 257; **10.** Ibid., 241; **11.** Ibid., 39; **12.** The AMA's success on the state level was bolstered when Congress passed the Comstock law in 1873. The law, advocated by moral crusader Anthony Comstock, secretary of the New York Society for the Suppression of Vice, banned "obscene" materials from the U.S. mail, including abortifacients and contraceptives and advertisements for such products. Among the first victims of the Comstock law was the abortion franchiser Madame Restell, who committed suicide in 1878 while awaiting prosecution; **13.** Mohr, *Abortion in America,* 245; **14.** In today's overheated abortion debate, there is a running argument over what happened in the last century. Historians and legal scholars in recent years have submitted friend-of-the-court briefs to the Supreme Court and published articles in professional journals arguing about public attitudes and legal views concerning abortion from colonial times until before the AMA campaign. Supporters of abortion rights argue the regular medical profession's antiabortion attitudes, encouraged by the AMA crusade, were an aberration. They said the framers of the Constitution tolerated abortion before quickening. On the other hand, pro-lifers argue there is evidence in the common law that antiabortion attitudes existed in America before the AMA crusade. They contend the AMA crusade merely toughened sanctions against abortion. They believe the doctors' campaign was more than a gimmick to professionalize medicine. Both sides think the group that owns the past may control the present by influencing the Supreme Court. There is no doubt, however, that the AMA provided a base from which Storer and like-minded colleagues helped shape public opinion and policy to criminalize abortion; **15.** The statistics on abortion practices are from the report of the AMA Committee on Human Reproduction, American Medical Association, *Proceedings of the House of Delegates,* 1967, 40; **16.** Ibid., 47; **17.** Ibid., 50–51; **18.** Ibid., 49; **19.** Dick Kirschten, "AMA Relaxes Stand for First Time Since 1871," *Chicago Sun-Times,* 22 June 1967, 26; **20.** "Abortion Change Proposed," *American Medical News,* 25 May 1970, 1; **21.** Richard D. Lyons, "Abortion Reform Debated by A.M.A.," *New York Times,* 24 June 1970, 1; **22.** Ibid.; **23.** "AMA Abortion Position Liberalized," *American Medical News,* 6 July 1970, 1; **24.** Interview with Stanton; **25.** Former AMA president Joseph Boyle estimated that about 8 percent of AMA membership quit in protest. The AMA itself had no figures. The proportion of physicians who were in the AMA had started to decline after the Medicare fiasco in the mid-1960s, a trend that accelerated after the abortion decision. See "Abortion Stand Stirs Resignations," *American Medical News,* 20 July 1970, 1; "AMA's Future Seen Bleak If Defection Rate Continues," Associated Press, *Boston Evening Globe,* 28 November 1972; **26.** *U.S. Law Week,* 23 January 1973, 4237; **27.** For a behind-the-scenes look at how Justice Harry Blackmun prepared *Roe v. Wade,* see Bob Woodward and Scott Armstrong, *The Brethren: Inside the Supreme Court* (New York: Simon & Schuster, 1979); **28.** *U.S. Law Week,* 4226; **29.** Ibid., 4229; **30.** Ibid., 4232; **31.** Ibid., 4221; **32.** Ibid.,

4239;   **33.** Ibid., 4233;   **34.** Ibid., 4246;   **35.** "Abortion Policy Reaffirmed; Alternatives Stressed," *American Medical News* 2/9 July 1973, 13;   **36.** Telegram to Senator Edward W. Brooke from Dr. James H. Sammons, AMA executive vice president, 19 July 1977; **37.** Letter to Dr. Joseph R. Stanton, president of the Value of Life Committee, from Dr. James H. Sammons, executive vice president, AMA, 29 August 1977;   **38.** Storer, "Criminality and Physical Evils of Forced Abortions," 720;   **39.** Dr. Joseph Boyle, chairman of the board of the American Medical Association, testimony presented to the Senate Judiciary Committee, Subcommittee on the Separation of Powers, S. 158 to Provide That Human Life Shall Be Deemed to Exist from Conception, 18 June 1981, 2;   **40.** Amicus brief filed in *Rust v. Sullivan* by AMA et al. on July 27, 1990. Standing apart from its fellow petitioners, the AMA said in the brief: "The AMA opposes the regulations at issue to the extent that they will force physicians to deviate from accepted standards of medical practice and conduct. The AMA has concluded that it is not necessary to reach the constitutional issues presented in this brief . . ." Other petitioners said the regulations interfered with health professionals' First Amendment rights and also with a woman's right to make an informed decision to terminate her pregnancy;   **41.** Johnson interview;   **42.** Pine interview;   **43.** Paul R. McGinn, *American Medical News,* "Delegates Support Woman's Right to 'Early' Abortion," 15 December 1989, 3;   **44.** Wolinsky, "Doctors Debate Abortion Policy; Parental Permission Called Unnecessary," *Chicago Sun-Times,* 23 June 1992, 5; **45.** "Pro-Lifers to Picket AMA Chicago Meeting," Pro-Life Action League, news release, 19 June 1992;   **46.** See note 44;   **47.** Wolinsky, "Abortion Without Consent Okd," *Chicago Sun-Times,* 24 June 1992, 14;   **48.** National Commission on America Without *Roe, Facing a Future Without Choice: A Report on Reproductive Liberty in America* (Washington: National Abortion Rights Action League and NARAL Foundation, 1992), 6;   **49.** Interview with Todd;   **50.** Storer, "Criminality and Physical Evils of Forced Abortions," 724; **51.** AMA Council on Scientific Affairs, Report H, "Induced Termination of Pregnancy Before and After *Roe v. Wade:* Trends in the Mortality and Morbidity of Women, 17.

CHAPTER 9: POLITICAL SCIENCE VS. MEDICAL SCIENCE

In addition to the sources listed below, the following were interviewed: Dr. Ronald Bayer, Columbia University; George Bergalis, father of AIDS victim Kimberly Bergalis; former California congressman William E. Dannemeyer; Dr. Leonard Fenninger, former AMA vice president of science policy; Larry Kramer, playwright; Dr. Sanford Kuvin, infectious disease specialist and consultant to the Bergalis family and vice chairman of the National Foundation for Infectious Diseases; Jeffrey Levi, government relations director, AIDS Action Council; Dr. Alvin Novick, past president, American Association of Physicians for Human Rights; Dr. Jane Petro, past president, American Association of Physicians for Human Rights; Dr. David Rogers, vice chairman of the National Commission on AIDS; Ben Schatz, executive director, American Association for Physicians for Human Rights; Dr. M. Roy Schwarz, vice president for science and medical education, AMA; Dr. Mervyn Silverman, executive director, American Foundation for AIDS Research.

1. Larry Kramer, *The Normal Heart,* (New York: New American Library, 1985), 80; **2.** Centers for Disease Control and Prevention, "AIDS Information, Cumulative Cases," 3 November 1993;   **3.** Denslow Lewis, M.D., "The Gynecologic Consideration of the Sexual Act," *JAMA* 8 July 1983, 222, 228, 224;   **4.** David Sanford, "The AMA and That Disease," *New Republic,* 18 September 1965, 10;   **5.** "AMA Bars Stand on Homosexuals," *New York Times,* 4 December 1974;   **6.** American Medical Association Council on Long Range Planning and Development, *Policy Compendium* (Chicago: American Medical Association, 1993), policy 270.997, 226;   **7.** The AMA in 1991 reaffirmed this policy. But the policy also angered many gays because it still supported the controversial concept of reversing homosexuality. Gays argued that the AMA was ignoring science, which shows that sexual orientation is as much a factor in a genetic inheritance as height and race. AMA Council on Long Range Planning and Development, *Policy Compendium,* policy 160.991, 127; Brian McCormick, "Organized Medicine's Open Door," *American Medical News,* 15 June 1992, 27. It was not until June 1993, after four failures to change its policy, that the AMA

House of Delegates inserted a disclaimer in its bylaws to explicitly ban discrimination against gays;   **8.** Dennis L. Breo, "AMA AIDS Expert's Grim Message," *American Medical News*, 5 December 1986, 32;   **9.** AMA Board of Trustees Report FF, December 1983; **10.** Fenninger interview;   **11.** Centers for Disease Control, "HIV/AIDS Surveillance Report," February 1993, 17;   **12.** Ibid.;   **13.** Brune and Wolinsky, "New Jab at AIDS Testing: Experts Out to Block AMA Plan," *Chicago Sun-Times*, 22 June 1987, 3;   **14.** Brune and Wolinsky, "Koop Endorses Proposal by AMA to Combat AIDS," ibid.;   **15.** See note 13;   **16.** *Hospital Ethics*, September/October 1987, 11;   **17.** Sari Staver, "Unethical to Refuse to Treat HIV-Infected Patient, AMA Says," *American Medical News*, 20 November 1987, 1;   **18.** Policy is quoted from Abigail Zuger, M.D., and Steven H. Miles, M.D., "Physicians, AIDS, and Occupational Risk: Historic Traditions and Ethical Obligations," *JAMA*, 9 October 1987, 1924–1928;   **19.** See note 17;   **20.** Zuger, 1926;   **21.** Interviews with Rogers and Levi;   **22.** Zuger, 1924–1928;   **23.** In addition to the Arline case, the AMA filed a number of other amicus briefs to defend patients with HIV against discrimination. It has also submitted amicus briefs opposing the exclusion from school of the Ray brothers, Florida hemophiliacs who had been infected with HIV from contaminated drugs used to treat their disease, and supporting Vincent Chalk, a teacher who had been fired because he had AIDS;   **24.** Marsha F. Goldsmith, "CDC Ponders New HIV Guidelines," *JAMA*, 5 September 1990, 1079;   **25.** Bonnie Johnson, "A Life Stolen Early," *People*, 22 October 1990, 78;   **26.** Interview with Schwarz;   **27.** Marlene Cimons, "Dentist with AIDS Was Likely Source of Infections in 3 Patients, Officials Say," *Los Angeles Times*, 11 January 1991, A27;   **28.** Sari Staver, "HIV-Infected Doctors Should Tell Patients, Stop Surgery—AMA," *American Medical News*, 4 February 1991, 42;   **29.** Dickey, AMA Statement to the Centers for Disease Control, "HIV Transmission During Invasive Procedures," 21 February 1991, 4;   **30.** *American Medical News*, 11 March 1991, 3; Marsha F. Goldsmith, "Physicians and Dentists Tell the CDC: 'Avoid Quick Fix for a Tough Problem,'" *JAMA*, 13 March 1991, 1221. The *JAMA* article said that "many speakers characterized the AMA-ADA response as a reaction to public fear and hysteria more typical of the early days of the 10-year-old pandemic rather than a proactive policy based on rational thought and scientific understanding of the disease";   **31.** Account based on Michael L. Millenson and Keith L. Alexander, "AIDS Group in a Clash with Police," *Chicago Tribune*, 25 June 1991, Section 2, 1; Wolinsky, "Quayle: Test MDs for AIDS; He Wants Patients Checked, Too," *Chicago Sun-Times*, 25 June 1991, 3; Jim Casey and Theresa Cameron, "AIDS Activists March on AMA; 27 Arrested," *Sun-Times*, 25 June 1991, 3;   **32.** Deborah Pinkney, "HIV Testing: Easier for Patients; 'Appropriate' for Doctors," *American Medical News*, 8/15 July 1991, 48; **33.** Statement, Dr. Nancy W. Dickey, AMA, "AMA Reaction: CDC Guidelines on HIV Transmission by Health-Care Workers," 15 July 1991;   **34.** Laurie Jones, "Murky Future on Penalties for HIV-Infected Doctors," *American Medical News*, 2 September 1991, 2; **35.** Notes on the closed meeting in Chicago, 28 August 1991, regarding exposure-prone procedures, Centers for Disease Control;   **36.** Sari Staver, "CDC's HIV Plan: Science or Politics? Medical Groups Split on Exposure-Prone List," *American Medical News*, 16 September 1991, 41;   **37.** Subcommittee on Health and the Environment, Committee on Energy and Commerce, House of Representatives, 102nd Congress, "Centers for Disease Control Guidelines for Health Professionals on the Prevention of Transmission of HIV During Exposure-Prone Invasive Procedures" (Washington: Government Printing Office, 1992) 19 and 26 September 1991, 128;   **38.** Lawrence K. Altman, "Dentists' Group Offers No List for AIDS Risk," *New York Times*, 11 October 1991, Section A, 12;   **39.** American College of Surgeons, "Position Statement on Surgeons and HIV Infection," 21 October 1991;   **40.** Rebecca Voelker, "Surgeons Join Opposition to 'Exposure-Prone' List," *American Medical News*, 4 November 1991, 4;   **41.** Bruce Lambert, "Kimberly Bergalis Is Dead at 23; Symbol of Debate Over AIDS Tests," *New York Times*, 9 December 1991, D9; **42.** Jane Anderson, "AMA Votes for AIDS Test Without Patient OK," *Chicago Sun-Times* 12 December 1991, 32. The confusion among health experts about what to do about HIV-infected doctors was reflected in the fact that Graduate Hospital in Philadelphia, where the unnamed surgeon also was on staff, did not conduct a lookback study. The hospital decided that it would notify patients only if a specific risk was discovered (Loretta Tofani, "3 Patients of HIV-Infected Surgeon Have AIDS Virus; Source Uncertain," *Philadelphia Inquirer*, 11 December 1991, B4);   **43.** Memo from Dr. Gary Noble, CDC, to senior staffers at

the Centers for Disease Control, 13 December 1991;   **44.** Interview with Schwarz;
45. These are the figures through June 1992, according to the CDC;   **46.** 18 June 1992
memo to state health officers from William L. Roper, CDC director;   **47.** Interview with
Silverman;   **48.** Interview with Petro;   **49.** Interview with Schwarz;   **50.** C. Everett
Koop, M.D., *Koop: Memoirs of America's Family Doctor* (New York: Random House, 1991), 207;
51. Interview with Schatz;   **52.** Interview with Kramer.

Index